Expertise in Physical Therapy Practice

Second Edition

D1516455

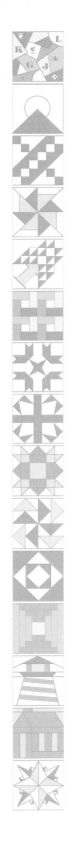

SECOND EDITION

Expertise in Physical Therapy Practice

Gail M. Jensen, Ph.D., P.T., FAPTA
Dean of the Graduate School and Associate Vice President for Faculty Development in Academic Affairs, Professor, Department of Physical Therapy, School of Pharmacy and Health Professions, and Faculty Associate, Center for Health Policy and Ethics, Creighton University, Omaha, Nebraska

Jan Gwyer, Ph.D., P.T.
Professor, Doctor of Physical Therapy Division,
Department of Community and Family Medicine,
School of Medicine, Duke University, Durham, North Carolina

Laurita M. Hack, D.P.T., Ph.D., M.B.A., FAPTA
Professor, Director of Ph.D. Program in Physical Therapy,
Department of Physical Therapy, College of Health Professions,
Temple University, Philadelphia, Pennsylvania

Katherine F. Shepard, Ph.D., P.T., FAPTA
Professor Emeritus, Founding Director, Ph.D. Program in Physical Therapy,
Department of Physical Therapy, College of Health Professions,
Temple University, Philadelphia, Pennsylvania

with six contributors

Forewords by
Ruth B. Purtilo, Ph.D., P.T., FAPTA
Jules Rothstein, Ph.D., P.T., FAPTA

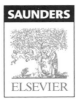

SAUNDERS

ELSEVIER

SAUNDERS
ELSEVIER

11830 Westline Industrial Drive
St. Louis, Missouri 63146

EXPERTISE IN PHYSICAL THERAPY PRACTICE   ISBN-13: 978-1-4160-0214-7
SECOND EDITION   ISBN-10: 1-4160-0214-6

Notice

Knowledge and best practice in this field are constantly changing. As new research and experience broaden our knowledge, changes in practice, treatment, and drug therapy may become necessary or appropriate. Readers are advised to check the most current information provided (i) on procedures featured or (ii) by the manufacturer of each product to be administered, to verify the recommended dose or formula, the method and duration of administration, and contraindications. It is the responsibility of the practitioner, relying on their own experience and knowledge of the patient, to make diagnoses, to determine dosages and the best treatment for each individual patient, and to take all appropriate safety precautions. To the fullest extent of the law, neither the Publisher nor the Author assumes any liability for any injury and/or damage to property arising out of or related to any use of the material contained in this book.

The Publisher

ISBN-13: 978-1-4160-0214-7
ISBN-10: 1-4160-0214-6

Publishing Director: Linda Duncan
Editor: Kathryn Falk
Developmental Editor: Andrew Grow
Publishing Services Manager: Melissa Lastarria
Project Manager: Kelly E. M. Steinmann
Designer: Ellen Zanolle

Printed in the United States of America

Last digit is the print number: 9 8 7 6 5 4 3 2 1

Working together to grow
libraries in developing countries

www.elsevier.com | www.bookaid.org | www.sabre.org

ELSEVIER   BOOK AID International   Sabre Foundation

The dedicated life is the life worth living. You must give with your whole heart.

Annie Dillard, *The Quotable Woman*, Running Press, 1991

To the therapists who have shared their lives with us and who lead the life worth living.

About the Authors

Gail M. Jensen, Ph.D., P.T., FAPTA, is Dean of the Graduate School and Associate Vice President for Faculty Development in Academic Affairs, Professor, Department of Physical Therapy, School of Pharmacy and Health Professions, and Faculty Associate, Center for Health Policy and Ethics, Creighton University, Omaha, Nebraska. She has a Bachelor of Science in Education from the University of Minnesota, and a Master's Degree in Physical Therapy and a Doctor of Philosophy Degree in Educational Evaluation and Curriculum from Stanford University. Her research interests, publications, and presentations span the areas of clinical reasoning, development of expertise, qualitative research, interprofessional education, and assessment. She has served on several editorial boards and is the deputy editor for *Physiotherapy Research International* and associate editor for *Physiotherapy Theory and Practice*. She is co-author of the *Handbook of Teaching for Physical Therapists* (with K. Shepard, 2nd ed., 2002) and *Educating for Moral Action: A Sourcebook in Health and Rehabilitation Ethics* (with R. Purtilo, C. Royeen, 2005). Over the past 10 years, she has been involved in initiating federally funded interdisciplinary grants supporting an academic–community partnership with the Native American communities in northeast Nebraska that has led to self-sufficient rehabilitation clinical services and ongoing interdisciplinary education. She received the American Physical Therapy Association's (APTA's) Golden Pen Award and is a Catherine Worthingham Fellow of the APTA.

Jan Gwyer, Ph.D., P.T., is Professor and Doctor of Physical Therapy Division, Department of Community and Family Medicine, School of Medicine, Duke University, Durham, North Carolina. She holds a Bachelor of Science degree from the Medical College of Virginia and Master's and Doctor of Philosophy degrees from the University of North Carolina at Chapel Hill. She has held several leadership roles in the APTA, serving on the board of American Physical Therapy Specialists, on the Clinical Instructors Education Board, and on the board of directors of the APTA. She has served on the Project Advisory Group for the *Guide to Physical Therapist Practice* and as a member consultant to the Clinical Research Agenda. In 1998 she received the APTA Lucy Blair Service Award. She also has written in the areas of clinical education, career patterns, and workforce issues in physical therapy.

Laurita M. Hack, D.P.T., Ph.D., M.B.A., FAPTA, is Professor and Director of the Ph.D. Program, Department of Physical Therapy, College of Health Professions, Temple University, Philadelphia, Pennsylvania. She received a Bachelor of Science in Biology from Wilmington College; a Master of Science degree in Physical Therapy from Case Western Reserve University; a Master of Business Administration in health care administration from the Wharton School, University of Pennsylvania; a Doctor of Philosophy degree in Higher Education from the University of Pennsylvania; and a doctor of physical therapy degree from MGH Institute of Health Professions.

She serves as a site team leader for the Commission on Physical Therapy Education and has served on the Central Panel of the Commission. She has served as president of the APTA's Community Home Health Section, of the Section on Health Policy, and of the Education Section, and as chief delegate of the Pennsylvania chapter, all components of the APTA. She is the recipient of the Carlin-Michels Award for Achievement from the Pennsylvania chapter and the APTA's Lucy Blair Service Award and the Baethke-Carlin Award for Teaching Excellence. She has also been named a Catherine Worthingham Fellow of the APTA. She has owned and managed a large physical therapy practice that included outpatient care, home care, and a membership-based exercise center. Throughout her career, she has written and lectured on many health services issues in physical therapy.

Katherine F. Shepard, Ph.D., P.T., FAPTA, is Professor Emeritus, Founding Director, Ph.D. Program in Physical Therapy, Department of Physical Therapy, College of Health Professions, Temple University, Philadelphia, Pennsylvania. She received a Bachelor of Arts in Psychology from Hood College, a Bachelor of Science in Physical Therapy from Ithaca College, and Master of Arts in Physical Therapy and Sociology and a Doctor of Philosophy degree in Sociology of Education from Stanford University. Her professional career in physical therapy spans more than 40 years, and she has published extensively in the areas of social science research related to physical therapy education and practice. She is co-author of the *Handbook of Teaching for Physical Therapists* (with G. Jensen, 2nd ed., 2002). She has taught graduate courses in qualitative research in the United States, Sweden, and South Africa. She is the recipient of the APTA Baethke-Carlin Award for Teaching Excellence, the APTA Golden Pen Award for outstanding contributions to physical therapy, and the APTA Lucy Blair Service Award. She is a Catherine Worthingham Fellow of the APTA and has been named the Mary McMillan Lecturer for 2007.

Contributors

IAN EDWARDS, Ph.D., P.T.
Lecturer, School of Health Sciences (Physiotherapy), Physical Therapist, Brian Burdekin Clinic, University of South Australia, Adelaide, South Australia

ANN JAMPEL, P.T., M.S.
Center Coordinator for Clinical Education, Physical Therapy Services, Massachusetts General Hospital, Boston, Massachusetts

MARK A. JONES, M.APP.SC., P.T.
Program Director, Senior Lecturer, Postgraduate Coursework Masters Programs in Physiotherapy, School of Health Sciences, University of South Australia, Adelaide, South Australia

ELIZABETH MOSTROM, P.T., Ph.D.
Professor, Director of Clinical Education Program, Physical Therapy School of Rehabilitation and Medical Sciences, Central Michigan University, Mount Pleasant, Michigan

MICHAEL G. SULLIVAN, P.T., D.P.T., M.B.A.
Director, Physical and Occupational Therapy, Massachusetts General Hospital, Boston, Massachusetts

LINDA RESNIK, Ph.D., P.T., O.C.S.
Assistant Professor (Research), Department of Community Health, Brown University, Providence, Rhode Island; Research Health Scientist, Providence VA Medical Center, Providence, Rhode Island

Foreword to the Second Edition

This second edition of *Expertise in Physical Therapy Practice* is a useful tool for the reader who is being introduced to the topic, as well as the one who has worn thin the pages of the first edition. From the earliest times, "expertise" in the health care professions has been characterized as excellence in the exercise of both the art and the science of practice. This book demonstrates how physical therapists can continue to develop so that both aspects can be realized in today's health care environment. It is an essential resource for all who want not only to practice physical therapy but also to continue to develop their expertise to its full potential.

The authors of *Expertise in Physical Therapy Practice* sound the encouraging note that the knowledge, skills, and decision-making abilities used by expert clinicians can be identified, nurtured, and taught. The authors' studied attention to how and why experts do the right thing at the right time is both timely and important: timely because individual expertise is under siege today, owing to a growing tendency to emphasize efficiency and measure therapeutic success largely, or even solely, on the basis of pooled data; and important because efficiency and outcomes measures are valid indicators of one dimension of therapeutic success—but a success that risks becoming vacuous and skeletal without the nourishment of human interaction. In short, this book has given thought to when and how a more adequate criterion of effectiveness is achieved, and the second edition provides additional strategies for successful applications in education and practice. It puts people back into the health professions, both as professionals and as patients.

Edmund Pelligrino, a health professional and humanities scholar, reminds us that the idea of a "profession" is that "one professes something." Health professionals profess something that goes straight to the heart of society's values by selling themselves as vehicles of healing and comfort! This, then, is what health professionals in general say they will do and are charged by society—and given license by it—to do. The technical competence of each profession must be combined with development and use of skills and other conduct that heals and comforts.

As the authors of *Expertise in Physical Therapy Practice* aptly highlight with their writing and examples the rehabilitation professions pose an interesting question about what effectiveness in the health professions entails. The traditional notions of healing and comfort were conceived in a time when the health professional (i.e., physician) was viewed in a priestly role as knowledgeable and powerful—the sole means to healing and comfort for the suffering of injury or illness. The art of medicine included an acknowledgment that it could not do everything to heal or alleviate suffering, but up to that point the power was in the physician's hand. In contrast, the rehabilitation professions were born in different times and places: partially in the ravages of war, when the human will to survive and thrive was far more central an agent of healing and comfort than the availability of health professionals or health care technology; partially in a secularized, individualized society that equated independence with well-being; and, at least partially, in cultures that had developed an understanding of human rights that gave the patient power to place a claim on the society for help. The idea of how the skills of healing and comforting should be applied had to be expanded, and the rehabilitation professions were one healthy offspring of the mating of tradition with these new social forces.

An expert clinician in the rehabilitation professions today is less priest than teacher, less parent than coach, less stranger than advocate. The effective rehabilitation professional can help heal (e.g., boost) a patient's flagging morale through instruction in exercise techniques designed to improve function; can help heal decreased self-esteem caused by the sudden onslaught of illness or injury by providing reassurance of the person's worth; and can help "cure" disabling social attitudes toward people challenged by impairment through advocacy, involvement in policy, and political action. "Comfort" (*com* + *forte* = with strength) can be more long-lasting if directed toward the ultimate goal of the patient's reintegration into her or his community of support and meaning than if directed solely toward the (also important) goals of reversing dysfunction. For example, a physical therapist may provide comfort through instruction about how to avoid work injury or by helping the patient endure work hardening after injury.

In viewing expert clinicians as those who effectively adapt more traditional approaches to healing and comforting while facing the demands of modern social conditions, the authors of this book help us to understand how physical therapists can continue to be relevant and how they also can become expert agents of transformation. The authors contribute to our understanding of specific developmental tasks clinicians have to undertake to become experts. Their definition of *expert practice* as being able to do the right thing at the right time acknowledges the deep well of information that always has been available in clinical experience within a given time and social and cultural context. They have bothered to tap it and show that there is much to sustain the rehabilitation professions—and individual professionals within them—today.

As an ethicist, I also am informed by their work regarding implications for a relevant professional ethic. A traditional health professions ethic justifiably emphasizes its ethical role as one that needs constraints on abuses of power. Students of ethics will recognize the ethical duties/principles such as do not harm, act to benefit the patient, be faithful to reasonable expectations, and be truthful as socially mandated guidelines that reflect society's anxiety about its dependence on physicians' knowledge, skills, and conduct.

But just as the study reported in this book shows an evolving model of the health professional and patient relationship, so, too, does it make good sense to include such insights in our understanding of physical therapists' ethical mandates. Insights from their stories enrich our appreciation of how story and viewpoint provide data for ascertaining a caring course of action in the years ahead. Such a course does not include the dumping of constraints embodied in traditional duties and principles, but the traditional ethic is malnourished as the sole approach.

In summary, in this second edition the authors leave intact fundamental concepts and illustrative material that skillfully introduces clinicians and educators to the whats, whys, and wherefores of expertise in physical therapy practice. At the same time, these well-established and respected physical therapy leaders have continued to listen skillfully and with due care to the stories of physical therapy professionals and to interact with the leading researchers and writers in this area across the health professions. Drawing on these essential resources, they have updated their initial contribution to make this second edition fully relevant to the ever-developing demands of professionalism in physical therapy today.

RUTH B. PURTILO, Ph.D., P.T., FAPTA
Director and Professor, Ethics Initiative
MGH Institute of Health Professions
Boston, Massachusetts

Foreword to the First Edition

The debate never seems to end, the arguments never seem to illuminate, and, in the end, the issues never seem to be resolved. When it comes to understanding what makes some practitioners better than others and to agreeing on a definition of a clinical expert, calm discussions give way to passions that rise to levels achieved not even in gothic romance novels. No wonder the questions remain. How do members of health care professions best provide their services? What is the "magic" of the successful practitioner? What is the nature of the expert practitioner, and how can we obtain more expert practitioners? The debate is often characterized by assaults on motives, and some discussants seek refuge by claiming they speak on behalf of patients. Who can argue with those who are cloaked with the best interests of those not participating in the debate? The problem, however, lies not in the questions, but in the false premises that often are used in these discussions.

We have heard people defend the artistry of the health care professional while they demean the science that is the right of patients who deserve the best care possible. They characterize science and quantification as being antithetical to humanistic practice and argue for vague, undefined constructs that obscure rather than define. Others argue that some practitioner skills are intuitive—almost genetically endowed—and are, therefore, either present or not. Some view the use of evidence and concerns for outcomes as non–patient focused behaviors and therefore, at best, as a technical requirement for reimbursement rather than an appropriate practice mode. Still others take refuge under the banner of unproven expertise to facilitate self-promotion and deflect inquiry and accountability. The outrage of self-appointed experts when they are denied the center stage is an ugly sight and as incongruous as Madonna singing lyrics that compare her to a virgin.

Until the pioneering work of the authors of this book, serious inquiry into the nature of expertise has been rare—and thoughtful discussion of how we can learn from our experts has been even more rare. The time has come for us to face the truth. Expertise in physical therapy *can* be studied and understood, just it has been in other professions and, I add with bemusement, just as it has been in the arts. A book that takes a scholarly look at expertise is long overdue in physical therapy.

Science can be used to study expertise, and a variety of research methods can be used to understand how experts function and how to enhance practice by mimicking some of their behaviors. But first we must define what it means to be an *expert*. We should realize that factors such as the numbers of courses taken, the number of continuing education courses taught, or the reverence of colleagues do not really identify an expert. In my view, true expertise means that a practitioner can do something better and data exist to support this contention. Wouldn't we all want experts to treat our ailments? Of course. But unless they provide better *care*, what would be the point?

The authors of this book have long been proponents of studying expertise. Once they were lonely voices; now others are beginning to see the benefit of research into the nature of practice and what differentiates more effective therapists from less effective therapists. In other words, who are these experts, and what are they doing? Studying something does not mean that we will understand it today or even in the immediate future—only that the journey toward understanding has begun. And studying expertise does not mean that we dehumanize this very human trait, but rather that we can use all of the research techniques available to us to capture the essential elements that can be understood, shared, and nurtured.

One of the most remarkable things I have ever seen on television was the master class of the cellist Pablo Casals. An elderly man at the time, he sat curved around his cello, holding his bow loosely but waving it as needed to illustrate a movement, underscore a point, or celebrate the achievement of a student. The master's instructions were being codified and passed on to a new generation. Casals was deliberate and communicated directly. He carried his remarkable burden with grace. What was the burden? It was the burden of the expert who is committed to his craft. Like any true expert, he not only excelled, but he also knew that he had a responsibility to understand the source of his own greatness so that he could attempt to pass on what was important, so that he could turn his students' attention toward the essential and away from the trivial or irrelevant.

Artisans have always been known for their ability to train future generations, yet so many physical therapists recklessly dichotomize practice into "science" and "art." This dichotomy allows them to hide behind the canard that artistry cannot be codified or studied. Thankfully, the authors of this book—and the authors of the articles on which they base much of their work—did not share in this fatalistic excuse that delays the development of more experts and in the end denies our patients the best possible care. The invocation of art is designed to provide a seemingly attractive substitute for meaningful discussion. Too many of us respond to this image much as a moth is attracted to a light bulb—and with equal effect. If you found out tomorrow that you had a malignancy, would you seek out an oncologist known for his or her artistic flair in applying treatments? Would you want a practitioner who likes to deviate from known protocols because this allows expression of individualism? As for me, I would go with the expert—and I define the expert as the practitioner known to achieve the best outcome.

Our need to understand and enhance expertise is particularly acute today because physical therapy finds itself among the health professions being challenged to provide evidence that our services meaningfully change people's lives. Now that we are under fire and some of us believe the job market is shrinking, I suspect we will see fewer therapists taking shelter under the specious claim that our results and practice behaviors cannot be studied. As can be seen from the primary research cited in this book, some techniques—such as qualitative methods that can be used in isolation from, in coordination with, or as precursors to quantitative methods—allow us to study more than can be imagined by those who would argue rather than engage in inquiry. When debate is stilled or illuminated by the power of data, knowledge grows, understanding increases, and new questions arise. As a result, we move forward.

Some see today's focus on outcomes and evidence as automatically turning practitioners' attention away from the individuality of patients and their unique needs. I believe this phenomenon occurs only when we fail to understand the nature of outcomes data and the role of expertise and individualism—individualism of both the patient and the therapist. David Sackett, who is often referred to as the father of evidence-based medicine, argues that expertise and individual characteristics of the patient and the practitioner are very important. He contends that evidence-based practice "is the conscientious, explicit, and judicious use of current best evidence in making decisions about the care of individual patients" (1).

He appears to be defining some of the characteristics of an expert. Experts, he contends, should be explicit in their use of evidence, they should know what is the best evidence, and they should make decisions about individual patients. Outcomes data and some related research usually focus on groups, but as Sackett clearly indicates, when it comes to evidence-based practice, the issue is the application of information to specific patients. Often, data on outcomes are designed to examine results in the aggregate and to judge how therapists and facilities compare with other therapists and facilities or with established standards. Groups of patients are considered, not the individual characteristics of those who may have been better served by physical therapy than others were.

Although outcomes data are important in today's world of health care accountability, in my view data do little for the therapist who is dealing with specific patients. The most useful data for the expert and for the application of evidence in practice are those which can be used by specific types of therapists on identifiable patients. That is why we need data that can be applied by therapists in specific settings to specific patients, and our research community should generate these data. Data, however, are insufficient. Who can best use the data? Who can be the role model for the application of science in practice? Our experts should be able to do both!

If any doubt exists about how expertise and evidence-based practice are complementary, consider another observation by Sackett: "External clinical evidence can inform, but can never replace individual clinical expertise, and it is this expertise that decides whether the external evidence applies to the patient at all, and if so, how it should be integrated into a clinical decision" (1).

Evidence without clinical expertise is as useful as a supercomputer in a rain-forest: The sight might be impressive, but it isn't useful. Sackett and other proponents of evidence-based practice realize that expertise is the key. Evidence in the hands of an expert is a powerful tool. We, however, must first know what defines an expert and how we can develop enough experts to serve our patients. This book turns us away from hero worship and false prophets who proclaim expertise based on pretense and self-promotion, and turns us toward experts whose expertise is based on evidence of achievement—experts whose credentials can be externally verified. Within the profession of physical therapy, many are experts, but they remain an untapped resource. With this volume, we turn toward this valuable commodity and seek to exploit it for the benefit of us all.

JULES ROTHSTEIN, Ph.D., P.T., FAPTA[†]

Professor and Head, Department of Physical Therapy, College of Health and Human Development Sciences and Professor, Department of Bioengineering, University of Illinois College of Medicine, Chicago; Chief, Physical Therapy Services, University of Illinois Hospital, Chicago; Editor, *Physical Therapy*, American Physical Therapy Association, Alexandria, Virginia

REFERENCE   1. Sackett DL, Richardson WS, Rosenberg, et al. *Evidence-Based Medicine: How to Practice and Teach EBM*. New York: Churchill Livingstone, 1997.

[†] Decreased.

Preface

This book is about expertise that is grounded in physical therapy practice. It is a reflection of clinical practice that is built from our observations and in-depth discussions with expert therapists about how they think, why they think it, and why they do what they do, rather than being a description of what clinical techniques they choose to apply to particular patients at particular times. Our approach is not without risk because much of the previous work in physical therapy centers on the application of clinical techniques. We believe there is tremendous value in the in-depth interpretative description of expert physical therapists in practice, especially at a time when changes in the health care system cause some to question the value of reflection and decision making in health care practice. We pose a grounded theory of expert practice in physical therapy that provides the profession with our first comprehensive understanding of the multiple dimensions of expertise. These insights include how expert practitioners develop, what knowledge they use, where they acquire that knowledge, how they think and reason, how they make decisions, and how they perform in practice. This book is a useful tool for validating elements of expert practice; generating new ideas for practice and education; and stimulating conversation and debate among faculty, clinicians, policy makers, and students in physical therapy and across the health professions.

Our book is also about collaboration and learning from one another on several levels. The initial level of observation and data collection begins by collaborating with colleagues in practice. We learned a great deal from them as we studied them working in the trenches of clinical practice. We began our observational work of physical therapy in the late 1980s, when three of us merely watched a therapist work with a patient. That initial 20-minute observation fueled a 3-hour debriefing discussion that led to multiple projects and funded research through the 1990s, as we continued to be fascinated by what physical therapists actually do in practice. What we found were practice elements that were broader, deeper, more profound, and more interconnected than we could have imagined.

Collaboration among a community of scholars is a central aspect of qualitative research. Insightful qualitative research is seldom accomplished working alone. Good conceptualization and theory development in qualitative research demands collaboration. Analysis and interpretation of data are very much a collaborative act. Our team of four researchers met extensively throughout the project to discuss, listen, analyze, agonize, and challenge to move the work forward. Working together requires more dialogue, more patience, more compromise (and sometimes more frustration) than individual research, but the whole is astonishingly greater than the sum of the parts. The quilt patterns at the beginning of each chapter and the resultant quilt are an appropriate metaphor for this work. Each individual pattern provides a visual display of each chapter's focus. Together, the 15 quilt blocks become a unit—a quilt with a clear design and purpose, representing the fullness of clinical practice.

When we wrote these words in the first edition of this book, we had no plans for writing a second edition. Our thoughts were that the first edition met our goal of sharing our findings about expert practice in physical therapy. We found, however, that as we continued to discuss elements of expert practice and ideas for professional development with our colleagues through publications, presentations, workshops, and conversations, we all continued to learn through this reflective process. Our work in expertise, grounded in physical therapy practice, has been enriched through our interactions and thoughtful comments from our colleagues. Our work appears to serve as a common ground for clinicians to discuss and learn from the expertise that is part of everyday practice. Although individual therapists carry the responsibility for practice, it is this community of practice in physical therapy that is critical to the profession's growth. Our work in expertise in physical therapy appears to serve as a common ground for clinicians to discuss and learn from the expertise that is part of everyday practice. This is a generative time for physical therapists as the profession moves rapidly toward having the Doctor of Physical Therapy (DPT) as the primary, and eventually only, preparation for practice. The responsibilities that accrue to a doctoring profession mean that, now more than ever, the profession must acknowledge the fundamental importance of development of expertise. We believe this edition extends the conversation on expertise and professional development by presenting new applications of our work to research, teaching, and practice in physical therapy.

G.M.J.

J.G.

L.M.H.

K.F.S.

Acknowledgments

The completion of this book was made possible through the support and encouragement of a number of individuals. First and foremost are the expert clinicians who patiently gave of their time; allowed us to interrupt their lives repeatedly to observe, interview, and videotape their interactions with patients; and thoughtfully shared their insights and reflections about their professional journeys and how they view clinical practice. We are also grateful to their patients and families who allowed us to observe and videotape their treatment sessions.

This research effort could not have been done without the financial support of the Foundation for Physical Therapy, and we are grateful for the funding of our research. We also appreciate the seed money provided by the Dean's Incentive Funds at Temple University. Our time and efforts also were supported by our respective institutions and department colleagues at Creighton University, Duke University, and Temple University. To our consultants, Arthur Elstein, Ph.D.; Lee Shulman, Ph.D.; Anna Richert, Ph.D.; and John Hershey, Ph.D., we owe great gratitude for helping us to see different views. Their conceptual and theoretical insights were invaluable to our work. We are grateful to our other contributors who shared their research on expertise with us. All of these contributors have challenged us to think more deeply about expert practice in physical therapy.

We thank Marion Waldman and Kathy Falk for their guidance and support of the second edition of this book. We are extremely grateful to Andrew Grow, our developmental editor, who has patiently prodded and enthusiastically supported our efforts in this revision.

We also thank our friends and families for their support, encouragement, and endurance of our writing time. Special thanks to Judy Gale, Jack Hershey, Sarah Hershey, and Rose Lopopolo, and in memory of Herbert L. Gwyer.

Contents

Part I

Studying Expertise: Purpose, Concepts, and Tools

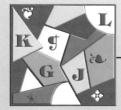

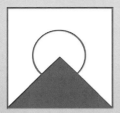

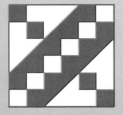

One of the recurring themes in our research and writing on expertise in physical therapy practice is the central role of context. Context includes understanding more about the human behavior and interactions, relationships, and belief systems that are part of physical therapy and expertise in physical therapy practice. We continue to assert that it is the uncovering and understanding of the contexts of physical therapy practices that are essential parts of our growing knowledge base in physical therapy. The role of qualitative research methods is critical in further exploring the context of physical therapy practice through description, explanation, understanding, and theory development. As we planned this second edition, we wished to continue to place our work in the larger context of the profession and professional life, research and theory development in expertise research, and the role of qualitative methods.

There has been tremendous growth and change in health care and the profession in the last few years from a stronger focus on health and wellness in a highly competitive health care environment to the acceptance of the role of the doctor of physical therapy degree for entry into the profession. Chapter 1 provides a critical reflective look at the current and future context of professional life across education, practice, and health care. In Chapter 2 we work to make meaningful connections between expertise research and theory and physical therapy. We explore the unique contribution of expertise research in physical therapy to expertise research across professions. We also embrace along with others the importance of seeing expertise as a continuous process, not a state of being, as an ultimate goal for professional development. In Chapter 3, we conclude this section with a succinct chronology of the conceptual models and theory development that underlies our work.

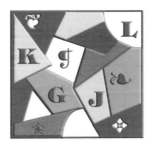

Crazy Quilt — An unstructured melding of diverse colors and textures, unified by embroidery and embellishments.

1 Professional Life: Issues of Health Care, Education, and Development

THE CURRENT CONTEXT OF PHYSICAL THERAPY PRACTICE

Physical therapy (PT) can be traced as far back as the ancient Greeks, who emphasized the healing properties of the sun's warmth and the value of exercise for producing sound minds in sound bodies. The profession of physical therapy, however, is a product of the twentieth century. Many of the defining events of the twentieth century allowed, and even fostered, its growth. Major strides in public health standards and the adoption of medical innovations have allowed people to benefit from rehabilitation services. Catastrophes such as world wars and epidemics have helped create a need for physical therapy, and social movements of the twentieth century can be credited with recognizing the needs of people with disabilities. All of these things contributed to nearly a century of continued growth for the practice of physical therapy. Physical therapy appeared to have escaped the almost regular cycles of surplus and shortage that have plagued medicine, and especially nursing, and has been generally in demand with a continuous upward trend, as events in the external environment conspired to create continual need (1).

Events of the late 1990s, however, created shifts that did change the demand for physical therapy for a period. The federal government, in its role as a major reimbursement source for health care services, made changes in its reimbursement for long-term care services in the Balanced Budget Act of 1997, which took effect in 1999. The response from the health care market was swift. Within days of the date the law went into force, skilled nursing facilities and outpatient practices began to limit their use of physical therapy. Within a few short months there was an almost complete freeze in the market for physical therapists and physical therapist assistants. The predictions that the demand for physical therapy would diminish, although based on entirely different reasons, appeared to be true (2).

These changes in the health care market, although not yet fully documented, were accompanied by all of the predictable changes in physical therapy. Physical therapists, and especially physical therapist assistants, reported decreased work hours and reductions in salary (3). Educational programs reported declines in applicant pools. These declines were sharp enough to result in a reduction in the number of physical therapist assistant programs (4). Yet indicators of recovery began within 5 years, and, as we move to the middle of the first decade of the twenty-first century, by all anecdotal accounts the demand for physical therapists has returned.

What lessons can be learned from this period? We have learned that changes in health care markets can have a swift and furious impact on the organization of care and the role of health care providers. Yet we have also seen a resilience in physical therapy demonstrated by the ability to return to a state of demand in 5 years. Only time will tell whether this temporary decline in demand will fade in its importance as the overall trend in the need and demand for physical therapy increases or whether it signals a different level of growth.

Physical therapy is practiced in the context of the health care market. All signs indicate that there continue to be concerns over the growth of health care as a portion of our economy. These concerns are fueled on one side by increasing demands for monies to be spent in other sectors and the perspective that we have not achieved the health care outcomes (e.g., decreased mortality and morbidity) that might be reflected by the current level of investment. There continue to be many suggestions that limits should be placed on the growth of health care and that more accountability must be demanded from professions that have previously been relatively autonomous.

Almost all of health care in the United States is paid for by third parties: employers, through their role as manager of benefits for their employees, and the federal government as an employer and as a source of health insurance for defined populations. The past 25 years have seen major changes in the expectations placed on health care providers by these third-party reimbursement sources. Most of these changes have been focused on decreasing costs through increased controls over the decisions made by individual health care providers. In response to these increased controls, practitioners have modified their behavior, with a general reduction in the amount of services provided, as measured by lengths of stay (5).

Known loosely as managed care, these changes have primarily resulted in a greater emphasis on using policies predetermined by the reimbursement sources and their agents (i.e., insurance companies) for decision making and much less reliance on decisions made by individual health care practitioners themselves. Managed care has many other features, many of which are focused on reducing costs to payers (e.g., employers, insurance companies, and governmental agencies). Although these cost-control strategies abound and become more complex with each new attempt to design appropriate incentives for payment, they are based on the belief that care can be more efficient if provided in a more uniform manner.

PHYSICAL THERAPISTS' PRACTICE

Who is the typical physical therapist dealing with these clinical realities? Analyzing simple descriptive data reveals that the typical therapist is a woman who is white, in her 30s, educated as a therapist with a bachelor's degree, and working in either a hospital or an outpatient practice. Identifying the "average" therapist is deceptive, however, particularly when health care is changing at an ever more rapid pace. Instead, the range of possibilities that more fully describes the multifaceted practitioners of today must be examined (6).

The face of physical therapy is really more diverse than can be seen in simple modal statistics. Although the average age is in the late 30s, the rapid expansion of new entrants into physical therapy between 1985 and 2000, followed by a decline in the number of graduates through at least 2010, means that there are several age-based cohorts making up the distribution of therapists. Although most physical therapists are women, more than 30% are men; although most are white, almost 8% are from ethnic groups normally underrepresented in physical therapy (6). Based on the demographics of enrolled students, the numbers of entrants from underrepresented groups is growing (4).

Career patterns of physical therapy as a predominantly female profession reflect attempts to meet the dual responsibilities faced by women in today's society—career and family. To retain a license to practice physical therapy, one must meet variable state government requirements, which might include annual continuing education courses or documentation of continued active practice. Both of these requirements present challenges for women who wish to interrupt their careers to raise children. Historically, the profession has experienced a significant rate of attrition that has been higher for women than for men (1).

Perhaps most markedly, describing a model site for practice is nearly impossible. In a profession whose members were once almost exclusively in the employment of hospitals, remarkable shifts occurred in the 1980s and 1990s and continue today. Many therapists choose to own or work in practices owned by physical therapists. There has also been a fairly rapid shift in the ownership of practices to corporately held chains and health care systems (7). Major changes in the provision of care to acutely ill patients have occurred. Rapidly declining lengths of stay have moved those patients, whose physiologic ability to heal has not changed, from acute care hospitals to other sites of care, such as skilled nursing facilities and homes. To meet the demands of managed care, hospitals have redefined themselves and formed partnerships with these other sites, creating larger systems through mergers, acquisitions, and alliances. Physical therapists have responded to these changes by following the patient. Therapists have changed their employers and their employment relationships to continue to gain access to patient care.

Additionally, therapists have identified "niche" markets, with a focus on specific patient populations, such as women's health and prevention. Concurrently, there has been an increase in the acceptance of self-pay as a form of reimbursement (8). All of these changes mean that a great deal of diversity exists in both current practitioners and current practice of physical therapy.

Until very late in the twentieth century, not enough physical therapists were available to meet the needs of the patient population of the United States. In response, the number of educational programs preparing new therapists increased, the average size of graduating classes grew, and reliance on internationally educated therapists and on other providers (e.g., physical therapist assistants, athletic trainers, and occupational therapists) also increased.

The changes at the end of the 1990s, documented earlier, which include actual reductions in care and perceptions of uncertainty and volatility, have resulted in the need for new analyses of this situation. Any study of the balance of supply and demand for a particular occupation is always subject to being quickly rendered obsolete as market forces respond to the very changes being predicted in the study. At best, these studies are snapshots; what is most needed to help guide health personnel decisions is real-time video. Such research, however, can help identify the factors that contribute to balance by asking questions such as, "What is the demand or need for physical therapy?" "What controls the supply of physical therapists and their substitutes in the labor market?" and "How are practitioners distributed, both geographically and by specialty?"

What will the twenty-first century reveal about physical therapy? How will the work of physical therapists be transformed? The answers to these questions can be found in the profession of physical therapy and in the external environment of physical therapy practice. Today's environment is changing so rapidly that details of such changes cannot be accurately illustrated in the confines of printed text. Yet, no matter the specifics of change, the overall impact is that care must be provided more efficiently, more quickly, more accurately, more cheaply, and with more accountability.

DESCRIBING PHYSICAL THERAPY SERVICES

As in many other health care professions, models of disability have been used in physical therapy to help describe who we are treating and why. In the past, patients have been described almost exclusively by their diagnoses. For example, a system of classifying diseases, known most commonly as the International Classification of Diseases (ICD), was developed and has been used in the United States as the principal means of categorizing patients for reporting and reimbursement (9). This classification was based primarily on the types of diagnoses of pathology usually made by physicians. When the major goal of health care intervention is removal of the disease, this system works relatively well. However, it is increasingly clear that describing patients based on disease entities is insufficient for making a prognosis and predicting resource allocation. Disease-based classifications may also not be useful in identifying the full range of a patient's needs. As the ability to prolong people's lives improves and the number of people with chronic diseases and people living with permanent sequelae increases, this system begins to not work as well. Instead of concentrating on the precipitating event, health care practitioners should focus on the results of the event.

In response to these concerns, disablement models have been proposed (10,11). One such model is the Nagi model, as adapted and promulgated in the American Physical Therapy Association's (APTA) *Guide to Physical Therapist Practice* (Figure 1-1) (12). Although the initial disease, syndrome, or traumatic event begins the cascade of decision making, it is only the beginning.

Disablement models recognize that each disease results in certain impairments to systems or organs, that these impairments can lead to a decrease in functional ability, and that this decline in function can result in disability or a reduction in the ability to fully engage in one's role in society. The models also identify physical, psychological, and social factors that either can diminish or increase impairments, functional limitation, and disability. All of these disability models are rooted in the context of the biopsychosocial model for understanding health, illness, and well-being that has been put forth by the World Health Organization (WHO) (13). WHO has also sponsored the development of a new means of classification in health care, the International Classification of Functioning, Disability, and Health, known as the ICF. This classification differs from the ICD by adding emphasis on chronic conditions versus acute, by focus on function rather than disease, and by recognizing the impact of the environment on people with disabilities (14).

By adopting such models and systems for classification for describing care, health care practitioners are able to focus on the ongoing needs of patients in the context of the patients' lives. Prognosis and resource allocation become clearer, and the fact that, in addition to physicians, many participants in health care (e.g., other health care providers, insurance companies) make decisions about classification of patients by impairment, limitation, or disability becomes evident. The adoption of a disability model to provide a context for thinking about health care changes everything about how relationships to patients and colleagues are defined. For example, the label stroke does not define very much

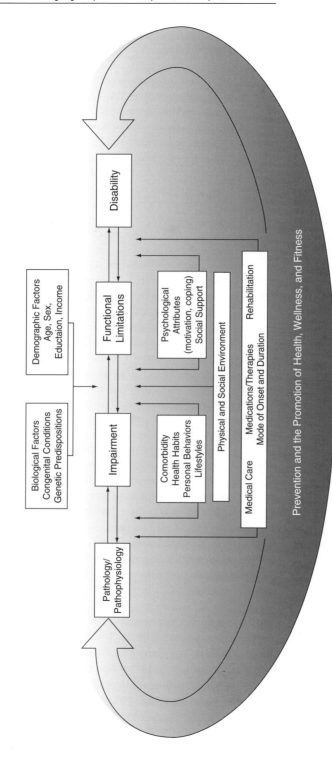

Figure 1–1 ■ The Nagi Model for the Process of Disablement. (Adapted from Guccione A. Physical therapy diagnosis and the relationship between impairments and function. *Phys Ther* 1991; 71:499–504.)

about the rehabilitation programs that are designed with and for patients who have had a stroke. Identifying the impairments and functional limitations of defined groups of patients who have had a stroke, however, can clearly identify the prognosis and the resource allocation needed to meet that prognosis.

The adoption of such a model has helped create the *Guide to Physical Therapist Practice* (12), which identifies patterns of care for groups of patients who benefit from the intervention of physical therapists and provides a common language for physical therapists to use in describing and documenting care that actually reflects our contributions to the health and wellness of our patients. The ICF, which is compatible with the assumptions used in the *Guide*, has extended this ability to converse across the world (15).

PHYSICAL THERAPISTS' EDUCATION

Education in physical therapy has progressed through four distinct phases in the nine decades of the profession's history: 1) postgraduate specialty training (1920s to 1950s) to 2) baccalaureate programs (1950s to 1980s) to 3) master's level programs (1970s to 1990s), and most recently to 4) doctoral programs (1990s to present). This last period has also seen the rapid shift from master's level programs to doctoral level programs.

Today, of the 214 physical therapist educational programs, more than 40% are at the doctoral level. Surveys of the remaining master's degree programs indicate that more than 90% of all physical therapist educational programs will be at the doctoral level by 2013. This represents a much more rapid shift from master's to doctoral level than from baccalaureate to master's, which took almost 25 years (4).

The type of student attracted to a career in physical therapy has also changed. In the first phase, almost everyone who entered the profession was female and had previously received training as a nurse or teacher. In the second phase, the majority of entrants were women who chose physical therapy while in high school and were educated at the baccalaureate level (16). In the beginning of the third phase, a higher number of applicants had previous employment and career experience and represented an increasing diversity in sex, race, and age (17,18). The fourth phase has also coincided with a decrease in the size of applicant pools, with fewer nontraditional students represented. However, the changes in the health care market that signify an increase in the demand for physical therapists have also caused an increase in the size of applicant pools.

The most typical format of professional education for the 214 accredited programs in physical therapy is a 2- to 3-year program of education at the master's degree level, with a number of 3-year postbaccalaureate professional doctoral degree programs emerging.

Although applicants to physical therapy programs share a comprehensive background in basic science and social science prerequisites similar to that of medical school applicants, they also bring diversity to the professional education curriculum through their areas of study and life experiences. The curricula for preparation of physical therapists in programs across the country are planned to achieve a required set of outcome expectations for graduates, as articulated in the Evaluative Criteria for Accreditation of Physical Therapist Educational Programs developed by the Commission on Accreditation in

Physical Therapy Education. These evaluative criteria provide the assurance that a minimum level of clinical competence can be anticipated for graduates of all accredited programs. The evaluative criteria used for accrediting educational programs are reviewed continuously for currency of the practice expectations for new entrants to the profession (19). A nationwide consensus project to develop curricular content and practice expectations for postbaccalaureate curricula in physical therapy has helped lend consistency to the curricular development process in many schools (20).

The curriculum content in physical therapy educational programs is presented in both didactic and clinical formats. Faculty members in the academic setting prepare students for phases of clinical education conducted under the supervision of clinical education faculty in a variety of practice settings that reflect current physical therapy practice. The didactic content includes current information in the following areas: basic sciences of anatomy, physiology, histology, pathology, and neuroscience; clinical sciences of kinesiology, arthrology, human development, motor control, and pathokinesiology; medical sciences of surgery, medicine, radiology, pharmacology, and nutrition; social sciences of psychology, sociology, ethics, research, and teaching/learning theory; and physical therapy sciences of examination, evaluation, diagnosis, prognosis, interventions, and outcome assessment. Didactic and clinical phases of the curriculum usually are integrated to allow progression of the student through successively more complex performance challenges with patients. At the conclusion of the professional education program, graduates must successfully complete a standardized national licensure examination before being admitted to practice.

Although standards for accreditation and licensure lend consistency to the preparation of physical therapists, an examination of the variety of educational programs also would reveal considerable diversity. Diversity among programs is found in the educational settings of physical therapist programs (ranging from liberal arts colleges to academic medical centers in universities), the sequencing and integration of the didactic content, and the length and breadth of the clinical education component (4).

Certainly, the shift to doctoral level education will mean changes in applicant pools, in faculty responsibilities, and in the physical therapy curricula. Yet this shift has occurred at the same time that market forces have affected the size of applicant pools and class sizes. Only time will tell how the shift in PT education to doctoral level will affect practice.

CONTINUED MATURATION OF THE PROFESSION

In the midst of all of these changes in practice setting, models for describing practice, and physical therapist education, the profession of physical therapy has also adopted activities that demonstrate a true commitment to patients and a willingness to accept the accountability required of professionals.

GROWTH IN SCHOLARSHIP, EVIDENCE-BASED PRACTICE, AND OUTCOMES MEASUREMENT

The amount of research being done to provide insight on the theory and practice of physical therapy continues to grow, as is documented by the increased number and quality of journals in the field and the increased number of articles in other journals that have specific application to physical therapy (21). The spectrum of research approaches and designs also has increased. It is now much easier to find qualitative work that helps us understand the perspectives of practitioners and patients at a much deeper level. We are also seeing an increase in epidemiologic and health services research that helps us learn about our practices by analyzing large databases and examining population-based risks. Finally, there has been an increase in the amount of research that is being done to measure the effectiveness of diagnostic and prognostic tools and interventions in actual patient populations. All of this expansion means that we have available to us an almost unmanageable amount of information that can help us improve care.

Over the past 10 years a new force has been active in the way clinicians think about and provide their care, which also gives us a means to manage this massive amount of information. This is the concept of evidence-based practice (EBP) (22–24). EBP was developed to help clinicians bring the results of current research (evidence) together with the patient's values and circumstances, to make decisions using their clinical expertise, thereby forging a therapeutic alliance with the patient. The proponents of EBP believe that using the processes of EBP can improve care. There is a growing body of evidence that supports this view (25,26).

One of the outcomes of EBP is to engage in careful analyses of individual research studies. An example of a resource that supports such analyses is the Hooked on Evidence project of the APTA (27). Another of the outcomes of EBP is to arrive at conclusions (clinical bottom lines) about preferable modes of treatment based on a systematic review of the current evidence. The Evidence in Practice feature in *Physical Therapy* is an example of such reviews (28). EBP's origins are found in the British Commonwealth countries; there are also numerous examples of resources found around the world (29,30).

The assumptions are that by using evidence from research, literature clinicians can identify a recommended course of action for similar patients and that clinicians can expect that a majority of their patients will benefit from application of these patterns. Because much of physical therapy, as is true across all health care, does not yet have specific research evidence to support it, expert opinion also becomes a source of guidance. Therefore, one of the major evaluative decisions made by clinicians in this mode of practice is to decide if the patterns apply to a particular patient presenting to the practitioner. This is quite different from the more traditional process of clinical decision-making, which focused much more on patient differences than on commonalties.

Choosing an appropriate pattern of care for a patient requires understanding how to classify that patient into a specific group and being assured that the patterns chosen are based on patients' full needs, addressing impairment, limitation, and disability. *Guide to Physical Therapist Practice* (12) offers more than 30 patterns of care for patients with problems in the four systems within the physical therapist's scope of practice: neurological, musculoskeletal, cardiovascular/pulmonary, and integumentary.

Changes in the health care system also have required the development of what is known as the outcomes movement, which focuses on better measuring outcomes at all levels, especially those related to functional ability and quality of life. As health care outcomes become more clearly explicated, practitioners can be expected to turn increasingly to evidence-based practice. In other words, learning more about what is actually achieved with interventions encourages using only those interventions that have clear documentation of success. This is a laudable goal but one that will take much time to achieve and will depend heavily on wise clinical input.

All health care practitioners grapple with the issue of how to adequately identify and measure the outcomes of their work. For outcome measurement to be successful, such measurement must meet the requirement of all sound measurements: It must be valid. Among other things, these measures must relate to the world in which patients live, reflect the roles patients have chosen in their lives, and be both sensitive and specific enough to provide information that helps validate our diagnostic and prognostic decisions. This is a difficult task that is made even harder when the process of care is not fully understood. A clear understanding of how therapists interact with patients to make individual decisions during the course of care is essential for capturing the full picture of all outcomes addressed by care (whether disease related, impairment based, or related to functional limitations), for identifying the variables that affect these decisions, and for developing measures that capture all aspects of care. The absence of such an understanding forces therapists to rely on gross measures that may easily miss the most important contributions they make to patients' lives.

For example, most physical therapists consider teaching patients to make good decisions about their own behavior one of the most important things therapists do. If research does not focus on the long-term effects of physical therapy, the effects of patient education on lifelong health cannot be measured. As another example, although most therapists believe that their individual interventions are different from each other because they provide different physiologic and anatomic benefits, developing specificity of intervention selection and intensity of service guidelines is impossible if all interventions are identified simply as physical therapy.

The trend toward better understanding outcomes also moves closer to evidence-based practice. Evidence-based practice requires health care practitioners to look to many sources of evidence to determine their choices in clinical decision making. These sources certainly include quantitative studies on efficacy, especially controlled clinical trials. Research should be designed to help improve decisions to define options and the results of specific choices. Another source of evidence is documentation of best practice based on expert opinion, such as the *Guide*. Evidence gathered in a systematic way on a case-by-case basis from each patient is also a source of guiding information for evidence-based practice (31). Therapists participate in evidence-based practice when they reflect on each patient and what can be learned from that patient about subsequent patients. This is in contrast to therapists who make decisions because of expediency, lack of knowledge, personal comfort with a type of intervention, or any other reason that does not arise from what is learned about patients and their responses to interventions.

DEVELOPMENT OF PROFESSIONAL CORE VALUES

There is a continued call across health professions for a set of core competencies that are seen as critical for reform of health professions education. The 2003 Institute of Medicine report, "Health Professions Education: A Bridge to Quality," proposes these five core competencies for all health professions: provide patient-centered care, work in interdisciplinary teams, use evidence-based practice, apply quality improvement, and use informatics (32).

In 2002 the APTA undertook a project to identify the core values that underlie physical therapists' behaviors as professionals committed to the welfare of their patients and clients. Two of the authors of this text were among the group convened to review the work that had been done in identifying these core values and to prepare a document for review across the profession. After widespread dissemination, the APTA Board of Directors adopted the Core Values. These value statements have since been integrated into normative descriptions of physical therapy education and into accreditation standards, as seen in Box 1-1 (19,20,33,34).

BOX 1–1   *The Seven Core Values*

> *Accountability*. A physical therapist (PT) demonstrates accountability by acknowledging and accepting the consequences of his or her actions, by responding to the patient's or client's goals and needs, and by maintaining membership in APTA and other organizations.
>
> *Altruism*. A PT demonstrates altruism by placing the patient's or client's needs above those of the PT, by providing *pro bono* services, and by providing services to the patient or client that go beyond expected standards of practice.
>
> *Compassion and Caring*. A PT demonstrates compassion and caring by being an advocate for patients' or clients' needs, understanding an individual's perspective and the various influences on that person's life in his or her environment, and demonstrating respect for others and considering them as unique and of value.
>
> *Excellence*. A PT demonstrates excellence by internalizing the importance of using multiple sources of evidence to support professional practice and decisions, seeking out and acquiring new knowledge throughout his or her professional career, and demonstrating high levels of knowledge and skill in all aspects of the profession.
>
> *Integrity*. A PT demonstrates integrity by abiding by the rules, regulations, and laws applicable to the profession; adhering to the profession's highest standards (in practice, ethics, reimbursement, and other

(Continued)

areas); confronting harassment and bias in oneself and others; being trustworthy; and choosing employment situations that are congruent with practice values and professional ethical standards.

Professional Duty. A PT demonstrates professional duty by facilitating the achievement of each patient's or client's goals for function, health, and wellness; promoting the profession; mentoring others; and getting involved in professional activities beyond the practice setting.

Social Responsibility. A PT demonstrates social responsibility by promoting cultural competence within the profession and the larger public; promoting social policy that affects the function, health, and wellness needs of patients and clients; promoting community volunteerism; and working to ensure the blending of social justice and economic efficiency of service delivery.

From Bezner J. Board perspective: getting to the core of professionalism, *PT Mag.* 2004;12(1).

PROFESSIONAL DEVELOPMENT OVER ONE'S CAREER

Informal and formal opportunities for continued development over a therapist's career have increased in the past 25 years and are expected to grow in the future. Self-directed, nonmandatory opportunities for professional development have significantly expanded, with continuing education courses available on a wide range of topics, in a variety of settings, and delivered both in person and through distance communication techniques.

The American Board of Physical Therapy Specialties of APTA sponsors a certification process for physical therapists who have specialized their practice in one of seven areas: 1) cardiopulmonary therapy, 2) clinical electrophysiology, 3) geriatrics, 4) neurology, 5) orthopedics, 6) pediatrics, or 7) sports. This rigorous program of self-assessment and standardized testing has been successful, with more than 6,000 board-certified specialists currently practicing (35).

Additional opportunities for continued professional development in a mentored, planned clinical format, termed "residency," exist for physical therapists who have selected a specialty area of practice. Residency training requires the therapist to be in residence for at least 6 months at a residency-training site for a combined program of didactic and clinical advanced education. There are 18 residency programs in four clinical areas: geriatrics, neurology, orthopedics, and sports (36).

More formalized, advanced programs provide opportunities for physical therapists to update and deepen their clinical knowledge base by earning an advanced master's or doctoral degree. There are more than 75 such programs in physical therapy departments (37) in the United States, with many more available in related basic and behavioral science fields.

The past 10 years have also seen the growth of programs termed transitional-Doctor of Physical Therapy (DPT) programs. These programs are available for practicing physical therapists and are therefore an opportunity for professional development. They are also designed to help practicing therapists match the level of current entry level, so they can be seen as part of entry-level preparation. There are more than 60 such programs, with almost 10,000 therapists enrolled or graduated from such programs (38).

Fellowship programs have also developed to further practice, research, and educational skills for therapists who have already completed doctoral degrees, residencies, or specialization. There are 15 fellowship programs in four clinical areas: hand therapy, movement science, orthopedics, and sports (39).

VISIONS FOR THE FUTURE

The APTA has set forth its view of what the future should be for physical therapy in what is termed Vision 2020:

> *By 2020, physical therapy will be provided by physical therapists who are doctors of physical therapy, recognized by consumers and other health care professionals as practitioners of choice to whom consumers have direct access for the diagnosis of, interventions for, and prevention of impairments, functional limitations, and disabilities related to movement, function, and health.*

APTA has identified that, to reach this Vision, physical therapists will be doctors of physical therapy who practice in an autonomous manner through direct access to their services, using EBP principles, adhering to professional core values, and thereby being practitioners of choice among health care consumers (40).

The growth that has been achieved in physical therapy practice and education has resulted only because of the work of leaders in physical therapy practice. Health care practitioners should continue to seek the judgment of such people to respond to the challenges in practice and education that lie ahead, especially if the vision described is to be achieved. The decisions that are made regarding where and how therapists practice will influence the ultimate ability of physical therapy to contribute to the care of patients. The ultimate answer to the economic analysis of surplus versus shortage depends on society's perception of its need for physical therapy and the translation of that need into demand. The choices therapists make regarding appropriate clinical care determine how many therapists are needed and where they need to practice. The advocacy exerted with patients, payers, and policymakers will affect the demand for this care. Professional expectations for quality can set the necessary limits on the cost reductions that can be derived from the system. The quality of education of new practitioners will determine these practitioners' ability to meet these challenges. Given the incredible rate of change in the health care system and the remarkable advances in physical therapy, perhaps it has never been more important to understand how our colleagues achieve expertise.

OVERVIEW OF THE BOOK

In the intervening years since we first presented our research on expertise in physical therapy, much has changed, but much has remained the same. We believe that the lessons we learned, and the work that has built on research, can continue to provide useful perspectives for the future.

The remaining chapters of Part I, Studying Expertise: Purpose, Concepts, and Tools, set forth a description of the research done in many fields to explain and define expertise, followed by a review of the specific research techniques used in our study of expert clinicians. The chapters in this section are designed to explain the theory and processes that guide reflections and research on expertise.

Part II, Portraits of Expertise in Physical Therapy, presents the cases and detailed stories of 12 expert clinicians in four clinical areas of practice. These chapters (4–7) deal with real clinicians and their patients as the clinicians make good decisions, make mistakes, learn from their mistakes, teach others, and reflect on their practice. Chapter 8 contains the synthesis of our cross-case analysis for the four clinical specialty areas and tells the greater story of what we learned from the 12 therapists that defines what it means to be a physical therapist striving to be the best clinician possible. The section closes with a postscript on our experts over the intervening years since they last shared their reflections with us.

We are excited by the addition of Part III, Lessons Learned and Applied, which sets forth the work of four groups of researchers and practitioners who have built on the premise of our work. In Chapter 9, Resnick connects concepts of expert practice to patient outcomes by using data from large databases. Edwards and Jones, in Chapter 10, add an international dimension with their work examining clinical decision-making in therapists in a variety of clinical settings in Australia. In Chapter 11 Mostrom updates her contribution from the first edition, adding elements about patient-centered reasoning and the role of the practice community. Chapter 12 is a presentation by Sullivan and Jampel about the application of what we know about expertise to the development of a practical system for professional development and recognition in practice.

Part IV, Pursuing Expertise in Physical Therapy, offers our views about how the work done explaining and understating expertise in physical therapy can be applied to future research (Chapter 13), education (Chapter 14), and practice (Chapter 15). We see the growth of physical therapy and the understanding of expertise in clinical practice as a grand journey. We invite the reader to join us on this journey, which started with profound respect for the work done by physical therapists and with inquisitiveness about how the best therapists think. Our collective journey has not ended; it continues because of the wonderful therapists we have met who have shown us an exciting, adventurous path toward high-quality, compassionate, and efficacious care.

REFERENCES

1. Gwyer J. Personnel resources in physical therapy: an analysis of supply, career patterns, and methods to enhance availability. *Phys Ther.* 1995;75:56–67.
2. American Physical Therapy Association. 2000 and beyond: the work-force study. *PT Mag.* 1998;1:46–52.
3. American Physical Therapy Association. *2005 median income of physical therapists summary report.* Alexandria, VA: APTA; 2005.
4. American Physical Therapy Association. *2004 fact sheet physical therapist education.* Alexandria, VA: APTA; 2004.
5. Agency for Healthcare Research and Quality. Reducing Costs in the Health Care System. Learning from what has been done. *Research in Action.* 2002;(9).

6. American Physical Therapy Association. *Physical therapist member demographic profile 1999–2004.* Alexandria, VA: APTA; 2005.
7. American Physical Therapy Association. *The APTA employment survey.* Alexandria, VA: APTA; 2005.
8. Hack LM, Konrad TR. Determination of supply and requirements in physical therapy: some considerations and examples. *Phys Ther.* 1995;75:47–55.
9. National Center for Health Statistics. *Classifications of diseases and functioning & disability.* Available at: http://www.cdc.gov/nchs/icd9.htm. Accessed February 2, 2006.
10. Jette AM. Physical disablement concepts for physical therapy research and practice. *Phys Ther.* 1994;74:380–386.
11. Guccione A. Physical therapy diagnosis and the relationship between impairments and function. *Phys Ther.* 1991;71:499–504.
12. American Physical Therapy Association. *Guide to physical therapist practice*, ed 2. Alexandria, VA: APTA; 2002.
13. Preamble to the Constitution of the World Health Organization as adopted by the International Health Conference, New York, 19–22 June, 1946; signed on 22 July 1946 by the representatives of 61 States (Official Records of the World Health Organization, no. 2, p. 100) and entered into force on 7 April 1948. Available at: http://www.who.int/about/definition/en/. Accessed February 2, 2006.
14. International Classification of Functioning, Disability, and Health. Available at: http://www.who.int/icf/icftemplate.cfm. Accessed February 2, 2006.
15. Reed G, Harwood K, Brandt D, et al. *International Classification of Functioning, Disability, and Health: A manual for health professionals.* American Physical Therapy Association Annual Conference, 2004.
16. American Physical Therapy Association. *1979 active membership profile report: a summary report.* Alexandria, VA: APTA; 1979.
17. American Physical Therapy Association. *1993 active membership profile report.* Alexandria, VA: APTA; 1994.
18. Pinkston D. *A history of physical therapy education in the United States* [PhD dissertation]. Cleveland, OH: Case Western Reserve University; 1978.
19. Commission on Accreditation for Physical Therapy Education. *Evaluative criteria for accreditation of education programs for the preparation of physical therapists.* Alexandria, VA: Commission on Accreditation for Physical Therapy Education; 2005.
20. American Physical Therapy Association. *A normative model of physical therapist professional education*, Version 97. Alexandria, VA: APTA; 1997.
21. Miller PA, McKibbon KA, Haynes RB. A quantitative analysis of research publications in physical therapy journals. *Phys Ther.* 2003;83:123–131.
22. Straus SE, Richardson WS, Glasziou P, Haynes RB. *Evidence-based medicine*, ed 3. New York: Churchill Livingstone; 2005.
23. Bury T, Mead J. *Evidence-based health care: a practical guide for therapists.* Oxford: Butterworth-Heinemann; 1998.
24. Geyman JP, Deyo RA, Ramsey SD. *Evidence-based clinical practice.* Boston: Butterworth-Heinemann; 2000.
25. Mikhail C, Korner-Bitensky N, Rossignol M, et al. Physical therapists' use of interventions with high evidence of effectiveness in the management of a hypothetical typical patient with acute low back pain. *Phys Ther.* 2005;85:1151–1167.
26. Ring N, Malcolm C, Coull A, et al. Nursing best practice statements: An exploration of their implementation in clinical practice. *J Clin Nurs.* 2005;14(9):1048–1058.
27. American Physical Therapy Association. *Hooked on evidence.* Available at: http://www.hookedonevidence.com/. Accessed February 2, 2006.
28. Smith B, Cleland J. Clinical question: Is radiologic examination necessary for a 9-year-old girl with a knee injury? *Phys Ther.* 2004;84(11):1092–1094.
29. www.nettingtheevidence.org.uk. *A ScHARR introduction to evidence based practice on the internet.* Available at: http://www.shef.ac.uk/scharr/ir/netting/. Accessed February 2, 2006.
30. PEDro. *Physiotherapy evidence database.* Available at: http://www.pedro.fhs.usyd.edu.au/index.html. Accessed February 2, 2006.

31. McEwen I (ed). *Writing case reports: a how-to manual for clinicians*, ed 2. Alexandria, VA: APTA; 2001.
32. Greiner A, Knebel E (eds). *Health professions education: a bridge to quality*. Washington, DC: Institute of Medicine of the National Academies, National Academies Press; 2003.
33. American Physical Therapy Association. *Professionalism in physical therapy: core values*. Alexandria, VA: APTA; 2003.
34. Bezner J. Board perspective: getting to the core of professionalism. *PT Mag*. 2004;12(1).
35. American Physical Therapy Association. *American Board of Physical Therapy Specialties*. Available at: http://www.apta.org/AM/Template.cfm?Section=ABPTS1&Template=/TaggedPage/TaggedPageDisplay.cfm&TPLID=42&ContentID=14391. Accessed February 2, 2006.
36. American Physical Therapy Association. *Residencies*. Available at: http://www.apta.org/AM/Template.cfm?Section=Residency&Template=/TaggedPage/TaggedPageDisplay.cfm&TPLID=118&ContentID=15371. Accessed February 2, 2006.
37. American Physical Therapy Association. *Post-professional degrees*. Available at: http://www.apta.org/AM/Template.cfm?Section=Post_Professional_Degree&TEMPLATE=/CM/ContentDisplay.cfm&CONTENTID=27838. Accessed February 2, 2006.
38. American Physical Therapy Association. *Transition-DPT programs*. Available at: http://www.apta.org/AM/Template.cfm?Section=Post_Professional_Degree&CONTENTID=28221&TEMPLATE=/CM/ContentDisplay.cfm. Accessed February 2, 2006.
39. American Physical Therapy Association. Fellowship web site. Available at: http://www.apta.org/AM/Template.cfm?Section=Residency&CONTENTID=28129&TEMPLATE=/CM/ContentDisplay.cfm. Accessed February 2, 2006.
40. American Physical Therapy Association. *Vision 2020*. Available at: http://www.apta.org/AM/Template.cfm?Section=About_APTA&TEMPLATE=/CM/ContentDisplay.cfm&CONTENTID=19078. Accessed February 2, 2006.

Moon over the Mountain — A traditional folk pattern with the brilliant moon illuminating the land below.

2 Understanding Expertise: Connecting Research and Theory to Physical Therapy

What is our fascination with expertise? We are quick to claim that we want to facilitate rapid development of novice practitioners toward professional competence and expertise, yet the focus on evidence-based practice has led to continued debate about the relative importance of "expert opinion" as an important source of evidence (1,2). This debate has been fueled, in part, by our own misconceptions of expert opinion, what counts as evidence, the dimensions of expertise and expert practice, and the assumption that research and theory on expertise and expert practice can be applied across health professions.

In the first edition of this book, we provided a basic overview of the literature on expertise and proposed a prototypical model of expertise. In this revised chapter, we take a bolder stand to explicitly make meaningful connections between theory, research, and physical therapy. We believe that the continued growth and acceptance of the Doctor of Physical Therapy (DPT) degree in physical therapy education signals a readiness of the profession to understand and use theoretical work in our thinking, in deliberations, and across settings (education, research, and practice).

This chapter begins with "coming to terms" with the terms and concepts. Why is this important? We use this introduction to lay the foundation for the importance and practical relevance of research in expertise for the profession of physical therapy. In this section, we explore the meaning of expertise, novice and expert differences, and novice development as it relates to contemporary definitions of professional competence. The middle section of the chapter focuses on an overview of predominant theories in expertise research. One of our challenges in this chapter is finding the right balance between sharing the research and supporting literature in a way that is relevant, is practical, and contributes to the physical therapy knowledge base. We hope we have found the right balance that will inform education and practice and facilitate the profession's intellectual growth. We believe that exposure to the breadth of expertise research and theory is important because it helps us understand how expertise research in physical therapy (3–16) contributes to the identity of the profession of physical therapy among other professions.

Finally, we conclude the chapter with a revised prototypical model of expertise that highlights the core dimensions of developing expertise. In this revised chapter, we embrace, along with others (17,18), the assumption that expertise should be seen as a continuous process, not as a state of being, because the ultimate goal of studying expertise is enhancing the professional development of novices and lesser-skilled practitioners.

"COMING TO TERMS": TERMS AND CONCEPTS IN EXPERTISE

What does it mean to be an expert? What is the relationship between professional competence and expertise? Why have we continued to see research and discussion about expert practice in physical therapy? These are questions we will begin to address in this section.

The simple definition of an expert is as follows: "an expert is capable of doing the right thing at the right time" (19, p. 308). In research on expertise there are several variations on this definition of an expert. An expert can be defined as someone who *performs* at the level of an experienced professional, such as a master or grandmaster in chess or a clinical specialist in medicine

(20,21). Experts also can be defined as top performers who excel in a particular field, such as elite athletes or musicians. Finally, experts can also be seen as those who achieve at least a moderate degree of success in their occupation (22). Another view or conception of expertise is that it is not just a cluster of attributes such as knowledge and problem-solving skills or high-level performance; expertise needs to be seen as a process rather than a static state or label (23). This does not mean that the process of moving toward expertise is based merely on the gathering of years of experience. Without learning mechanisms or reflection used to mediate improvement from experience, there will be little acquisition of expertise (17). If our definition or conception of expertise is seen more as a process than a state to be achieved, then we begin to see the critical importance of learning in the context of professional development. This includes broadening our discussion to additional considerations such as understanding expert–novice differences to facilitate novice development, professional learning, and the development of professional competence.

NOVICE–EXPERT DIFFERENCES

In more than 40 years of expertise research, there remains strong consensus in how experts differ from novices (18–26). The case examples in this chapter highlight key characteristics and differences in how a novice and an expert may handle a patient case.

CASE EXAMPLE

The patient is a 70-year-old man who is referred to physical therapy with right hip pain and a diagnosis of osteoarthritis of the hip.

1. Experts bring more knowledge to bear in solving problems within their clinical specialty area or domain of practice. This knowledge is highly organized, accessible, and integrated.

NOVICE: Forms immediate working hypothesis that the patient's primary problem is osteoarthritis of the hip, given the patient's age and history of arthritis.

EXPERT: Knows that hip pain may be referred from the low back and asks specific, directed questions in the patient interview to obtain a better understanding of the symptom patterns with activity and with rest. Given the presentation of pain in the L3 dermatome and relief the patient experiences with sitting, the expert is suspicious of an L3 spinal problem.

2. Experts figure things out. They solve problems more efficiently and monitor, adapt, and revise their approaches to problems with ease.

NOVICE: Does not discover the patient's symptom of radiating pain down the leg with specific lumbar movements and thinks the hip is the main problem.

EXPERT: Immediately shifts thinking in the physical examination process to include the lumbar spine and works quickly examine the hip.

3. Experts continue to learn through experience by monitoring their actions and evaluating ongoing efforts of problem solving. These actions are called *higher-order (metacognitive) skills* or *reflective processes.*

NOVICE: Uses an evaluation framework and emphasizes data collection. A novice's thinking process is governed by application of rules.

EXPERT: Thinks about and interprets the evidence as the evaluation progresses. When a special clinical test turns out negative and does not seem to fit with the working hypothesis, an expert reevaluates the techniques used to perform the test. An expert draws on a rich background of clinical knowledge by recalling experiences with patients who had, for example, initial diagnoses of hip pain but who, in fact, had spinal problems.

4. Experts continually develop skills through intense, focused, deliberate practice.

NOVICE: Has learned hip mobilization treatment techniques in the laboratory, practiced a few times, and feels fairly confident to do these with patients.

EXPERT: Has engaged in long hours of self-directed study, worked with mentors, and constantly practiced to learn and refine mobilization skills. An expert continually works to learn more and perfect manual skills.

5. Experts are insightful and investigate not only the stated problem but also factors that may affect the specific problem. Discovering these factors and issues is part of what is called *clarifying the context* of the problem.

NOVICE: Focuses on the hip problem and gathers limited contextual data. Limited insight is gained into other aspects of the patient's life.

EXPERT: Listens to the patient intently and with focus. An expert gathers data on the patient's family, beliefs about exercise, fears about loss of mobility, and concerns that can affect the patient's outcome throughout the evaluation.

Although there is strong evidence supporting the distinguishing aspects of experts from novices, how does this knowledge translate into more effective education or training? This is where we begin to see expanded discussions about the importance of professional learning as it relates to novice development and an expanded definition of professional competence.

NOVICE DEVELOPMENT TOWARD PROFESSIONAL COMPETENCE AND EXPERTISE

In professional education, we are concerned about novice development toward professional competence and development of expertise. In physical therapy, the profession's vision for increased autonomy brings with it increased responsibility and therefore greater accountability (27). In both academic and clinical settings there will continue to be increasing emphasis on demonstrating accountability for competent performance. For educational programs, this means we must be able to demonstrate that our graduates are competent and ready to begin practice. In practice, this means we must continue to show that professionals remain competent over time. Therefore when we talk about expertise we must also consider the steps or stages toward the development of expertise that include novice development and demonstration of professional competence. Concerns with the health care system place increasing emphasis on accountability for competent performance, and in turn our discussions in professional education and practice must also consider the interrelationships of competence, novice development, and expertise (28,29).

In medicine there have been two well-known models of professional competence described. In 1985 Norman (28) performed a methodological review and proposed the following categories as components of professional competence in medicine: clinical skills (patient interview and examination), knowledge and understanding, interpersonal attributes, problem solving and clinical judgment, and technical skills. More recently, Epstein and Hundert (29) proposed this expanded definition of professional competence for medicine:

> *Professional competence is the habitual and judicious use of communication, knowledge, technical skills, clinical reasoning, emotions, values and reflection in daily practice for the benefit of the individual and the community being served. (p. 226)*

Epstein and Hundert argue that competence builds on a foundation of basic clinical skills, scientific knowledge, and *moral development* (29). Dimensions of professional competence include the traditional elements of cognition and technical skills, but they also require integrative skills and behaviors involving context, relationship, affective/moral, and habits of mind (Table 2-1) (29,30).

Table 2–1. Dimensions of Professional Competence

Dimension	Examples, skills, or behaviors
Cognitive	Core knowledge, basic communication, information management, problem solving, generating questions, learning from experience
Technical	Physical examination skills, procedural skills
Integrative	Integrating scientific, clinical, and humanistic judgment; applying clinical reasoning strategies; managing uncertainty; linking basic and clinical knowledge
Context	Varying contexts of clinical delivery, use of time
Relationship	Communication skills, handling conflict, teamwork; teaching
Affective/moral	Tolerance for ambiguity, emotional intelligence, respect, caring, responsiveness to patients and society
Habits of mind	Observations of one's own thinking (metacognitive skills), critical curiosity, recognition and response to cognitive and emotional biases, willingness to acknowledge and correct errors

Adapted from Epstein RM, Hundert EM. Defining and assessing professional competence. *JAMA* 287. 2002;226–235.

A critical assumption here is that professional competence is developmental and context dependent.

Competence means connecting the person and his or her abilities with the performance of tasks in a specific clinical context. So, rather than seeing competence as simple possession of knowledge, skills, and attitudes that are presumed to work for most patient situations, Epstein and Hundert would see that caring for a patient with similar physical symptoms in different delivery settings requires different skills and abilities. They further assert that scientific, clinical, and humanistic judgments are all essential parts of clinical reasoning. This expanded view of professional competence requires us to also reconsider the traditional approaches to assessment of learning such as multiple-choice examinations, objective structured clinical examinations, or standardized patient assessments. They propose consideration of new learning assessment formats that also consider assessing clinical reasoning, expert judgment, management of ambiguity, professionalism, time management, learning strategies, and teamwork (29).

NOVICE LEARNING

What can teachers and schools do with curricula, classroom settings, and teaching methods to enhance student learning? The National Academy of Sciences, National Academy of Engineering, Institute of Medicine, and National Research Council, in their book, *How People Learn* (24), took several key findings from research on expertise integrated with research on learning to generate recommendations for teaching and learning. A central premise of this book is critical examination of key research findings along with application of these findings to classroom practices and learning behavior. In Table 2-2 we highlight key principles from research on expert knowledge and demonstrate an application to teaching and learning environments in physical therapy. One of the challenges for educators in an age of rapid development and transfer of information is decisions about time, content, and learning experiences in the curriculum. The research evidence here on learning supports providing novices with learning experiences that help them build a scaffold or conceptual understanding of their knowledge, that facilitate linking basic science concepts to clinical signs and symptoms, and that demonstrate the importance of understanding the conditions or context of the situations or problems they are trying to solve.

THEORIES OF EXPERTISE: MAKING MEANINGFUL CONNECTIONS

As we have stated before, one of the most compelling reasons for understanding expertise and expert practice is that we want to prepare students for the *profession* in ways that will facilitate the development of expertise. The primary goal of a profession is service to society, which involves broad and complex knowledge not readily available to the public. A profession is a practice that is grounded in bodies of knowledge that are created, tested, elaborated, refuted, and transformed by the profession. The profession needs both research and theory development. "Professions change, not because the rules of practice change or policies change, but they should change because of the process of knowledge growth, criticism, and new understandings that come through research and theory development" (31). One of the challenges in physical therapy has been the

Table 2–2. Principles of Experts' Knowledge and Implications for Teaching and Learning

Principle	Expert–novice difference	Learning strategy for novice development
Meaningful patterns of information	Experts recognize features or patterns not recognized by novices	Provide novices with learning experiences that enhance ability to link what they know to meaningful patterns (e.g., link basic science concepts to specific clinical signs and symptoms of a patient case)
Organization of knowledge	Knowledge for experts is not a list of facts or formulas but is organized around core concepts and "big ideas"	Consider building conceptual understanding as a critical element in curriculum design; teach for depth and not breadth of knowledge
Context and access to knowledge	Experts do not have to search through everything to know and identify relevant knowledge	Design learning experiences that help students learn about the conditions of application to specific cases or problems (not just the automatic application of information from a textbook)
Fluent retrieval	Experts work toward understanding the problem rather than jump to solution strategies and engage in a process of problem solving	Instruction and testing should also focus on fully understanding the problem and the situation, not just on accuracy
Adaptive expertise	Experts use metacognitive strategies and the ability to self-monitor own level of understanding; recognize their limits of knowledge and take steps to remedy	Help novices understand that an expert is not someone who knows all of the answers; help develop metacognitive skills through teaching and assessing self-awareness; promote intellectual humility

Adapted from Brandsford J, Brown A, Cocking R (eds). *How People Learn: Brain, Mind, Experience and School.* Washington, DC, National Academy Press; 2000.

significant focus on the scientific method that assumes the core tenets of the biomedical model as the most highly valued forms of knowledge generation. For example, we are more likely to see support in terms of grant funding and publication for a quantitative approach to research is which the evidence of clinical success is quantifiable and measured, such as the effects of a specific intervention on patient outcome. This intervention is more likely to be a modality or exercise than any consideration of the teaching skill and ability of the therapist. This quantitative approach is in contrast to more methodologically diverse approaches, such as qualitative exploration of the patient–clinician interaction that may have a significant and meaningful impact on patient outcome and function (32). You might be asking: Why is this knowledge and theory discussion important to understanding expertise? The answer to this question is twofold: 1) Physical therapy continues to have a paucity of conceptual models, frameworks that link research to the realities of clinical practice, and 2) understanding the theory development in expertise research is extremely helpful in seeing the important contribution that expertise research in physical therapy makes to knowledge generation and theory development.

THEORIES OF PROFESSIONAL EXPERTISE

EXPERTISE AS MENTAL PROCESSING

Initial work in expertise concentrated on mental processing, or, more simply, the conceptualization of problem solving. Newell and Simon suggested that reasoning brought progressive expansion of knowledge of a problematic situation that continued until the problem was solved (33). They proposed that general methods or heuristics could be used for problem solving or information processing in all fields. An expert was someone who was particularly skilled at doing this heuristic search (19,21,34). Investigative work required experts and novices to think aloud, or verbalize, as a way to explore thought processes and assess problem-solving skills. Subsequent studies in areas such as chess (34) and physics (35) revealed that expertise depended not only on the method of problem solving but also on the expert's detailed knowledge in a specific area, ability to memorize, and ability to make inferences (34,35).

Elstein et al.'s (36) well-known research in medical problem solving was based on elements from early cognitive work in clinical reasoning and problem solving. They used various methods to analyze the subject's reasoning process, including the use of simulated patients, recall tasks, and verbalization. Several major findings from this work have had strong influences on education in medicine and other health professions (36–39). A four-stage general model of medical inquiry, the hypothetico-deductive method, was generated from their research and has been used extensively in medical education (Table 2-3). Variations of the hypothetico-deductive method have been incorporated into models that represent the clinical reasoning process. Figure 2-1 is an example of a representation of the clinical reasoning process for physical therapists (39–42). The process of collecting data or cues from the patient and generating hypotheses is considered a technique for transforming an unstructured problem (e.g., a patient presenting with several complications) into a structured problem by generating a small possible set of solutions.

EXPERTISE AS KNOWLEDGE AND CLINICAL REASONING

As work progressed in investigating clinical reasoning processes of physicians, ability to determine the proper patient diagnosis was discovered to be highly dependent on the knowledge the physician held in a particular clinical specialty area, called *case specificity* (37,38). *Case specificity* means that a successful reasoning strategy in one situation may not apply in a second case because the practitioner may not know enough about the area of the patient's problem. Identification of case specificity increased attention to the role of knowledge in expertise. Experts appear to have not only methods of problem solving but also the ability to combine these methods with knowledge and an understanding of how the knowledge necessary to solve the problem should be organized (43,44). In a test of diagnostic reasoning, both successful and unsuccessful diagnosticians

Table 2–3. Four-Stage Model of Medical Inquiry

Stage	Definition	Application and skills
Cue acquisition	Gathering of cues without evaluation or generation of hypotheses	Gathering multiple cues from observation, history, or physical findings Cues weighted according to importance Cue recognition influenced by prior knowledge
Hypothesis generation	Generation of several hypotheses that pose a relationship between the cues and conditions and diagnoses	Holding multiple hypotheses; could be casual relationship, association, situational, or a null hypothesis
Cue interpretation	Assessment of the cues and formation of patterns of cues that appear to fit together	Formulating patterns of cues, sifting through positive and negative evidence
Hypotheses evaluation	Assessment of the hypotheses for viability	Application of cues to the hypotheses and evaluation of competing hypotheses

Adapted from Elstein AS, Shulman LS, Sprafka SA. Medical problem solving: a ten year retrospective. *Eval Health Professions.* 1990;13:5–36; and Elstein AS, Shulman LS, SA Sprafka. *Medical Problem Solving: An Analysis of Clinical Reasoning.* Cambridge, MA: Harvard University Press; 1978.

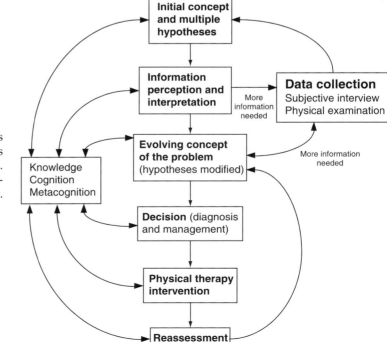

Figure 2–1 ■ Clinical reasoning process proposed by Jones based on elements of the hypothetico-deductive model. (Adapted from Jones MA. Clinical reasoning in manual therapy. *Phys Ther.* 1992; 72:875–884.)

used a hypothesis-testing strategy (38). Research on the clinical reasoning of expert physicians demonstrated that, in familiar situations, experts did not display hypothesis testing; instead they used rapid, automatic, and often nonverbal strategies. Expert reasoning in nonproblematic situations is similar to pattern recognition or retrieval of a well-structured network of knowledge. This process is called *forward reasoning*, which means clinicians see patterns from cues gathered from patients in interviews or data collections (37,44).

Forward reasoning is used by experts for solving routine cases in their own areas of specialty. Experts can make connections or inferences from the data by recognizing the pattern and links between clinical findings and a highly structured knowledge base. Novices and intermediate subjects tend to use hypothetico-deductive processes, which involve setting up hypotheses and gathering clinical data to prove or disprove the hypotheses (also called *backward reasoning*) (44,45). The following case example compares an expert's method for evaluating a patient with that of a therapist with little experience or expertise in the expert's field.

CASE EXAMPLE

The case is the evaluation and examination of a 1-year-old child who is being screened for possible motor delays. Following are the differences between the approaches of a pediatric specialist (expert) and a therapist with little recent experience in pediatrics (novice).

> **EXPERT:** The pediatric clinical specialist collects multiple and selective cues through observation, handling of the child, and conversation with the mother. The mother has noticed that the child always rolls to the right, although he can roll both ways when encouraged. The expert begins to see a pattern of motor delay that appears to be mild and knows the child would benefit from being encouraged to make specific movements.

> **NOVICE:** The physical therapist applies an evaluation framework, testing reflexes that he can remember. He tests the child in sitting, supine, and prone positions, looking for abnormal responses to the specific tests. He does not observe any abnormal responses to the tests he applies, nor does he solicit any information from the mother about her observations of the child's movement. He does not see any problems with the child based on his examination.

When experts work outside their area of expertise, they tend to use a mixture of forward and backward reasoning, using forward reasoning to account for the part of the problem that are solvable and backward reasoning to tie up loose ends. (Figure 2-2). This process is summarized well by the following passage (44):

> *The primary goal of diagnostic reasoning is to classify a cluster of patient findings as belonging to a specific disease category. From this perspective, diagnostic reasoning can be viewed as a process of coordinated theory*

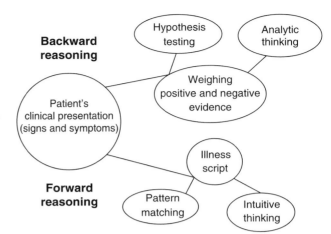

Figure 2–2 ■ Key concepts in forward and backward clinical reasoning.

2

(hypothesis) and evidence, rather than one of finding fault in the system. As expertise develops, the disease knowledge of a clinician becomes more dependent on clinical experience, clinical problem solving is increasingly guided by the use of exemplars and analogy, and is less dependent on a functional understanding of the system in question.

Investigators have also explored the development and changing form of medical students' knowledge structures as they develop initial expertise through professional education (46). Knowledge structures are mental representations that are a fundamental dimension of cognitive science. Mental representations help preserve information about and interpretations of objects and events. These are critical aspects of student learning because they help students move from memorization of facts or information to understanding key concepts and structure of knowledge (46,47). For example, if a student can grasp the critical concept of testing muscles in gravity and antigravity positions and knows muscle structure and function, memorizing specific tests is unnecessary. Instead, the student can rely on knowledge structures or understanding of critical concepts to determine the testing position. Based on work done with medical students, four developmental stages of knowledge acquisition have been described (22,48).

Stage one involves the development of elaborate causal networks that students use to explain the causes or consequences of disease in terms of pathophysiology. A clinical application is recognizing that rheumatoid arthritis results in changes in synovial fluid and that joint capsule and soft tissue change from an inflammatory process.

Stage two involves the transformation of elaborate causal network into an abridged network in which information about clinical signs and symptoms is subsumed under diagnostic labels. In a student clinical application, patients with rheumatoid arthritis may present with hand involvement specifically in the metacarpophalangeal joints and have an elevated erythrocyte sedimentation rate.

The first two stages evolve throughout the initial professional education. The third stage comes with accumulated experience with patients when clinical signs and symptoms are integrated with the didactic knowledge.

Stage three involves a transition from a network of knowledge organization to an illness script. The illness script requires three components: 1) enabling conditions of the disease (e.g., personal, social, medical, hereditary, and environmental); 2) the fault of the disease, which is the pathophysiologic process taking place; and 3) the consequences of the fault, which are the signs and symptoms (22,48). Illness scripts are activated as a whole and provide a list of phenomena that the clinician looks for during the examination. Less experienced clinicians recall information more effectively when it is presented in the order of a script, whereas more experienced physicians do not generally require a scripted order.

CASE EXAMPLE

A student on her last clinical rotation sees a patient with a fractured hip in a home health care setting. Although the patient case is fairly straightforward and the student does well when discussing the pathology, the surgical approach, and movement precautions with the clinical instructor, the student is less clear when discussing exactly how to implement a home program focused on functional activities.

Stage four of development involves the use of memories of previous patients and instantiated scripts. Clinicians can activate one or more of these illness scripts when dealing with a case. This process is often automatic and unconscious (22,48).

Referring to the previous case example, an experienced clinical instructor who had worked in home health would likely plan the home program as the evaluation proceeded and might actually use assessment of functional activities as a central aspect of the evaluation.

There has been continuing controversy in the literature about the role of basic science knowledge in expert diagnostic thinking. Patel and colleagues (44,45,49) have argued that when diagnosing a clinical case, medical experts mainly activate clinical knowledge and only in cases of uncertainty do they revert to biomedical knowledge. They see clinical knowledge and biomedical sciences as two distinct worlds. They further argue that students have difficulty transferring knowledge across contexts (basic science to clinical cases) and that traditional instruction fails to promote such transfer. Therefore, their recommendation is that medical schools develop ways to do both forward-reaching transfer (applying basic science knowledge to clinical cases) and backward-reaching transfer (moving from the clinical case back to the particular principles). A parallel theory here is the theory of knowledge encapsulation, in which basic science knowledge is seen as a critical element of the development of clinical knowledge. The example of medical student knowledge development across four stages (from knowledge networks to illness scripts) is an example of knowledge encapsulation (20). With the knowledge encapsulation area, the recommendation for teaching and learning is similar. Students should be introduced to clinical phenomena earlier in the professional curriculum. Introduction of clinical cases will stimulate students to find connections between patient findings and thereby begin to enhance the construction of a scaffold or conceptual basis for their knowledge that includes linking basic foundation science concepts to clinical presentations.

The chapter thus far has discussed expertise theory that focused on general problem solving and studies that emphasize the essential link between problem solving and knowledge. Experts use specific knowledge to solve problems, and their knowledge changes as they learn from their practice experience. These two general approaches to expertise, however, do not explain variations sometimes seen between experts and novices (Table 2-4). The lack of consistencies in expertise theory has led to continued work in what Holyoak calls the third generation of theory development in expertise (19). He and others call for an increased focus on integrating theoretical ideas drawn from models in earlier theory generation, looking at case studies, and using a combination of methods for research in practice environments to examine how experts think and use knowledge in normal situations (22,37,44).

EXPERTISE AS EVERYDAY PRACTICE

The clearest way to grasp the insufficiency of the positivist model of professional expertise is to notice what the positivist account of knowledge leaves out but must take for granted. (50, p. 242)

This quote represents well the current focus on everyday practice using qualitative methods that is seen in investigative work and theoretical writing done in several applied professions such as nursing (51–53); teaching (17,54,55);

Table 2–4. Comparison of Uniformities and Inconsistencies among Experts

Uniformities	Inconsistencies
Perform complex tasks in their areas of expertise (domain) more accurately than novices	Sometimes achieve mediocrity and are not always more accurate than novices
Solve problems in their domain with greater ease	Sometimes feel more pain and work harder than nonexperts
Have superior memory for information related to their area of expertise	Sometimes expertise and memory are not linked
Are better at perceiving patterns among the cues in their data gathering than are novices	Sometimes the search strategies for data gathering are highly varied and not identical for all novices and all experts
Hold knowledge in a highly specific area; their expertise is domain specific	May transfer knowledge across domains

Adapted from Holyoak KJ. Symbolic Connectionism: Toward Third-Generation Theories of Expertise. In Ericsson KA, Smith J (eds). *Toward a General Theory of Expertise.* New York: Cambridge University Press; 1991.

occupational therapy (56,57); and, more recently, physical therapy (3–16). These studies represent work done in the spirit of the third generation of theory in expertise where the theories emerge from research grounded in the context of practice. We will begin this section with an overview of two well-known models: the Dreyfus model of skill acquisition (58) and Schön's model of reflective practice (59,60).

Dreyfus Model of Skill Acquisition. The Dreyfus model of skill acquisition was developed by brothers Hubert Dreyfus, a philosopher, and Stuart Dreyfus, an industrial engineer in mathematical modeling and artificial intelligence (58). Their model originally developed from an effort to attack claims in artificial intelligence that facts and rules were the only things necessary for understanding the world. The Dreyfus model maintains that skill development involves elements of both analysis and intuition, as described in the following excerpt (52):

> *Even though computers can store far more facts than any human can remember and can apply inferential rules thousands of times more rapidly and with more accuracy than can human beings, programs optimistically called "expert systems" consistently fail to perform at the level of human experts in areas such as nursing, in which people learn with experience to make rapid, effective decisions.*

In her qualitative study of nurses' critical incidents, Benner used the Dreyfus model of skill acquisition in the analysis of her data and description of expertise in nursing practice (51). Her book *From Novice to Expert*, published in 1984, contains powerful narratives of clinical practice told by nurses. Benner explored the knowledge that was embedded through the practice of nursing. She applied the Dreyfus model to the interview data gathered from her sample of practicing nurses.

The Dreyfus model proposes five stages of skill acquisition passed through from novice to expert (Table 2-5). It emphasizes individual perceptions and decision-making abilities rather than just the performance of the skill. Skill is identified as an overall approach to professional action that includes both perception and decision making, not just what we would think of as technical skill or technique (59–61). The knowledge necessary to perform the skill is called practical knowledge (i.e., knowing how to perform a skill in its real setting). Practical knowledge contrasts with knowing material in a textbook or theoretical knowledge that is learned in the classroom (61,62).

CASE EXAMPLE

Mary has just finished her first year in the physical therapy program. She is an excellent student and has performed exceptionally well in her course work. She is teaching a patient how to use a walker on a curb or step. She remembers all the steps for teaching this gait activity but finds herself at a loss as the patient begins to fatigue and become anxious because Mary cannot figure out what to do with the patient and the walker. Fortunately, her clinical instructor is watching from a distance and comes to her rescue by providing the patient the correct verbal cue to move safely off the step.

Table 2–5. Dreyfus Model of Skill Acquisition

Stage	Knowledge use	Action	Orientation	Decision making
Novice	Factual	Given rules for actions	Cannot see whole situation	Rule-governed Relies on others
Advanced beginner	Objective facts More sophisticated rules	Begins use of intuition in concrete situations	Limited situational perception Relies on others	Less rule-governed
Competent	Hierarchical perspective	Devises new rules based on situation	Conscious of situation	Makes decisions Feels responsible
Proficient	Situational Can discriminate	Intuitive behavior replaces reasoned responses	Perceives whole situation	Decision making less labored
Expert	Knows what needs to be done based on practiced situational discrimination	Intuitive and deliberate rationality Where intuition not developed, reasoning applied	Can discriminate among situations and know when action is required	Knows how to achieve goals

Adapted from Benner P. *From Novice to Expert: Excellence and Power in Clinical Nursing Practice.* Menlo Park, CA: Addison-Wesley; 1982.

Students are proficient with theoretical knowledge and often apply this knowledge successfully in uncomplicated situations. Students are generally far less competent, however, when the situation is unanticipated or does not resemble examples in textbooks. Experienced practitioners are usually proficient and may not even be aware of how much they know until a student questions them. In the case study, the student was stuck not knowing how to teach a functional activity. The clinical instructor came to her rescue by quickly solving the problem. Polyani suggests that "We know more than we can tell" (63). For practicing professionals, this is tacit understanding of knowing and doing (59–61).

In the Dreyfus model, a novice moves from being rule governed and having poor situational perception to increasing his or her ability to recognize features of practical situations, discriminate, and perform routine procedures at a competent level. Proficiency develops only if experience is assimilated. Rule-governed behavior is replaced by situational discriminations as the novice learns to recognize features of practical situations.

CASE EXAMPLE

Mary knows the exact steps for transferring a patient between a treatment mat and wheelchair, but when confronted with a bed-to-wheelchair transfer in a home health setting, she was stuck because the steps she learned did not directly apply. She should assess the situation and adapt the transfer, while ensuring that the transfer is safe.

Over time, experienced practitioners replace reasoned responses to situations with more intuitive behavior because they have learned from their experience. Intuitive behavior replaces reasoned responses until, at the expert level, a therapist uses a more refined and subtle discrimination ability. An expert knows what needs to be achieved and how to achieve it (51–53). The strength of the Dreyfus model comes from its focus on tacit knowledge and the role of intuition in the development of expertise. The following describe how elements of the Dreyfus model apply to teaching novices (64):

1. Expertise is acquired step by step. One must learn components explicitly and learn to act with them analytically. Experience allows thinking to become more intuitive.
2. Novices should avoid trying to think intuitively without experience and analytic foundation because intuitive performance can be poor. Only experts have the privilege of not using rules.
3. Novices should practice intensively using rules and logic and not rely on rule-based expert systems. Students should be allowed the opportunity to develop expertise.

Model of Reflective Practice. Another well-known model of expertise comes from the influential writings of Donald Schön (59,60,65). In his book *The Reflective Practitioner* (59), Schön argues for a new approach to professional education that places less emphasis on a view of professional knowledge as a "model of technical rationality." Technical rationality is knowledge generated through basic and applied research, traditionally within university settings and outside professional practice. He argues that problems professionals encounter are often badly structured and defy solutions through application of traditional knowledge—technical rationality. Professionals must use practical experience, intuition, and quick thinking to solve complex practice problems. Schön developed a model of professional practice based on his study of several professions (e.g., architecture, psychology, and management). He sought to understand the artistry of professional practice—that is, the thinking used in practice (59,60).

Schön believed that the knowledge professionals use is not the same as the knowledge taught in professional schools and that the use of research-based knowledge is not what distinguishes excellent from average practitioners. The wise actions that professionals use involve practical knowledge. As discussed, practical knowledge is the knowledge of knowing how (also called *procedural knowledge*). Practical knowledge is distinguished from declarative knowledge, or "knowing about" (59, 61–63). Declarative knowledge involves knowing facts and knowing about things, which is similar to emphasizing teaching didactic information. Health professions education traditionally has placed most of the teaching and testing emphasis on declarative knowledge. Procedural knowledge, however, is not exclusively recall of information; rather, it is knowing how to do something. In health professions education, students are usually challenged to use procedural knowledge in clinical practice settings or clinical education. A difference between experts and nonexperts is that experts have more procedural knowledge (55, 59, 66).

A central concern for Schön is how practitioners gain practical knowledge. He asserts that practitioners add to a practical knowledge base not merely through experience but through a process of reflection (58,59). Reflection is triggered by recognition that a particular situation is not routine. The following processes are present in reflection:

1. Initial doubt and perplexity as the situation is identified as not routine but problematic (What is going on here?).
2. Questioning the thinking or action that caused the problematic situation (How did I get here?).
3. Working for problem resolution by trying new actions (What can I do to resolve the problem?).

Professionals learn from experience by using reflective inquiry to think about what they are doing, what worked, and what did not work as they are doing it. Schön considers the process of identifying the problem (problem setting) more critical than problem solving. Problem-setting activities allow experience and practical knowledge to influence current action. Professionals build their practical knowledge through a repertoire of examples, images, illness scripts, and understanding learned through experience. This knowledge is best learned through practice and reflection (60,61). Schön sees practical reasoning as a central component of reflection in action. The reflection is not only a psychological process but also a social process that is action oriented (60,61). Figure 2-3 is a representation of the arbitrary separation that occurs in professional education; teaching is often done in one world and practice is done in another. Schön's plea is to bring these two worlds together through more realistic laboratory experiences, teaching methods that facilitate reflection, and more "good studies of actual practice" (60).

Figure **2–3** ■ Arbitrary separation between knowledge used in education and practice.

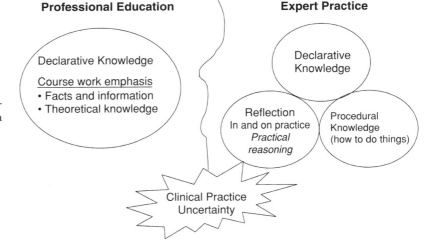

Learning from Practice: The Critical Role of Practical Reasoning. Benner and colleagues' work in *Expertise in Nursing Practice: Caring, Clinical Judgment and Ethics* (1996) (52) and *Clinical Wisdom and Interventions in Critical Care: A Thinking-in-Action Approach* (1999) (53) represents the richness and the relevance of "learning from practice" to improve understanding of expert practice. Their work is consistent with Schön's writings (59,60) that emphasize the importance of artistry in practice and the limits of the technical–rational model for learning and developing expertise. Benner and colleagues (51–53) use observations and narrative accounts of actual clinical examples as primary tools for understanding everyday clinical and caring knowledge and practical reasoning that occurs in nursing practice. Although their work is based on a large representative sample of critical care nurses, the use of the term "expert" does not refer to a particular nurse or specific role; the focus is the expertise found in the practice of experienced clinicians.

Important findings from this work include the following six aspects of clinical judgment and skillful comportment of experienced nurses: (53)

1. *Reasoning-in-transition.* This refers to practical reasoning in an evolving or open-ended clinical situation. The clinician is always interpreting the present clinical situation in terms of the immediate past condition of that particular patient. There is evidence of ongoing clinical problem solving applied to the situation of that particular patient rather than a strict focus on the pathophysiology of the condition.
2. *Skilled know-how.* This refers to the skillful performance of interventions done by practitioners visible through observation. For example, one would see differences between novices and experienced therapists in how they position themselves in guarding and guiding a patient in a transfer.
3. *Response-based practice.* Excellent clinicians are able to read a situation and engage in proactive, response-based actions. In physical therapy we see this kind of proactive, response-based action frequently in the management of patients in acute care settings when early ambulation is a critical element in the rehabilitation effort. The skilled therapist must read the patient and situation carefully to facilitate early cooperation and movement for the patient. This is in contrast to a more "parental approach" to the patient that ends in refusal of therapy for the day.
4. *Agency.* Agency refers to moral agency seen through the practitioner's ability to act on or influence a situation. It is not enough to just go through the routine clinical actions based on objective findings. The practitioner must be engaged in the clinical situation demonstrated through action, reasoning, and the relationship with the patient and family. Here one would see the therapist taking a stand in promoting what he or she considered to be in the patient's best interest. Agency is seen as a critical component of expertise.
5. *Perceptual acuity and skill of involvement.* This component of clinical judgment links two essential, linked attributes. The first refers to the perceptual acuity necessary to frame and reframe the problem. This attribute is consistent with Dewey and Schön's notion of problem identification or

setting (59,70). If you are not aware that you have a problem situation, your handling of the situation is likely to be misguided. To have perceptual acuity you must have skillful engagement with both the problem and the person. Emotions play a key role in the perception of the problem, and Benner suggests that they may even act as a moral compass in learning a practice. The interpersonal skills of engaging with the clinical and human situation are called the skills of involvement. There is an important distinction here as the emotional engagement element is not interpersonal engagement, but it does require establishing boundaries between self and patient.

6. *Links between ethical and clinical reasoning.* Finally, Benner and colleagues argue that it is not possible to separate clinical and ethical reasoning because good clinical judgments reflect good clinical practice.

Although biomedical ethical principles and procedures such as ensuring autonomy of the patient, informed consent, justice, beneficence, and nonmaleficence are important, they must be translated into good practice. Expert practitioners are motivated to do excellent work along with their moral obligation to help other human beings.

> *Learning to make good clinical judgments and be a good practitioner requires ongoing experiential learning, reflection, and dialogue with patients and their families...Nursing, like teaching, medicine and social work, and other helping professions, depends on solidarity with one's fellow human beings and on professional standards of beneficence and nonmaleficence for helping people during periods of vulnerability and distress—this is what it means to be "good" at one's work. (53, p. 17)*

DIMENSIONS OF DEVELOPING EXPERTISE

We began this chapter with the assumption that we see expertise as a continuous process, not merely a state of being achieved through certification or years of experience. We conclude this chapter by revisiting the core dimensions of expertise that are critical to thinking more deeply about facilitating the development of expertise. These dimensions of expertise will be helpful for analyzing the profiles of our clinical experts in Chapters 4–8 (Figure 2-4).

KNOWLEDGE: WHAT DO EXPERTS KNOW?

One of the fundamental differences between experts and novices is depth and use of knowledge. Experts bring more specific knowledge to problems and handle problems more effectively. Knowledge has long been a critical dimension of what constitutes a profession. The knowledge base of a profession should be specialized, specific to the discipline, scientific, and standardized. The focus on a scientific knowledge base fueled the development of university professional schools in which professional knowledge was the foundation science, applied science, and the clinical component that emphasized skills and aptitude development. This is the model of technical rationality that Schön argues has created a crisis in professional education (59,60).

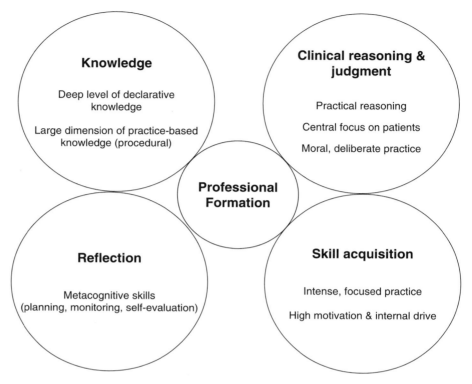

Figure 2–4 ■ Dimensions of developing expertise.

Creation and validation of a knowledge base is considered a critical component for faculty who teach in professional education programs at universities, and this approach still has great appeal. For example, in physical therapy, the move to house educational programs in university settings has allowed the field the opportunity to enhance credibility as a profession. Faculty who teach students must be prepared to be members of the academy and contribute to the creation of knowledge. This affects educational preparation of the next generation of professionals. In physical therapy, an increased emphasis on creation and validation of a knowledge base is visible through a number of mechanisms, such as an increase in the number of textbooks now written by physical therapists for physical therapists, expansion of the literature in both the quantity and quality of papers published, and an increase in the number of journals specific to physical therapy.

Current pressure in the health care delivery system for evidence to demonstrate the effectiveness of clinical interventions on patient outcome (1,32) may emphasize the central importance of technical rationality. If the focus of investigations is on cause-and-effect relationships, the potential importance of the clinician's practical knowledge may be missed. Care must be taken to acknowledge and investigate the essential role of practical or procedural knowledge that is part of expert practice. Both declarative knowledge (i.e., the knowledge of facts, rules, definitions, or strategies) and procedural knowledge (i.e., the knowledge that consists of skills and cognitive operations of how to do things) must be investigated because both are essential for skill performance (55,67).

What types of knowledge can be identified in the domains of declarative and procedural knowledge that are necessary for expert practice in physical therapy? This is a primary research question addressed in Chapters 4–7, which focus on clinical experts. Investigations done with teachers demonstrate a useful model for discussion. Expert teachers must have content knowledge (i.e., the knowledge of subject matter to be taught). They must also have pedagogic knowledge, knowledge of how to teach, and knowledge of how to teach that is specific to what is being taught (i.e., pedagogic content knowledge) (24,31).

Although experts possess more knowledge, it is the organization of that knowledge that is critical. Experts understand how knowledge is structured—that is, experts understand the structure underlying this declarative knowledge. This includes ideas, facts, and concepts in the content area and relationships between them. For example, a student struggles to know how to perform all the cranial nerve tests by memorizing the order of the tests, the number of the cranial nerves, and the tasks required. A clinical specialist in neurology, however, holds a deeper understanding of the functional anatomy, functional application, and meaning of these tests for evaluating the patient.

The expert prototype thus far has a well-organized framework and holds a deep level of understanding of declarative knowledge. What about procedural knowledge? Is this merely knowing how to do a task or skill? Investigations of the knowledge physicians use indicate that this is integrated knowledge, or wisdom, of practice. This knowledge goes beyond medical knowledge and knowledge gained from experience, such as knowledge of patients and communication issues (29,30,68,69). Physical therapists must not only know the subject matter of physical therapy but also the techniques for "doing" physical therapy—that is, how to apply their knowledge and work with patients. This is likely to include communicating with patients, interpreting and understanding clinical signs and symptoms, applying intervention techniques, and working with patients to solve problems. The work of therapists involves cognition and psychomotor and affective skills.

Knowledge used by experts in practice is not simply direct application of declarative knowledge. Instead, it is knowledge combined with the practical reasoning that transforms what the expert knows. This practical knowledge base of the expert is often tacit. Tacit knowledge is not taught explicitly, nor is it often verbalized. This is the knowledge practitioners learn through experience. Research on tacit knowledge has demonstrated that it generally increases with experience on the job, is unrelated to IQ (intelligence quotient), and predicts job performance better than IQ. Tacit knowledge is thought to be an important component of expert performance (55).

Recognition of practice as a legitimate source of knowledge comes from Dewey (70). Schön's writings have continued to advocate a well-defined epistemology (i.e., study of knowledge) of practice knowledge that demonstrates the relationship between scientific knowledge and professional practice (59,60,65). The tacit or implicit knowledge of experts develops as a result of an ability to reflect. Tacit knowledge is continually built through the practitioner's actions and reflection. Benner and colleagues' work (51–53) discussed earlier in this chapter are good examples of research focused on the knowledge embedded in practice.

In their classic text, *Theory in Practice*, Argyris and Schön call tacit knowledge *theories in use* (71). Theories in use contrast with established or espoused theories (i.e., the theories used to teach students). For example, motor learning theory provides a framework for designing and implementing exercise programs with patients. A therapist asked why he or she gives feedback to the patient in a particular way would likely respond with an espoused theory—most likely some element from motor learning theory. If the same therapist is working with a patient, however, something more than application of timed feedback may be observed that is based on the therapist's theory-in-use or tacit knowledge. One way to uncover this knowledge is to promote reflection or discussion of what is being done and why. Theories in use can be uncovered through observation of behavior and dialogue consistent with what is done in qualitative research (32,71,72).

In their qualitative study of clinical reasoning in occupational therapy, Mattingly and Flemming focused on identification of theories in use by occupational therapists (56). Theories in use represent tacit knowledge and are what may guide practice and fill the deficiencies and gaps between espoused theories and practice. This tacit understanding of knowing and doing is something that experienced practitioners implicitly trust. They know that they "know what they are doing. They have the confidence that they can assess a situation quickly and accurately and quickly come up with the right answer or do the right thing" (56).

Many terms have been used to describe the "elusive knowledge of practice," including *craft knowledge, practical knowledge,* and *wisdom of practice* (31,66,67). The basic distinction, however, is that something different exists between factual, information knowledge (declarative knowledge) and knowledge that is necessary to practice (procedural knowledge) (see Figure 2-3).

Chapters 4–8, which examine expert practice in each of the clinical specialty areas, provide further explication of the practical theories that are part of expert practice in physical therapy.

CLINICAL REASONING AND JUDGMENT: HOW DO EXPERTS SOLVE PROBLEMS?

Experts solve problems most efficiently within their area of expertise (21,25,26). They can plan, monitor, and revise their approaches to solving problems as they go. Understanding that not all experts use a hypothetico-deductive approach (backward reasoning) is important. In problem-free cases, experts made fast and almost automatic decisions that looked more like pattern matching (forward reasoning). The method selected depends on the complexity of the problem.

Work done on clinical reasoning in female-dominated health professions, such as nursing and occupational therapy, also has important applications for work in physical therapy. As discussed with the work of Benner and colleagues (51–53), this research represents a third generation of theory in expertise development that involves investigating practice settings (19). Studies in nursing and occupational therapy have investigated the practical reasoning that is part of clinicians' practice using qualitative research methods. These interpretive studies provide new insights into how skilled clinicians make judgments. One aspect of this work is the central role of knowing the patient as part of the clinical judgment process. The clinical reasoning process begins with understanding and knowing the patient and treating that patient as a unique individual.

Benner et al. (51) added to their original work (52) with a 6-year investigation of the nature of clinical knowledge, clinical judgment, clinical inquiry, and expert ethical comportment. They assert that clinical judgments of experienced nurses resemble practical reasoning (knowing how) rather than more rational, theoretical approaches advocated by cognitive psychologists. Benner et al. identify the following interrelated aspects of nurses' clinical judgments:

1. Not only individualized assessment of what is good and right, but also actions that humanize and personalize care particular to each clinical situation.
2. Caring practices that reveal knowing and that preserve the identity of the patient as a person.
3. Knowing the patient, understanding the patient's illness, and responding to the disease process. Knowledge includes specific local knowledge about particular patient responses, functions, and physical presentations.
4. Use of practical knowledge about particular patient populations.

In occupational therapy, Mattingly and Flemming's ethnographic investigation of clinical reasoning among occupational therapists reveals a similar focus on the central importance of the patient (56). Mattingly and Flemming were interested in how therapists think when they treat patients and in what therapists think about their practice as a practice. They discovered that therapists used different reasoning strategies for different purposes or in response to particular problems. They identified three different reasoning strategies:

1. Procedural reasoning. Procedural reasoning is similar to hypothetico-deductive reasoning identified in early work done in medical problem solving and expertise. This type of reasoning occurs when therapists treat physical problems by applying knowledge of clinical conditions.
2. Interactive reasoning. Interactive reasoning occurs when a therapist interacts with a patient as a person. The interaction is not simply idle conversation; it is done with purpose and structure to better understand the patient.
3. Conditional reasoning. Conditional reasoning occurs when a therapist thinks beyond specific concerns about a patient's physical problems by considering the patient in a broader social and temporal context. This includes the entire condition (e.g., person, illness, meanings of the disease for the person and family, and social and physical contexts).

In a synthesis of investigative work on clinical reasoning in physiotherapy, Jones et al. (73) proposed a model for clinical reasoning for physiotherapy that has a central hypothetico-deductive core and also emphasizes consideration of the context of the patient. They acknowledge the importance of theoretical and clinical knowledge integrated through reflective processes. More recent work and writing across the health professions support the central importance of the expert clinician perceiving the situation, the context, and understanding the patient as central to the clinical judgment process (14,16,74). The possible limitations of purely cognitive models are summarized well by Benner et al. (52) in the following excerpt:

> *The study of clinical judgment using cognitive models and methods has limited the possibility of seeing other important aspects of clinical judgment. By highlighting these aspects, we do not mean to say that rationality has no place. Calculated reasoning…consulting research and theoretical literature for possible interventions and solutions…does and should figure prominently in the practice of experienced clinicians. Our claim is that it is not the only form of reasoning, nor necessarily the best. Rather, the reasoning that is a significant part of everyday practice of expert clinicians is one that relies on intuition, including deliberative rationality, on a disposition toward what is good and right, on practice wisdom gained from experience, on involvement in the situation, and on knowing the particular patient through being attuned to his pattern of responses and through hearing narrative accounts of his illness experiences. (p. 12)*

The tension between a more rational model of reasoning involving analytical processes and more practical, engaged reasoning has been discussed for quite some time. Aristotle used the term *phronesis* to describe the virtue of practical wisdom (75). This was the capacity for moral insight and discerning what moral choice or action is most conducive to the good of an agent. The conflict between knowledge of the patient and knowledge of a disease has been part of medicine since its beginnings; much tension has existed between rationalism (e.g., focus on theory of disease, biological mechanisms, science) and empiricism (e.g., focus on patients, and their interaction with their environment and other people).

SKILL ACQUISITION: HOW DO EXPERTS ACQUIRE SKILLS?

Experts have the ability to perform specific technical tasks. An architect draws, a surgeon operates, and a physical therapist teaches and facilitates movement. Technical skills performed by an expert are not done in isolation of knowledge or judgment. The application of technical skill is integrated with practical knowledge, clinical judgment, and precise technique. The separation of skills from knowledge, theoretical principles, and clinical judgment is often used as a way of distinguishing traditional professions. In physical therapy, for example, the role of the physical therapist's assistant has a strong emphasis on application of technical skills that are given initial direction from the evaluation of the physical therapist. This is not to say that an assistant applies techniques without drawing on knowledge and thinking or using judgment. The role of a physical therapist is to analyze a situation critically, identify presenting problems, and prioritize solutions. An expert must use declarative knowledge and procedural knowledge as well as clinical insight and clinical reasoning skills.

An important dimension of expert skill is performance (20,26). Elite performers in various fields of expertise have been used to demonstrate that expert performance comes from acquired complex skills and physiologic adaptations. Expert level of performance requires mastery of knowledge and prerequisite skills in addition to deliberate practice. Deliberate practice is intense, focused practice intended to improve performance. Concentration is the most essential aspect of deliberate practice. Expert skills also require internal representations and feedback about performance. Frequently, expert performers receive inherent enjoyment from their practice activity. Experts are highly motivated and constantly strive to better themselves. Expert performers also remain highly active in their domains of expertise (20,26).

REFLECTION: HOW DO EXPERTS LEARN FROM PRACTICE?

Strong evidence suggests that experts differ from novices in the use of higher-order processes or metacomponents. These metacomponents are used to plan, monitor, and evaluate efforts at problem solving. Important metacognitive skills include problem recognition, definition, and representation; strategy formulation; resource allocation; monitoring; and evaluation of problem solving (47,55). Experts spend a large percentage of solution time trying to understand the problem, whereas novices tend to be more involved in trying different solutions (22,24). Experts also engage in reflective processes—that is, they monitor solution attempts, check for accuracy, and continue to learn through thinking about their experience (47,55). Sternberg's (55) model of developing expertise (Figure 2-5) provides evidence of the central importance of reflection and metacognitive skills in novice development.

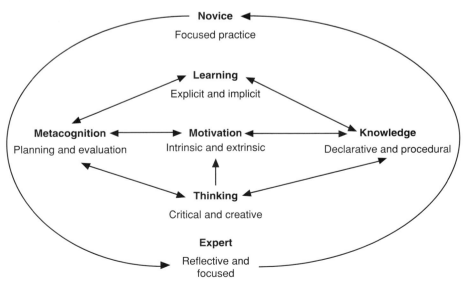

Figure 2–5 ■ Model of developing expertise. (Adapted from Sternberg R. Abilities are forms of developing expertise. *Educational Researcher*. 1998; 28:11–20.)

PROFESSIONAL FORMATION: WHAT IS THE ROLE OF ENCULTURATION?

We are proposing here in our revised chapter one final dimension for consideration, the process of professional formation. As seen in Figure 2-4, this is a dimension that is critical to our assumption that expertise is a continuous process and that there is an important moral dimension of professional competence. We began this chapter with a discussion of terms including "experts," "expertise," "novice," "expert differences," and "novice development" as it relates to the development of professional competence. These terms are not mutually exclusive; they are all part of an important, renewed discussion among health professions on the role of the professional in the larger society (50,76). A fundamental premise in these discussions is the development of professional competence that is grounded in the developmental progression of a novice through a process of professional formation.

Professional competence is seen as a foundation of basic clinical skills and scientific knowledge and a foundation of moral development that is critical to those "habits of mind" that allow the practitioner to be self-aware, attentive, and engaged. Novice development is a learning process that is both a process of change within the individual (knowledge, skills, and thinking) and an enculturation process as a professional that has a social context. The community of practice plays a critical role as they continue to learn from experience, which includes evidence gathered from diverse sources including research, reflection on their own work, and more fully understanding the context of patients and communities they serve (22,31,50). Research that focuses on the problems in one's own practice is central to what it means to profess (31). The goal of professional formation and learning must include considerations well beyond knowledge and decision making. As Sullivan states:

> ...real expertise is never entirely separable from a community of practice, it is never purified of social or moral engagement....The great promise of the professions has always been that they can ensure the quality of expert services for the common good. (50, p. 255)

This chapter provided a foundation for understanding the importance, relevance, and application of expertise research and theory to physical therapy and to our research. We propose a broadening of our conception of expertise from core components such as knowledge, reasoning, or skill to also include a developmental process (formation) with strong moral grounding. The model of expertise we propose in this chapter includes knowledge, clinical reasoning and judgment, acquisition of skill, reflection, and professional formation. Chapters 4–7 provide our evidence of expertise in physical therapy practice, and in Chapter 8 we discuss evidence across chapters in further developing a grounded theory of expert practice. In Part III (Chapters 9–12), we have four invited chapters, in which authors will be sharing their research and applications to practice that address and further develop one or more components of the grounded theory in expert practice.

REFERENCES

1. Sackett DL, Strauss SE, Richardson WS, et al. *How to practice and teach evidence-based medicine.* New York: Churchill-Livingstone; 2000.
2. Tonelli MR. In defense of expert opinion. *Acad Med.* 1999;74:1187–1192.
3. Payton OD. Clinical reasoning process in physical therapy. *Phys Ther.* 1985;65:924–928.
4. Jensen GM, Shepard KF, Hack LM. The novice versus the experienced clinician: insights into the work of the physical therapist. *Phys Ther.* 1990;70:314–323.
5. May BJ, Dennis JK. Expert decision making in physical therapy: a survey of practitioners. *Phys Ther.* 1991;71:190–202.
6. Jensen GM, Shepard KF, Gwyer J, Hack LM. Attribute dimensions that distinguish master and novice physical therapy clinicians in orthopedic settings. *Phys Ther.* 1992;72:711–722.
7. Embrey DG, Guthrie MR, White OR, et al. Clinical decision making by experienced and inexperienced pediatric physical therapists for children with diplegic cerebral palsy. *Phys Ther.* 1996;76:20–33.
8. Martin C, Siosteen A, Shepard K. The professional development of expert physical therapists in four areas of clinical practice, *Nordic Physiother.* 1995;1:4–11.
9. Jensen G, Gwyer J, Hack L, Shepard K. *Expertise in physical therapy practice*, Boston: Butterworth-Heinemann; 1999.
10. Mostrom E. Wisdom of practice in a transdisciplinary rehabilitation clinic: situated expertise and client centering. In Jensen G, Gwyer J, Hack L, Shepard K (eds). *Expertise in Physical Therapy Practice*, Boston: Butterworth-Heinemann; 1999.
11. Shepard K, Hack L, Gwyer J, Jensen G. Describing expert practice. *Qual Health Res.* 1999;9:746–758.
12. Jensen G, Gwyer J, Shepard K, Hack L. Expert practice in physical therapy. *Phys Ther.* 2000;80:28–52.
13. Resnik L, Hart D. Using clinical outcomes to identify expert physical therapists. *Phys Ther.* 2003;83:990–1002.
14. Resnik L, Jensen G. Using clinical outcomes to explore the theory of expert practice in physical therapy. *Phys Ther.* 2003;83:1090–1106.
15. Gwyer J, Jensen GM, Hack L, Shepard KF. Using a multiple case-study research design to develop an understanding of clinical expertise in physical therapy. In Hammell KW, Carpenter C (eds). *Qualitative research in evidence-based rehabilitation.* New York: Churchill-Livingstone; 2004.
16. Edwards I, Jones M, Carr J, et al. Clinical reasoning strategies in physical therapy. *Phys Ther.* 2004;84:312–330.
17. Tsui A. *Understanding expertise in teaching.* New York: Cambridge University Press; 2003.
18. Ericsson KA. Recent advances in expertise research: a commentary on the contributions to the special issue. *Appl Cognit Psychol.* 2005;19:233–241.
19. Holyoak KJ. Symbolic connectionism: toward third-generation theories of expertise. In KA Ericsson, J Smith (eds). *Toward a general theory of expertise.* New York: Cambridge University Press; 1991.
20. Rikers R, Paas F. Recent advances in expertise research. *Appl Cognit Psychol.* 2005;19:145–149.
21. Ericsson KA, Smith J (eds). *Toward a general theory of expertise.* New York: Cambridge University Press; 1991.
22. Boshuizen H, Bromme R, Gruber H (eds). *Professional learning: gaps and transitions on the way from novice to expert*, Norwell, MA: Kluwer Academic Publishers; 2004.
23. Bereiter C, Scardamalia M. *Surpassing ourselves—an inquiry into the nature and implications of expertise.* Chicago: Open Court Press; 1993.
24. Brandsford J, Brown A, Cocking R (eds). *How people learn: brain, mind, experience and school*, Washington, DC: National Academy Press; 2000.
25. Chi MT, Glaser R, Farr M. *The nature of expertise.* Hillsdale, NJ: Lawrence Erlbaum; 1988.
26. Ericsson KA (ed). *The road to excellence.* Mahwah, NJ: Lawrence Erlbaum; 1996.
27. American Physical Therapy Association Vision Statement for Physical Therapy 2020. Available at: http://www.apta.org. Accessed December 23, 2005.
28. Norman GR. Defining competence: a methodological review. In Neufeld VR, Norman GR (eds). *Assessing clinical competence.* New York: Springer Publishers; 1985.
29. Epstein RM, Hundert EM. Defining and assessing professional competence. *JAMA.* 2002;287:226–235.

30. Epstein RM. Mindful practice. *JAMA*. 1999;282:833–839.
31. Shulman LS. *Teaching as community property: essays on higher education*. San Francisco: Jossey-Bass Publishers; 2004.
32. Hammell KW, Carpenter C. *Qualitative research in evidence-based rehabilitation*. New York: Churchill-Livingstone; 2004.
33. Newell A, Simon H. *Human problem solving*. Englewood Cliffs, NJ: Prentice-Hall; 1972.
34. Chase WG, Simon HA. Perception in chess. *Cognitive Psychol*. 1973;4:55–81.
35. Chi MT, Feltovich PJ, Glaser R. Categorization and representation of physics problems by experts and novices. *Cognitive Sci*. 1981;5:121–152.
36. Elstein AS, Shulman LS, Sprafka SA. *Medical problem solving: an analysis of clinical reasoning*, Cambridge, MA: Harvard University Press; 1978.
37. Elstein AS, Shulman LS, Sprafka SA. Medical problem solving: a ten year retrospective, *Eval Health Prof*. 1990;13:5–36.
38. Elstein AS, Schwartz A. Clinical reasoning in medicine. In J Higgs, M Jones (eds). *Clinical reasoning in the health professions*. Boston: Butterworth-Heinemann; 2000.
39. Rothstein JM, Echternach JL. Hypothesis-oriented algorithm for clinicians. A method for evaluation and treatment planning. *Phys Ther*. 1986;66:1388–1394.
40. Jones MA. Clinical reasoning in manual therapy. *Phys Ther*. 1992;72:875–884.
41. Jones MA, Rivett D. *Clinical reasoning for manual therapists*. Philadelphia: Butterworth-Heinemann; 2004.
42. Barrows HS, Pickell GC. *Developing clinical problem-solving skills: a guide to more effective diagnosis and treatment*. New York: Norton; 1991.
43. Patel VL, Groen GJ. Knowledge-based solution strategies in medical reasoning. *Cognitive Sci*. 1986;10:91–116.
44. Patel V, Kaufman D, Magder S. The acquisition of medical expertise in complex dynamic environments. In KA Ericsson (ed). *The road to excellence*, Mahwah, NJ: Lawrence Erlbaum; 1996.
45. Patel VL, Groen GJ. Developmental accounts of the transition from medical student to doctor: some problems and suggestions. *Med Educ*. 1991;25:527–535.
46. Schmidt HG, Norman GR, Boshuizen HP. A cognitive perspective on medical expertise: theory and implications, *Acad Med*. 1990;65:611–621.
47. Sternberg RJ, Horvath JA. A prototype view of expert teaching. *Educ Res*. 1995;24:9–17.
48. Boshuizen H, Schmidt HG. The development of clinical reasoning expertise. In J Higgs, M Jones (eds). *Clinical reasoning in the health professions*, Boston: Butterworth-Heinemann; 1995.
49. Patel V, Kaufman D. Clinical reasoning and biomedical knowledge: implications for teaching. In J Higgs, M Jones (eds). *clinical reasoning in the health professions*. Woburn, MA: Butterworth-Heinemann; 2000.
50. Sullivan W. *Work and integrity: the crisis and promise of professionalism in america*. San Francisco: Jossey-Bass; 2005.
51. Benner P. *From novice to expert: excellence and power in clinical nursing practice*. Menlo Park, CA: Addison-Wesley; 1982.
52. Benner P, Tanner CA, Chesla CA. *Expertise in nursing practice: caring, clinical judgment and ethics*. New York: Springer; 1996.
53. Benner P, Hooper-Kyriakidis P, Stannard D. *Clinical wisdom and interventions in critical care: a thinking-in-action approach*, Philadelphia: WB Saunders; 1999.
54. Berliner D. In pursuit of the expert pedagogue. *Educ Res*. 1986;15:7:5–13.
55. Sternberg R. Abilities are forms of developing expertise. *Educ Res*. 1998;28:11–20.
56. Mattingly C, Flemming MH. *Clinical reasoning*. Philadelphia: FA Davis; 1994.
57. Fleming MH, Mattingly C. Action and narrative: two dynamics of clinical reasoning. In J Higgs, M Jones (eds). *clinical reasoning in the health professions*. Woburn, MA: Butterworth-Heinemann; 2000.
58. Dreyfus HL, Dreyfus SE, Athanasiou T. *Mind over machine: the power of human intuition and expertise in the era of the computer*. New York: Free Press; 1986.
59. Schön DA. *The reflective practitioner: how professionals think in action*. New York: Basic Books; 1983.
60. Schön DA (ed). *The reflective turn: case studies in and on educational practice*. New York: Teachers College Press; 1991.

61. Eraut M. *Developing professional knowledge and competence*. Washington, DC: Falmer; 1994.
62. Ryle G. *The concept of the mind*. Chicago: University of Chicago Press; 1949.
63. Polanyi M. *Personal knowledge: toward a post-critical philosophy*. Chicago: University of Chicago Press; 1962.
64. Hamm RM. Clinical intuition and clinical analysis: expertise and the cognitive continuum. In J Dowie, AS Elstein (eds). *Professional judgment: a reader in clinical decision making*. New York: Cambridge University Press; 1988.
65. Schön D. *Educating the reflective practitioner*. San Francisco: Jossey-Bass; 1987.
66. Higgs J, Titchen A. *Practice knowledge and expertise in the health professions*. Woburn, MA: Butterworth-Heinemann; 2001.
67. Harris I. New expectations for professional competence. In L Curry, J Wergin (eds). *Educating Professionals: responding to new expectations for competence and accountability*, San Francisco: Jossey-Bass; 1993.
68. Irby D. What clinical teachers in medicine need to know. *Acad Med*. 1994;69:333–342.
69. Dunn TG, Taylor CA, Lipsky MS. An investigation of physician knowledge-in-action. *Teaching Learning Med*. 1996;8:90–97.
70. Dewey J. *How we think*. Buffalo, NY: Prometheus Books; 1991.
71. Argyris C, Schön DA. *Theory in practice: increasing professional effectiveness*. San Francisco: Jossey-Bass; 1974.
72. Jarvis P. *The practitioner-researcher: developing theory from practice*. San Francisco: Jossey-Bass; 1999.
73. Jones M, Jensen GM, Edwards I. Clinical reasoning in physiotherapy. In J Higgs, M Jones (eds). *Clinical reasoning in the health professions*. Boston: Butterworth-Heinemann; 2000.
74. Higgs J, Jones M (eds). *Clinical reasoning in the health professions*. Boston: Butterworth-Heinemann; 2000.
75. Pellegrino ED, Thomasma DC. *The virtues in medical practice*. New York: Oxford University Press; 1993.
76. Leach D. Professionalism: the formation of physicians. *Am J Bioethics* 2004;4:11–12.

2

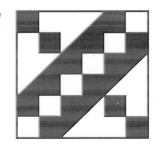

3 Methods for Exploring Expertise

In Chapter 2 we assert that it is important for the profession of physical therapy to make meaningful connections between theory, research, and practice. Let us return to the discussion of the role of expert opinion in our practice. Evidence-based practice is an important element in helping clinicians make decisions about the care of individual patients. After initial challenges about the deemphasis of clinical expertise, Sackett and colleagues did redefine evidence-based practice as "the integration of best research evidence with clinical expertise and patient values" (1, p. 1). What does this recognition of clinical expertise and patient values have to do with our research on expert practice in physical therapy? Although experimental designs for clinical studies are important for demonstrating a specific link between intervention and an outcome, there is much to be understood in exploring the context of clinical practice in physical therapy. This exploration of context is best done through the use of qualitative methods. Morse states it well here:

> …*epidemiological and experimental designs for clinical drug trials seek to decontextualize, qualitative research asks them to consider the context. We have different definitions and agendas for "providing care": their focus is on the pill and if it works; our focus is different—why patients might decide whether to swallow the pill or to accept, reject, or modify the prescribed treatment, or how it affects patients' lives. (2, p. 3)*

This chapter provides an overview of our qualitative research methods used to study expertise in physical therapy practice. We discuss the intent and outcomes of a series of research studies that advanced our thinking and ongoing development of our conceptual models; frameworks; and, ultimately, grounded theory about expert practice in physical therapy. This overview of our theory development is an important element, because our grounded theory work provides a scaffold for others to build on (3). In Part III, Lessons Learned and Applied, are examples of continued research and writing in physical therapy that has been influenced by our original work.

Our work began with two questions: Do differences exist between the ways expert physical therapy clinicians and novice physical therapy clinicians practice, and, if differences do exist, how do they develop? After several years, we turned our focus exclusively to clinical reasoning, performance behaviors, attitudes, philosophies, and professional development of expert clinicians. A grounded theory approach guided a series of research studies that spanned 8 years (4–8).

GROUNDED THEORY

Chenitz and Swanson describe grounded theory as a "highly systematic research approach for the collection and analysis of qualitative data for the purpose of generating explanatory theory that furthers the understanding of social and psychological phenomenon" (9). Grounded theory has its roots in the symbolic interaction traditions of sociology and social psychology (10) and is similar to naturalistic traditions in which researchers seek to understand human behavior from the subject's point of view. According to Morse, grounded theory should be used for examining a phenomenon that is a process or extended experience (11). Research conducted using grounded theory does not begin with speculating about theories; it proceeds inductively to study human experiences from which theories are subsequently developed.

True to the grounded theory approach, we gathered data, made theoretical interpretations, and then returned to the field to collect more data to reaffirm our interpretations and investigate new areas suggested by the data analysis. We read everything we could find on expertise to help us understand our work and place it in a larger context of understanding how health professionals gain and use expertise (12–17).

FIRST CONCEPTUAL FRAMEWORK: UNCOVERING ELEMENTS OF EVERYDAY PRACTICE

Our earliest conceptual framework, drafted in 1988, explored the very basic elements of physical therapy practice (Figure 3-1). The framework identified four parts of clinical practice that affect therapeutic intervention and patient care: 1) professional and personal characteristics of the therapist; 2) personal characteristics of the client or patient; 3) factors related to the organizational setting in which physical therapy is delivered; and 4) tools and treatment techniques, including communication skills, manual skills, and modalities. The reason for studying these factors is that identifiable differences between expert and novice clinicians may have effects before and after patient–therapist interaction, therapeutic intervention, and patient care outcome.

The most interesting part of our framework was the therapist–patient interaction during the therapeutic intervention—that is, what physical therapists specifically did during evaluations and treatment sessions. Therapeutic intervention continued to be a focus of a number of our studies. Related studies

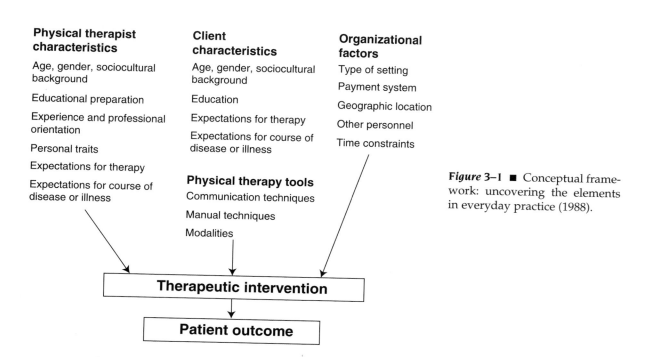

Physical therapist characteristics

Age, gender, sociocultural background

Educational preparation

Experience and professional orientation

Personal traits

Expectations for therapy

Expectations for course of disease or illness

Client characteristics

Age, gender, sociocultural background

Education

Expectations for therapy

Expectations for course of disease or illness

Physical therapy tools

Communication techniques

Manual techniques

Modalities

Organizational factors

Type of setting

Payment system

Geographic location

Other personnel

Time constraints

Therapeutic intervention

Patient outcome

Figure 3–1 ■ Conceptual framework: uncovering the elements in everyday practice (1988).

include the Dreyfus model of skill acquisition (17), Benner's work on novices and experts in nursing (12), and information on hypothetico-deductive models of clinical reasoning studies in medicine (18) and physical therapy (19,20). As is common for researchers involved in the study of phenomena, we grappled with whether to use previously identified models of expertise and practice to guide our data collection and analysis. In accordance with the grounded theory approach, we decided to use available literature to help us understand and interpret our research but did not use it as a framework for conducting our work (21). Robrecht has noted that the "[g]rounded theory method stresses that theory must come from the data, not prior knowledge, and that the operations leading to theoretical conceptualizations must be revealed" (22). Thus, each time data were gathered, the literature was consulted to determine how our findings and interpretations compared with those of other researchers and whether our work fit with other midrange or grand theories (23).

DISCOVERY OF THEMES AND ATTRIBUTE DIMENSIONS: REFRAMING THE ELEMENTS IN EVERYDAY PRACTICE

Our work began in 1989 with the collection of data on eight physical therapists who had varying levels of experience, ranging from less than 2 years to more than 20 years (1). Participating therapists worked predominantly with orthopedic patients in a variety of settings. Field notes and audiotape recording were used to document observations of treatment sessions. The original themes developed from these data are shown on the left side of Figure 3-2. The first observations of novice and experienced clinicians at work revealed differences related to working with patients, eliciting and using information, and managing the chaos of a clinical setting.

The data from our next study, in 1991, were collected by observing three novice clinicians and three expert clinicians who practiced in orthopedic outpatient settings (expertise was defined by length of experience and identified competence) (2). This time, the data collection included observation of each clinician treating at least three patients, patient interviews, interviews with clinicians regarding perceptions of their decision-making and clinical skills, and reviews of patient records. Analysis of these data suggested a reaffirmation and a revision

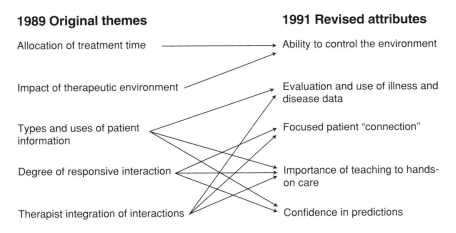

Figure **3–2** ■ Struggle to reconceptualize themes: reframing the elements in everyday practice.

1989 Original themes

Allocation of treatment time

Impact of therapeutic environment

Types and uses of patient information

Degree of responsive interaction

Therapist integration of interactions

1991 Revised attributes

Ability to control the environment

Evaluation and use of illness and disease data

Focused patient "connection"

Importance of teaching to hands-on care

Confidence in predictions

of original themes, shown on the right side of Figure 3-2. The arrows in Figure 3-2 illustrate our struggle to progress from our original themes to increasingly definitive concepts, which we began calling *attribute dimensions*. We consulted the work of Livingston and Borko, who were studying novice and expert teachers in classroom settings, to help us organize attribute dimensions (24). Similar to novice and expert teachers, novice and expert physical therapists differed in both knowledge held (knowledge dimension) and in interaction with patients (improvisational performance). Attribute dimensions are displayed in Figure 3-3.

The following are brief examples of how the observational and interview data were used to inform the identification of these attribute dimensions.

EVALUATION AND USE OF PATIENT ILLNESS AND DISEASE DATA

EXPERT: I try to think of the patients in their environments, about their work and recreational activities. Then I think about structural and functional considerations.

NOVICE: I have a standard routine: observation, palpation, posture, gait, manual muscle testing, range of motion, and any special test for each joint. Then, of course, some functional activities. . . . I'm constantly taking objective data—maybe too much of it.

IMPORTANCE OF HANDS-ON TEACHING

EXPERT: I think I'm good at teaching them what to do and impressing on them that they have to do it. I never, never let them think that I am going to make them better. They have to make themselves better. All I can do is be their coach and cheerleader.

Attribute dimensions
Improvisational performance

Attribute	Master	Novice
Evaluation and use of patient data	Dynamic; specific to each patient	Routine; use of standardized forms
Importance of teaching	Teaching seen as essential	Focus on hands-on skills and patient rapport
Ability to control the environment	Interruptions controlled	Responds to all interruptions; unsure of what is important
Focused communication	Intense; patient-centered	Unfocused; medley of approaches

Figure 3–3 ■ Attribute dimensions that distinguish between expert and novice clinicians.

Knowledge

Confidence in predicting outcomes	Elaborate; comfortable	Shotgun approach; seeks help

NOVICE: I explain to them all the machines I am using. I try to develop a good rapport with them to develop their trust. I try to act interested in something they did outside of therapy.

ABILITY TO CONTROL ENVIRONMENT

NOTES MADE DURING OBSERVATION OF EXPERT: The expert clinician used time efficiently by maintaining focus on patient evaluation and treatment regardless of ambient noise and confusion inherent in a busy clinical setting.

NOTES MADE DURING OBSERVATION OF NOVICE: The novice clinician appeared very distracted by ambient noise and inevitable treatment interruptions that occur in the clinic. She appeared unable to distinguish between what was important to respond to and what was not important and thus frequently lost her focus on the patient she was treating.

FOCUSED COMMUNICATION

NOTES MADE DURING OBSERVATION OF EXPERT: The clinician's attention to the patient during evaluation sessions is intense. She directs her questions in a pattern to determine the source of the patient's problem. Her body language demonstrates complete attention to the patient, from sitting on a stool directly at the feet of the patient to take his history to keeping physical contact with the patient throughout the examination.

NOTES MADE DURING OBSERVATION OF NOVICE: The novice therapist's focus on trying to fill out an evaluation form dominated her interactions with patients. At times, her questions were long and involved, but she paid little attention to the answers.

CONFIDENCE IN PREDICTING OUTCOMES

EXPERT: I try to correlate subjective and objective data. I also try to think about patients in their environments, about their work and recreational activities.

NOVICE: I'm continually taking objective data—maybe too much of it— but I feel like right now I have to do it. I'm not comfortable enough with knowing what will happen.

INITIAL CONCEPTUAL FRAMEWORK

In 1992 we began videotaping treatment sessions of experienced clinicians. While they watched the videotaped sessions, we asked them to discuss what they were thinking as they proceeded with treatment. We began to realize how limited our interpretations were because they had been based predominantly on *our* observations. The data from these clinical reasoning interviews provided an entirely new understanding of what clinicians were thinking and how they made clinical decisions. This new understanding facilitated movement of the attribute dimensions into a more complex conceptual framework, as illustrated in Figure 3-4.

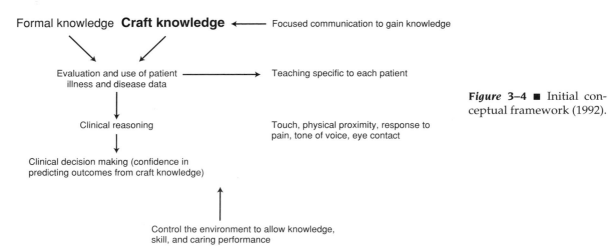

Figure **3–4** ■ Initial conceptual framework (1992).

Attributes were grouped into two dimensions: 1) knowledge and skill and (2) interpersonal skills and caring. The knowledge and skill dimension was expanded after we realized how much and what kinds of knowledge developed as a result of clinical experience. Expert clinicians appear to reflect constantly on accumulated clinical knowledge (often called *craft* or *tacit knowledge*). Craft knowledge is accumulated through focused verbal and non-verbal communication with a succession of patients. The size of craft knowledge relative to formal knowledge demonstrated the importance of craft knowledge for clinical reasoning and decision making. In addition, a close relationship exists between having a skill in evaluation and use of patient illness and disease data and having a skill in teaching—that is, teaching was specific to each patient problem and to patient–family needs based on the illness and disease data obtained. The amount of close physical contact and nonverbal as well as verbal responsiveness to patient needs exhibited by experts represented an additional attribute dimension, identified as *caring*. The theme of controlling the environment was positioned at the lower edge of the conceptual framework to demonstrate that this ability should be fully engaged with the patient to allow successful performance within the two dimensions of practice. At this point, no differences between novice and expert clinicians were evident in any of these areas.

REVISION OF CONCEPTUAL FRAMEWORK: MOVING TO EPISODES OF CARE

The weakness of our research in 1992 was that we had observed experts and novices treating patients only in single treatment sessions. We had limited knowledge of how they evaluated, progressed, and reevaluated patients over the course of a treatment program. Looking at single instances of patient treatment was abandoned in favor of examining treatment across an episode of care (Figure 3-5).

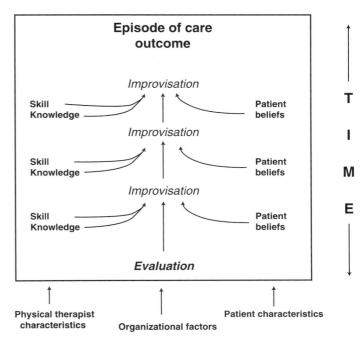

Figure **3–5** ■ Revision of conceptual framework: looking at treatment outcomes across episodes of care (1993).

An *episode of care* was defined as all physical therapy visits for one patient (or up to 3 months for patients with permanent or chronic impairments and related functional limitations). Focusing on an episode of care provided excellent information for understanding how expert clinicians practice. *Practice* included skill and knowledge used while working with a patient's disease characteristics and illness beliefs exhibited in sequences of improvisational performances, from initial evaluation to discharge (outcome).

CASE STUDY GROUNDED THEORY RESEARCH

By the end of 1993, enough preliminary data and theory development were available to submit a funding proposal. After several failed attempts to convince physical therapy grant reviewers to fund our naturalistic methods (which appeared strange to them because the methods did not involve *a priori* hypotheses or statistically significant data outcomes), we received a 2-year grant from the Foundation for Physical Therapy. Our study, the first grounded theory research funded by the Foundation for Physical Therapy, was designed to look at expert practitioners in four clinical practice areas: 1) pediatrics, 2) geriatrics, 3) neurology, and 4) orthopedics. A qualitative case study design was chosen primarily because it permitted a focus on documenting, understanding, and making sense of the perspectives of the clinicians being studied with as little interference as possible from the researchers.

In each specialty area, data were collected on three expert clinicians working with two or more patients across an episode of care. The first and last evaluation and treatment sessions, as well as at least one treatment session per week, were videotaped. The expert clinicians reviewed the videotapes with investigators and responded to questions regarding information about their clinical reasoning and decision-making processes, identifying knowledge bases used to inform their reasoning processes. These interviews took place throughout the episode of care. The investigators also had access to notes recorded on patients' charts. These notes were used to reaffirm the information gathered and clinical decision-making style used by the clinician. In addition, experts participated in several interviews focusing on their professional development. Selected data collection strategies used in the funded research are more fully described in the Appendix. These included structured tasks, such as résumé sorts (25) and exemplars (26), and interview questions that were used to stimulate the expert's recall of professional development from novice to expert and document significant incidents in the development of professional expertise (26,27).

The interviews allowed investigators insights into the minds of expert clinicians. *Expertise* has been defined as having the ability to do the right thing at the right time (14). Examining what kinds of knowledge experts use, how they reason, what patient-care interactions they consider essential, and how they became experts is essential for understanding how expert clinicians know how to "do the right thing at the right time."

All interview, observation, and document data were transcribed and coded, and individual case reports were developed for each expert. Each case report identified themes, such as kinds of knowledge held by expert clinicians and where this knowledge came from, how experts engaged in clinical reasoning, how their practice of physical therapy was conceived and implemented, and what personal values and beliefs guided their practice.

The completed case reports were returned to the expert clinicians to be examined for accuracy and possible researcher misinterpretation. Triangulating data from multiple sources, using member (participant) checks, and incorporating peer evaluation were three techniques used to ensure the credibility and trustworthiness of data. As data began to be compiled for the second and third therapists in each clinical area, we started to look for similarities and differences in the case reports of the three therapists in each clinical area. Then, for each clinical area, we wrote a composite description of expert practice in that clinical area. At this point, the unit of analysis was the composite case study.

The basic research design of our study involved using multiple qualitative case studies that incorporated within- and cross-case analyses. The following cognitive processes, outlined by Morse, are used to understand datasets (21) (Figure 3-6):

- *Comprehending*: obtaining enough data to write a complete, detailed, coherent, and rich description.
- *Synthesizing*: merging stories; separating significant data from insignificant data; forming categories and looking for similarities.
- *Theorizing*: linking data or themes in an explanatory model.
- *Recontextualizing*: examining a theory's application to other settings and populations.

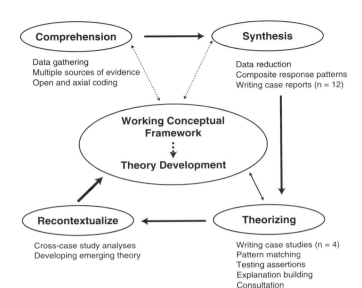

Figure **3–6** ■ Cognitive process involved in qualitative data analysis. (Adapted from Morse J. Emerging from the data: the cognitive processes of analysis in qualitative inquiry. In J Morse (ed). *Critical issues in qualitative research methods*. Thousand Oaks, CA: Sage; 1994, 23–43.)

3

CONCEPTUAL FRAMEWORK: BUILDING THE SCAFFOLD FOR THE GROUNDED THEORY

By 1996 we had identified 19 themes that were common to all or nearly all 12 experts. Some of these themes reaffirmed the work we had done. Many themes were new to us, however, because they came from deeper and richer data acquisition and analysis. The 19 themes were summarized and placed in one of three content areas: 1) knowledge, 2) clinical reasoning, or 3) philosophy.

KNOWLEDGE THEMES

The experts studied appeared to be continually learning—they seemed to have a passion for knowledge. The types of knowledge they held included fundamentals of natural and behavioral sciences and knowledge of movement dysfunction, especially as it related to their clinical specialty area. They also had knowledge of patients, which they used when treating patients who had similar physical impairments and functional limitations. They sought knowledge of patients as people. This knowledge was used in their therapeutic encounters with patients and in patient education. They had knowledge of the operation and resources of the health care system. They moved themselves and patients safely and with an ease that illustrated knowledge of their own bodies and motor planning to facilitate, guide, and support patients during hands-on treatment. They also understood the limits of their own knowledge—both what they did know and what they sought to learn.

CLINICAL REASONING THEMES

Clinical reasoning abilities of these expert clinicians focused on patient-specific functional outcomes. Each had devised a personal framework for collecting data that helped him or her discover useful patterns of clinical problems on which to focus. These clinicians engaged in very little writing when they worked with patients. The personal frameworks they had devised to collect data also helped them store data until they had an opportunity to do their charting. The evaluation and treatment was iterative and interactive—that is, the clinicians constantly moved between evaluation and treatment of the clinical problems on which they were working. The patients were intimately involved in this process and shared in clinical problem solving and decision making. The experts relied little on instruments or data collection forms or chart data. They emphasized letting patients describe problems to clinicians. They asserted that listening to patients and observing what they do tells the clinician everything he or she needs to know.

PHILOSOPHY THEMES

The personal philosophies the experts followed at work were remarkably similar. They believed people should become healthy by taking responsibility for their own health. They believed that all physical therapists have a moral responsibility to use their knowledge and skills to their full extent on behalf of the patient and to administer therapy with compassion. They were reluctant to impose judgments on patients and exhibited true modesty—that is, they were quietly confident in what they did know and unafraid to clearly state what they did not know.

The three areas of knowledge, clinical reasoning, and philosophy change in relation to each other as therapists develop from students to expert clinicians (Figure 3-7). Students bring budding philosophies with them when they begin their physical therapy education. At this point, they have little knowledge and thus few clinical reasoning skills. After graduation from physical therapy

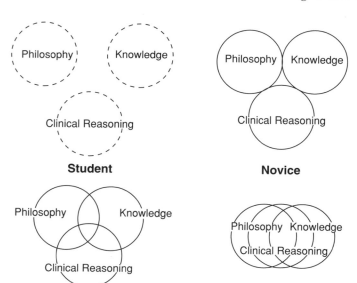

Figure 3–7 ■ Conceptual framework: building the scaffold for the grounded theory (1996).

programs, they enter the field as novices. As novices, they hold more information and have more insight into their philosophies, knowledge, and clinical reasoning skills. The three thematic areas begin to be related to each other. This closer relationship is depicted in Figure 3-7. Competent practitioners demonstrate a coherent overlap of philosophy, knowledge, and clinical reasoning skills in clinical areas that they enjoy and are consequently successful with patients. The skills of expert clinicians who have, for example, 30 years of experience have a remarkable overlap over these three areas. Their daily practice is infused with all three thematic areas to such a degree that extricating their philosophies of practice from their knowledge and clinical reasoning is difficult, if not impossible.

MOVEMENT COMPONENT: "THE IMPLICIT DIMENSION"

Throughout our research, we had used three consultants from outside the physical therapy profession who have written about expertise in their own professions (i.e., medicine, education, and business). These consultants responded to our methodologic questions and reviewed and commented on each analytical phase of the study. They were enormously helpful, especially in noticing deficiencies in our data collection and analysis. For example, they helped us identify an implicit (missing) dimension of expertise—that is, the movement component. Because what the experts were actually doing with patients, such as performing mobilization techniques or teaching functional activities, was so obvious to us as physical therapists, we forgot to address this movement and task data in our study. Movement and task data have subsequently been entered into the final conceptual model, illustrated and explained in Chapter 8.

CONCLUSIONS

Using grounded theory as a guide for a research program helped develop a rich and well-grounded analysis of what expert physical therapy clinicians do; how and why they do it; and how they have acquired knowledge, insight, and skill. Morse (3) proposes three suggestions for incorporating the research of others in your own research: 1) deconstruct the concept/phenomenon, 2) develop a skeletal framework, and 3) develop a scaffold. We believe that our grounded theory work demonstrates those three key elements. The application and growth of our work can be seen in the continued use, revision, modification, and expansion of our grounded theory in Part III, Lessons Learned and Applied.

REFERENCES

1. Sackett DL, Strauss SE, Richardson WS, et al. *How to practice and teach evidence-based medicine.* New York: Churchill-Livingstone; 2000.
2. Morse JM. Beyond the clinical trial: expanding criteria for evidence. *Qual Health Res.* 2005;15:1–2.
3. Morse JM. Theory innocent or theory smart? *Qual Health Res.* 2002;12:295–296.
4. Jensen GM, Shepard KF, Hack LM. The novice versus the experienced clinician: insights into the work of the physical therapist. *Phys Ther.* 1990;70:314–323.
5. Jensen GM, Shepard KF, Gwyer J, Hack LM. Attribute dimensions that distinguish master and novice physical therapy clinicians in orthopedic settings. *Phys Ther.* 1992;72:711–722.
6. Jensen GM, Gwyer J, Shepard KF, Hack LM. Expert practice in physical therapy. *Phys Ther.* 2000;80:28–52.
7. Shepard K, Hack L, Gwyer J, Jensen G. Describing expert practice. *Qual Health Res.* 1999;9:746–758.

8. Gwyer J, Jensen GM, Hack L, Shepard KF. Using a multiple case-study research design to develop an understanding of clinical expertise in physical therapy. In Hammell KW, Carpenter C (eds). *Qualitative research in evidence-based rehabilitation.* New York: Churchill-Livingstone; 2004.

9. Chenitz WC, Swanson JM. *From practice to grounded theory.* Menlo Park, CA: Addison-Wesley; 1986.

10. Strauss A, Corbin J. Grounded theory methodology: an overview. In Denzin NK, Lincoln YS, (eds). *Handbook of qualitative research.* Thousand Oaks, CA: Sage; 1994.

11. Morse JM. *Qualitative nursing research: a contemporary dialogue.* Rockville, MD: Aspen; 1989.

12. Benner P. *From novice to expert: excellence and power in clinical nursing practice.* Menlo Park, CA: Addison-Wesley; 1984.

13. Benner CA, Chesla CA. *Expertise in nursing practice.* New York: Springer; 1996.

14. Ericsson KA, Smith J. *Towards a general theory of expertise: prospects and limits.* New York: Cambridge University Press; 1991.

15. Ericsson KA (ed). *The road to excellence.* Mahwah, NJ: Lawrence Erlbaum; 1996.

16. Higgs J, Jones M (eds). *Clinical reasoning in the health professions.* Boston: Butterworth-Heinemann; 1995.

17. Dreyfus HL, Dreyfus SE. *Mind over machine.* New York: Free Press; 1986.

18. Elstein A, Shulman L, Sprafka SA. *Medical problem solving: an analysis of clinical reasoning.* Boston: Harvard University Press; 1978.

19. Payton OD. Clinical reasoning process in physical therapy. *Phys Ther.* 1985;65:924–928.

20. Thomas-Edding D. Clinical problem solving in physical therapy and its implications for curriculum development. In *Proceedings of the 10th International Congress of the World Confederation for Physical Therapy.* Sydney, Australia; 1987.

21. Morse JM. *Critical Issues in qualitative research methods.* Thousand Oaks, CA: Sage, 1994.

22. Robrecht LC. Grounded theory: evolving methods. *Qual Health Res* 1995;5:169–177.

23. Fawcett J, Downe FS. *The relationship of theory and research.* East Norwalk, CT: Appleton-Century-Crofts; 1986.

24. Livingston C, Borko H. Expert-novice differences in teaching: a cognitive analysis and implications for teacher education. *J Teacher Educ* 1989;40:36–42.

25. Grossman PL. *The making of a teacher: teacher knowledge and teacher education.* New York: Teachers College Press; 1990.

26. Benner P, Wrubel J. *The primacy of caring: stress and coping in health and illness.* Menlo Park, CA: Addison-Wesley; 1989.

27. Martin C, Siosteen A, Shepard K. The professional development of expert physical therapists in four areas of clinical practice. *Nordic Physiother.* 1995;1:4–11.

Part II

Portraits of Expertise in Physical Therapy

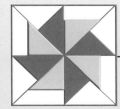

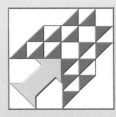

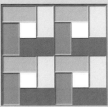

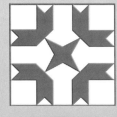

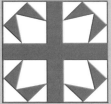

The core section of this book remains the portraits of our experts in pediatrics, geriatrics, neurologic rehabilitation, and orthopedics. We have found that these portraits of experts continue to represent a level of authenticity and credibility that is well understood by clinicians and students. Whether it is through presentations and discussion at professional meetings or use of these portraits in our teaching, we continue to see how these portraits are much like "exemplars" representing some of this first, rich description of expertise in physical therapy practice. We decided not to change the original set of cases, found in Chapters 4–7, Pediatrics, Geriatrics, Neurologic Rehabilitation, and Orthopedics. In Chapter 8, "Expert Practice in Physical Therapy," we have added a section that is a reflection on our model of expertise.

As a postscript to Part II and our case analyses, we elected to contact our experts again and have them reflect on their professional development and current practice, 10 years after our original data collection. Readers of the first edition of *Expertise in Physical Therapy Practice* will want to learn about the continued professional development of our inspiring subjects.

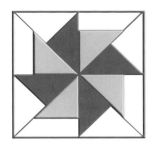

4

Expert Practice in Pediatrics: Playful Process

Jan Gwyer

LUCY: I guess I've stopped thinking of our information as treasured secret information, and I've stopped thinking of us as being people who have all the answers and speak in a secret language and will take their child and will tinker and give the child back—that whole very insular kind of [physical therapist] thing. I'm real up front with the parents about what's possible and what isn't. And I give them articles to read, or, you know, whatever they want; if it's research articles, I give them research articles or books or whatever. . . . They tell me what their goals are. . . . I'm there to consult with them on their goals, and I will share whatever information I have, but I certainly don't know everything, and I'm open to any other information. It puts you into different waters with respect to the families, and it makes it a lot easier in some ways. . . . There's a role that therapists have that I heard a parent allude to in a conference once. . . . She was talking about certain professionals that they valued in their life, and these were people who would walk through the valley of the shadow with them. . . . A lot of the times it's just, you know, things are really bad sometimes. . . . The children are . . . they're not getting any better and they're crying and they need operations and they're getting seizures and things are just getting awful, and if you will just go through it with them . . . it's important.

This interview excerpt illustrates major themes identified in our study of three expert pediatric physical therapists. The data from the qualitative case study indicate clinicians who have done no less than reinvent themselves on their paths to expert practice. The subjects described extensive processes of professional growth characterized by reevaluation of their roles with their patients, expansion and transformation of their knowledge bases, and acquisition of confident clinical decision-making and therapeutic treatment skills. During these processes, their individual virtues also strengthened. They have indeed become health care providers who can walk through the "valley of the shadow" with patients. The experts were remarkably reflective, and their stories—too numerous to include in their entirety here—provide vivid examples of the remarkable physical therapists they have become.

BACKGROUND

Elizabeth, a single, 37-year-old certified pediatric specialist, worked in the children's hospital of a university medical center, where she treated children as both inpatients and outpatients. Elizabeth earned a bachelor of science in physical therapy and completed a master of science degree and a fellowship in pediatrics. She has worked in pediatrics for her entire 15-year career and teaches part-time at several local universities.

Lucy is a 52-year-old single mother of an 8-year-old daughter. She has practiced physical therapy for 30 years, spending all but a few years specializing in pediatrics. She received a bachelor's degree, has since completed a master's degree, and is in the process of completing a doctor of philosophy (PhD) in special education. Lucy has worked in private practice settings and institution-based pediatric settings, including a long tenure with a university-affiliated facility for children.

Janis is a 46-year-old single woman who has practiced pediatrics for all but 2 years of her 24-year career. She also earned a bachelor of science degree in physical therapy but has since pursued both a master's degree in pediatric physical therapy and a PhD in motor control in addition to a postgraduate fellowship in pediatrics. Janis has practiced in institution-based and community pediatric settings and has held an academic faculty position for several years. She holds a grant-funded faculty position with a university, but she spends the majority of her time in an off-campus regional medical center outpatient clinic. In her practice, she treats infants in follow-up clinics and during inpatient stays in the hospital neonatal intensive care unit. (See Table 4-1 for a profile summary).

Table 4-1. Professional Profiles of Expert Pediatric Physical Therapists

	Elizabeth	Lucy	Janis
Years of clinical experience	15	30	24
Practice settings (past and present)	Pediatric clinic and school Pediatric inpatient and outpatient hospitals	Adult inpatient rehabilitation University-affiliated pediatric program Private pediatric practices	Adult long-term care Adult acute care hospital University-affiliated facility pediatric program Early intervention program State board of education consultant Medical center pediatric diagnostic clinic and neonatal intensive care unit
Education	Bachelor of science Master of science	Bachelor of science Master of science Doctoral candidate	Bachelor of science Master of science Doctorate
Advanced clinical education	NDT certification Continuing education PCS	Proprioceptive neuromuscular facilitation course Continuing education	NDT certification Continuing education
Teaching experience	University classroom Clinical education	University classroom Clinical education	University classroom Clinical education
Professional organizations	APTA NDTA	APTA	APTA NDTA

NDT = neurodevelopmental treatment; PCS = Pediatric Certified Specialist; APTA = American Physical Therapy Association; NDTA = Neurodevelopmental Treatment Association.

All three subjects were involved in various teaching activities in addition to direct patient care, including academic, clinical, and continuing education, and all three are white women. The patient subjects observed in this study ranged in age from premature infants to 10-year-old children. These patients primarily had neurologic diagnoses (e.g., cerebral palsy [CP], muscular dystrophy, autism, traumatic brain injury), but many also had secondary musculoskeletal or pulmonary dysfunction. They came from varied socioeconomic situations and had different ethnic backgrounds. The roles played by these therapists may not reflect the entire range of roles of pediatric physical therapists, but they closely reflect those of many pediatric therapists who treat children with neurologic dysfunctions.

Although all three subjects pursued advanced formal education in addition to their baccalaureate degrees in physical therapy, their assessments of the value of their professional educations varied; these assessments are discussed in Types and Sources of Knowledge in Practice. Each therapist began pediatric practice very early in her career. Elizabeth has worked with no other types of clients, and Lucy and Janis were attracted to pediatrics within the first few years of their practice. None have left pediatric practice since. This career pattern is typical for physical therapists who specialize in clients of a specific age group.

CLINICAL PRACTICE THEMES

PHILOSOPHY OF PEDIATRIC PHYSICAL THERAPY PRACTICE

Transformation over Time

Because she had practiced pediatrics for at least 15 years, each therapist was able to discuss how her concept of her role as a pediatric physical therapist had changed over time. Each described similar paths of moving from a framework focused on physical therapy treatment of a child's physical impairments to a much broader concept of her role with the patient and the patient's family. The two more-experienced subjects recalled early years of practice that were quite prescriptive, understanding that they were to treat children frequently in hospitals, rehabilitation settings, or outpatient offices.

> **JANIS:** I used to think "The more, the better."

The traditional scope of practice limited treatment to a child's physical impairments, such as muscle strength, tone, or flexibility.

Two of the experts traced their desire for careers with children to their preteen years and remember gaining a distorted conception of their roles as physical therapists with disabled children.

> **JANIS:** The Telethon was, like, this ideal thing that was baloney, really. Now it makes me mad when I watch it, you know? But when you are a child . . . boy, this is great: You're going to help all of these people and get them to walk and fix them right up.

Although the therapists' concepts of their roles with children changed somewhat during their formal educations, the first years of clinical practice provided the major impetus for redefining their roles in treating children with disabilities.

JANIS: Part of what I do is to help people accept that they have a child with a severe motor problem. I mean, you can't . . . I can't fix brains—though I'd like to.

The therapists stressed not being limited by traditional structures of physical therapy, illustrated by the following comments from Lucy:

LUCY: I started getting more tuned into families and how families work coping with the fact that they had a child with a disability. And that was another experience of breaking out of that little box where we're just somehow doing [physical therapy] in the clinic, and doing things, and then you give them back to the parents, and they go away, and next week, they come back, and you do some more things in the clinic. That whole system really broke up at that point, and I did home visits, and I think . . . I think I got very frustrated at my inability to really have much of an impact on the motor problems. And frustrated at . . . or feeling really, really powerless at being able to help the families. But I could see the kinds of problems that they were going through.

Lucy tells a beautiful story of her early years of practice with a patient that taught her quite a bit about the type of therapist she would become. The following example describes a novice physical therapist exploring multidisciplinary practice, learning to trust her own intuition, and breaking through social and professional mores that dominated her perception of how children should be treated.

LUCY: In working with Hansie, I would have him for an hour during the day, but then the rest of the time he was being treated in a very stimulating way. And so I did something that all the other therapists there thought was very weird because Holland was a very structured kind of place, and you didn't sort of go out of your own little level, and it was very hierarchical. But I . . . I had seen the nurses washing his hair, and giving him a bath, and scrubbing him up with shampoo, and dowsing him with hoses, and he was screaming his head off. So it seemed like the gains that I was making with him were just being negated, pretty much, throughout the rest of the day. So I started talking to them and asking my mom to send me one of those shower—you know, a shampoo protector—and then his bath time got to be nice, and so that was nice and . . . then a doctor . . . this was the worst thing I did there. The surgeons wanted to do a heel-cord lengthening because he walked on his toes. And every time they examined him, he would start screaming so he would get real stiff and they thought he had tight heel cords. And they actually had him in the operating room, and I went in, and—they hadn't sedated him yet—and I said, "Look. He has fine range of motion." And they said, "Oh, yes. He does." Picked him up and carried him back. Carried him back victoriously down the hall, and all the other therapists were cheering. . . . But only somebody who was outside that society could have ever done something like that because they would . . . they would never be able to get away with it. So maybe that was an early experience with seeing that you can't just think of what you do in your own little hour.

4

Focus on Families

Each expert experienced a similar period of growth that caused her to rethink what she actually did with children during therapy, who she should serve, and how she should serve them. Amazing similarities in concepts of care are shared by these three experts. The focus of care for these therapists is strongly centered on the child–family unit in the context of community. The rationale for this broadened concept has both ethical and practical reasons.

> **JANIS:** I think whoever's going to be the caretaker in life is going to make the biggest difference in the way they are treated. I feel more and more that pediatric therapists, especially working with children with neurological problems like that, that we can't make a difference, you know, by doing something one time a week with a child. I don't think that's going to do it.
>
> Watching babies and what things they're doing and what they do is they practice. All the time, normal children practice doing something. If you see them do anything—like, say, getting up into standing—when they first learn that, they do it all day long. So, think about how much practice that takes, and if I just help some child do that once a week, is that going to get carried over? Are they learning anything? You know, there's a big difference between practice and learning. So, yes, I've changed that way.

> **LUCY:** Your starting point for therapy is what's important to this family. And there's lots of really good reasons for that. One of them is just a kind of an ethical honoring of . . . that you are the consultant—that they're hiring [you] to do work for them—and it's not like you're a God-like creature who has curative powers in your hands to dispense out. You're just there to try to serve their needs, and so you have to know what their needs are. . . . If you want to get a good outcome, you really have to have enough intensity of intervention. And the only way that you can get that is if the parents have decided what it is that will be worked on because that's what they want and that's what they'll work on. And you get results much faster because they do it every day, especially if you're structured about it and specify what the goal is and show them how you take data and how you count things and how you measure things, then they have some kind of concrete feedback. And that's a whole other way of operating than eternal therapy, where you just kind of go on and on and on and on, and you don't really know exactly what you're doing. But the child still has cerebral palsy; therefore, you still have to keep doing the therapy.

> **ELIZABETH:** I have a strong preference that the parents are always there. Parents may need you to show them how to [perform the treatment] with their child, but to start off thinking that you know more about somebody else's child, I think, is a ludicrous starting point.

Transition from Treating to Teaching

Each therapist's time spent with children has expanded from just treating to treating and teaching. The therapists value the time they spend with patients.

They use their hands to assess and treat, believing something very powerful is associated with what they do with their hands. The information that they gain from these treatment sessions allows them to target and refine teaching elements of a child's treatment program. Their philosophy is to teach a child's caregiver to recognize and understand the expected motor, sensory, cognitive, and social development of the child to help the caregiver identify behaviors to reinforce and those to discourage.

What do these experts try to teach the families? They share a commitment to establishing goals with the family that are intensely functionally oriented and aimed at maximizing the child's potential, no matter the progressive nature of the diagnosis. This is accomplished by listening intently to the child and the family and by treating each with utmost respect.

4

> **JANIS:** Part of what I feel like I do is try to work toward whatever independence the child could have. So it was important for me to help the family deal with what's going on with the child all the time, not just some of the end results of CP. You know, when you work with somebody that closely—when you work with children with CP—it's not like you work with them for 3 months or 6 months, but you work with them over years. You're sort of developing, you're changing as the child changes and as the family changes, and you're helping the process, you hope.

> **LUCY:** I come from the background of respecting [the patient's parents] and their integrity, and whatever they say as goals, I just take at face value. And that's what we work on. I think one of the things I have learned over the past couple of years, in conjunction with the PhD studies, in a special education context, is that the parents' goals are *the* goals, and the child's goals are *the* goals. It's not that the therapist's goals are *the* goals.
>
> I'm trying to influence the dad's behavior because . . . it's kind of a conflict because a parent knows a child better than anybody who sees the child once or twice a week, and I really have to respect their instinctive ways of interacting with their children.

> **ELIZABETH:** You can't kid people about whether you respect them or not. And she [the mother] knows that I respect her knowledge of [her child], and she's more willing to put that out there.

> **JANIS:** There are interesting dynamics in the clinic because you know you're not just working with a patient, but you're working with a patient and a family and another family member. It's like this other family that comes: the mother comes, the grandmother comes, the grandfather comes, the baby comes, and I feel like I'm trying to balance everything—all the needs of everybody. Like the grandmother saying, "Do you think he's going to walk?"—she asks me that every time now—or, "You think if I just do this more he'll walk?" And then the mother says something else, and them talking to each other, and then the grandfather being there playing with the baby. It's like I'm trying to bring everybody into the action. . . . It's exhausting.

By including the child and family in such an important way in physical therapy, these experts express their desire to empower the child and family to take as much responsibility as they can for their own care. This is a well-founded principle in the promotion of health and wellness in the general population but one that is often overlooked in a client group that has never been treated as having usual patient concerns and often has very little control available to them.

The Importance of Fun

A striking similarity in each of the therapists' practices is the role of play in the physical therapy care of these children. Even an uninitiated observer might not be surprised to find physical therapists using play as part of their treatment or as a technique to persuade a child to perform a specific movement. On reflection, each of the therapists provided a much deeper explanation of the importance of play to patients and to her own sense of satisfaction with their care. All three subjects had a well-developed sense of humor and used it frequently during patient care and interviews. Each was able to create a playful environment for even the most distressed child, and all of the experts talked about learning to increase the "fun quotient" of therapy.

> **JANIS:** What I'm trying to do is help people learn how their baby moves, and ways that they can help their baby move easily, more easily, and prevent certain problems and, hopefully, sort of incorporate what I'm showing them into whatever they're doing so that it doesn't become such a burden. I try to say that this shouldn't be something that's really going to stress you. This should be something that you can do when you're playing, when you're diapering. . . . So I teach people to do a little bit of light stretching because it can just be incorporated into play.

> **ELIZABETH:** See, now he's starting to play with me. He's starting to play with my face. He wants me to, you know, puff air into my cheeks—you know that silly game children do. See, I feel that level of trust is just worth a million dollars. And now we are getting all the physical stuff we need. If I tried to force this on him, therapy would be this miserable thing in his life, and it's got to be in his life for all his life.

> **LUCY:** I've been thinking a lot lately about the fun requirements of childhood and how, as therapists, we really have kind of medicalized children with cerebral palsy. . . . They go into this whole other world of having their clothes off and being manipulated and exercised, and it's so abnormal for a child. . . . Therapists change the balance of fun. I mean, they're in the position of changing the fun quotient in a negative direction by making children do stupid, boring things that aren't fun. So, I think it has an effect—a psychological effect—on a developing child that can be bad when they're grown up. It's like bad memories. . . . I've really been working as hard as I can to try to make everything as much fun as I can.

> I feel more like I can give a real good justification for why I am [including fun in treatment], whereas when I started, I started out of boredom.

I was bored stiff with this treatment program and the little girl was bored stiff. . . . I can remember really clearly the day that I had her over the ball, and she looked up at me and I looked at her, and it was like, "This is disgusting, isn't it?," and she couldn't talk, and so I said, "Forget it. We're not going to do therapy anymore and we're gonna have fun." And so we started with ballet and some dramatics, making plays and things like that. And I was still doing the same therapy. I still had the same goals, but I felt kind of nontherapist like because I was doing it in that way.

JANIS: I think I don't play enough. When I look at those tapes I see that I need . . . I'm glad that I have the tapes because it makes me think that I need to play more. I get too serious with the child and the family, and I think that if it was more fun—if I could play more with the child—the child would be more receptive to me. I have always had a hard time playing. And it's a big deal because a lot of people interview adults who had therapy since they were very young, and a lot of them thought their physical therapists were terrible. They don't have that good feeling, going back to when they were children. I don't want someone to remember me as someone who only caused pain and aggravation! I think maybe that this has gotten better. As I feel more comfortable treating, I have more fun, so now it's a matter of having fun more often. . . . What I try to do with families is help them have more fun with their child, instead of therapy being another thing that has to be done, rather than another thing that they would want to do in their typical life with their children.

These comments describe gradual changes in the experts' philosophies, influenced by external environments and beliefs about appropriate roles for physical therapists with their patients and families. Prescriptive practice under the direction of a physician is now largely a memory. Two of the experts in this study were involved with this type of practice early in their careers and knew that it did not inherently fit with their philosophies of physical therapy care for children. Their personal philosophies and individual efforts, along with those of many colleagues, are responsible for the changed expectations of physical therapists in pediatrics.

These experts could not have so successfully implemented expanded concepts of their roles in practice without concurrently changing several major elements of practice, which emerged as the following clinical practice themes in the data: knowledge (type, source, and use), clinical reasoning, and skilled movement.

TYPES AND SOURCES OF KNOWLEDGE IN PRACTICE

The type of information found valuable by experts, sources of information, and methods of information use by experts are of considerable interest. Educators often have limited time with their students, both in professional education and continuing education. Consequently, they try to choose wisely from the myriad of detailed content when deciding what to teach.

Transformation of Content Knowledge

Each of the subjects demonstrated a broad and deep content knowledge of normal and abnormal human physical, psychological, and social development. This knowledge was much broader, they said, than was ever introduced in their professional education programs. Field notes and subject interviews also revealed that the therapists had a significant understanding of themselves and of patients as individuals. Most impressive, however, is the transformation of their depth of content knowledge and knowledge of themselves and the patient into the tacit knowledge that supports clinical decisions. How do they develop this ability to store, sort, secure, and use these types of knowledge? The process begins during professional education, but, as Elizabeth describes, the typical emphasis on memorization was useless when brought to the task of clinical problem solving with patients.

> **ELIZABETH:** The first year I was out of school, I immediately felt like I had to go back to the things I learned in physical therapy school and refile everything because I felt like everything I learned was from one perspective and I needed to immediately pull it out by diagnosis. When I started doing that—from my notes, say—I went back to my kinesiology course and they mentioned a couple of things for one diagnosis or another, I pulled that stuff out, and I realized when I did that, the net total of the packages I had for any given diagnosis were really incomplete to me. So I went to the library and just started looking up spina bifida or muscular dystrophy or any of the diagnoses and just [started] pouring through articles. Now, that time period I loved because I had never done anything like that before in terms of being completely self-initiated, completely for myself. I could follow my own criteria for what I thought was important. The contrast with learning in college struck me. This was a completely different type of learning and I just loved it! It was really addictive! That was the first level of learning that was directly clinically applicable and was driven by what I needed in the clinic, which was to pull things together in relation to any given child.

Elizabeth's example of reformatting, reindexing, and comparing content knowledge to the reality of the clinical experience describes the process of reflection that seems to guide these experts as they build their substantial frameworks of clinically useful knowledge. The paths these experts took to enriching their knowledge were similar, as all three initiated a process that led them to formal certification in the neurodevelopmental treatment (NDT) approach, to graduate school, or both. The path immediately out of professional education, however, was not as similar. Two subjects felt strongly that their professional education did not provide them with enough content knowledge to adequately treat children and began immediately identifying such sources of knowledge in continuing education and, rather quickly, in formal education programs. Lucy, however, recounts leaving professional education with an attitude of mistaken self-confidence, which quickly changed when she began graduate education.

LUCY: At that point in my life, I had no doubt that I knew everything that there was to know. . . . I mean, I didn't hesitate to take on anything (laughs). I guess it was youthful "ignorance is bliss" or something like that. But, no, it never occurred to me that there could be anything at all that you couldn't just show me one time and I would know how to do it. But, mostly, I came into the program thinking again . . . I mean, that I pretty much had it and I just needed the credential. Hubris plays a very large role in my life (laughs). So I started the program and . . . and ran right smack dab into [teacher Jan Wilson], who was a huge influence. First semester: One of the first courses that I took was with Jan Wilson, and I thought I knew [the subject matter] because I knew how to do the Milani Comparetti. And so I remember, the first day, she asked us what questions we had about reflexes, and . . . nobody had any questions—we knew how to do the Milani Comparetti! And I remember the last day of class she said, "Well, *now* do you have any questions about reflexes?" And she started writing on the board all the questions that we had, and she had to get out the stool and stand up so she could get more room at the top of the board. Every blackboard on three sides of the class was covered with questions that we had about reflexes. That was the real opening up of the fact that there aren't any answers, that there's always more questions. And that . . . that was the death of the idea that I knew what I was doing.

Career Mentors

Career mentors become a significant source of knowledge and motivation for these therapists. Each recounts stories of individuals who encouraged them to return to school, learn more, or study harder. Although the therapists mentioned some academic instructors as individuals who challenged them to think critically, most of the mentors discussed were clinical therapists, colleagues, or recognized experts with whom they had crossed paths and whose skills and knowledge impressed them and motivated them to expand their own knowledge. In graduate school, these experts found a much wider range of topics available and of interest to them. This branching out into content areas that they knew to be important to their practice is the basis of their broad conception of their practice with children. In addition to content knowledge in pediatric physical therapy, they have evidence of expanded content knowledge in pediatrics, biomechanics, cognitive development, psychological development, and language and communication.

LUCY: I became very enamored of [teacher Margaret Rood's] ideas . . . and really started reading journals—doing things that I had never done before, like reading journals, starting to read books. She was the person who got me back to studying. I had not cracked a book since I had gotten out of [physical therapy] school because I thought I knew everything and I could just kind of fly by the seat of my pants in any problem that I ran into.

The therapists had the following comments about returning to graduate school:

> **LUCY:** It was such an opening up of . . . of new worlds of literature—that people had actually thought about these things and written about them . . . and written books about them and written articles about them and done research on them. . . . It was amazing to me how much there actually was. Margaret Rood had her little box of articles that we pulled from, but now we actually went to the library and found our own articles!

> **ELIZABETH:** The things that strike me about the influence it had was again the sorting out about what information you wanted to keep and how you looked at information and that to me, what was most important was content. And I didn't necessarily get the content I wanted always in the [physical therapy] department, and so I took courses in other departments and it was really nice to have the option to do that.

> **LUCY:** But today, I was doing [consultation] with a much richer background of knowledge—not just about child development but about family issues, about adulthood interactions, about early intervention policy at a national level, about . . . the school system situation—you know, resources versus demands in the school system and how that relates to private practitioners—and also a general theoretical base about seeing the child as an integrated whole. So all of those things that I was reading about were kind of floating around, and that influenced how I structured the conversation with the mother.

> **JANIS:** I appreciate [graduate school] now, and I'm glad that I went through that hassle, and I'm glad that I learned the things I did. I think that it has helped me do clinical work because I think that the process teaches you to sort of analyze at a different level.

Patient as Source of Knowledge

The youngest expert, Elizabeth, described a process of reflecting on and integrating content knowledge with the knowledge she gains every day from her clinical work. She trusts her knowledge gained from her patients and tends to distrust more formal sources of knowledge if information from a patient contradicts it.

> **ELIZABETH:** The importance is to have a continual building, and because my heart is in the clinic, everything I would hear . . . struck some connection to what I knew to be true of children in the clinic, that stuff really caught my attention, and when I hear stuff that conflicts with what I feel I've known to be true when I actually have watched a child, then I do question it. . . . I do want to explore it further before I just take it. I can't take it on the assumption of someone . . . if it really conflicts with what I've experienced in the clinic.

> I think part of it is a personal thing in that I don't trust. I have never trusted that I understood something unless I understood it in context. . . .

I always felt that I could never understand anything until I walked all the way around it. . . . You know, if you walk around the corner and look at that thing from behind, it could be completely different, and so somehow context has always been really important to me.

Each expert emphasized the respect she has for the learning that can take place in the clinical setting, with the patient as the source of the most useful kind of knowledge. This has provided the therapists with the antidote to boredom in practice. They clearly value what they can learn from every patient encounter.

LUCY: One thing that I think I've really improved on with practice, and because of specific course work I've had with specific people, is shutting up and listening, and that was real hard for me to do. I just always want to jump in there with a solution no matter what it is. . . . I've gotten much more information from listening than I ever did from structuring my questions. . . . It really isn't a problem getting the parents to tell you about the child. . . . It's mostly just giving them the permission to tell you . . . and acknowledging—honoring—what they say.

These experts also possessed important knowledge about their current patients (e.g., a child's personal tastes, temperament, and family issues that might be affecting therapy).

LUCY: With Amy, I had intended to offer dance as an option, and I was going to do ballet. But she didn't want that because her sister does that, and she wanted something different than her sister. So we switched to tap, so that she had different kinds of shoes. . . . Respecting the desires of the child and the fantasies of the child is the starting point.

CLINICAL REASONING

Several of these expert clinicians found motivation to participate in this study because it allowed them to observe their own clinical reasoning skills. Perhaps this uncertainty is a residual effect of what the subjects agreed was a lack of any instruction in a systematic clinical decision model in their professional education programs.

LUCY: When I went to school they didn't talk about systems. They just said do this and this and this and this. And so that was how I was operating, and I think that gave me the illusion that I . . . kind of knew everything.

JANIS: I don't think they taught us any processes when I went to school, that I can remember. There was a lot of memorizing.

Types of Clinical Judgments Required in Practice

Lucy and Janis, the two therapists with the most experience, were able to recount a progression in the types of clinical decisions demanded of them over the years, from early positions characterized by prescriptive care requiring few clinical decisions to the positions they find themselves in today. Each subject discussed her broad systems approach to patient problem solving and dissected her clinical reasoning process during treatment when watching her videotape. Although the experts may have varied theoretical preferences in the care of children with central nervous system dysfunction, they each articulated the use of an expansive system of evaluation that guided each clinical problem.

The types of clinical decisions required of the subjects during this study spanned the continuum of decisions that arise in a pediatric physical therapist's practice, including minute-to-minute treatment decisions required by a patient with a rapidly fluctuating central nervous system, consultative meetings with parents regarding the appropriate type of day care, and important diagnostic decisions (e.g., Does this child have CP?) performed in collaboration with neonatologists and others on the team. The subjects believe that each type of clinical decision requires a different type of knowledge applied in a specific context.

Integrated Evaluation and Treatment Decisions

Understanding clinical decisions that take place on a moment-to-moment basis during treatment requires careful examination of the extraordinarily fluid movement seen in each therapist–child interaction. In videotaped debriefing sessions, the therapists elucidated the activities that were occurring at any moment (e.g., observation, evaluation, or treatment). What was striking was that the task of dissecting the practice of an expert pediatric clinician was as difficult for a novice physical therapist or student as picking the second violin line out of a Beethoven concerto would be for a beginning violinist. On the surface, an expert's evaluation appears as a graceful dance or one continuous motion. The subjects agreed that their treatment-session decisions are heavily influenced by verbal and tactile input from patients. None of these experts routinely took any notes during treatment sessions of 1 hour or longer. They have tremendous powers of concentration and trust their evaluation skills and memory.

> **ELIZABETH:** I learned to evaluate as you go, paying attention to what the child wants and trusting what your hands are telling you, and you trust the child's response and you let the child's response motorically or emotionally drive how you're trying to do what you want to do with them. Really good therapists do this. I think that they are always watching. They are always paying attention to how they're handling or doing it instinctively. . . . I think the terrible thing is if you ever see a pediatric physical therapist who's treating and they're not paying attention to their hands and they're not watching any of it. . . . I think it is a bad sign.
>
> I think [NDT is] really important in terms of the way it teaches you to pay attention to the job because one of the basic premises is you let the child lead you. . . . You listen with your hands, and you go by what's right in front of your face in the clinic, and I feel like the importance of that is huge.

> **JANIS:** I have a tremendous memory for how a child feels in my hands, and I often don't see these children for 6 months. I make notes after an examination. I'm glad to have my notes, but I trust my memory.

ELIZABETH: I can tell with my hands immediately that his tone is totally different. There is no dynamic response with this. The speed with which I can move him into his range without resistance is completely different from before.

Elizabeth continues her reflection as she views a videotape of her treatment of an 8-year-old child with CP, illustrating the fluid movement between evaluation and treatment and the demands that places on her ability to recall a treatment session:

ELIZABETH: I had to remeasure his ankles at this point because I couldn't tell whether the range I was getting before was accurate. So now that he's really calm, I am going to remeasure. It seems he had more. Now I should stop and write this stuff down, but there's no way I'm going to stop. See, now I'm pretending to him that I'm taking turns, but I what really want him to know is that he can go into that position without hurting.

Developing a Broad Systems Approach to Clinical Decisions

Each subject recounted instances in her career in which she broadened her approach to defining a child's problem, pursued additional knowledge to support a larger systems approach to care, and consequently expanded the nature of her clinical decisions. The therapists believe that an effective pediatric physical therapist cannot view children's physical performance problems in isolation; each learned this lesson over and over from patients and families. Lucy's career path crossed with several significant clinical masters, each of whom influenced her thinking but stimulated her to move further in her development of her own systems approach.

LUCY: Margaret Rood came for some workshops, and she was a huge influence because she was an incredible therapist. And she had this system that was very elaborate. If you worked real hard, you could figure out what she was talking about and develop this nice little protocol that all had to do with, you know, the "We're gonna fix up the central nervous system" idea, but it was very attractive for two reasons. One of them was she was very specific about what she was doing, and so you could really understand it and follow a train of thought. And the other thing was she was an absolutely incredible therapist. When she worked with a child, you really saw changes.

I took a three-week course, [a proprioceptive neuromuscular facilitation] course, at Northwestern with Dorothy Voss, and she was quite impressive. . . . I remember being quite impressed because she had a system.

Getting back to Rood and her systems . . . yeah, it was another big swipe at "Okay, here's a way to organize information in a really big context" because she had a big, big, big context of the body. And she also had a big context of function. And she really looked at, you know, how people were able to garden and eat and enjoy life—that I really appreciated.

And she had the answers, by God—you know? I mean, there was nothing that woman wouldn't tackle—any patient, any problem. . . . She'd work up this map of their body and how she was gonna get in there . . . and tinker and then it was gonna be better. . . . I liked that a lot.

We were doing little study groups and pulling out journal articles and using it on our patients, and I considered myself to be sort of in [Rood's] camp. That was a time to, you know, pick a camp to be in. So the other thing . . . then there was this . . . there was this conflict that arose between NDT and Rood, and people at [the university] were very NDT-oriented, and I was very Rood-oriented. So, there was a certain amount of conflict there. I think what that did was . . . to again push me into a position of saying, "You can't just toe a party line." You have to really think about what you're doing and be able to have sensible explanations for what you're doing.

There's all these different levels of subsystems. You can tease out and try and look at how they interact and then what you can change, and that gets to be real complex because you have the basic elements in a dynamic action model: the performer, the task, and the environment. And so you could take any one of those and just tease out a million different things and subcircles within the big circle. . . . After I've figured out what the issues are in a particular environment around a particular task, then I do an exam of the child and the subsystems of the child, which is basically a pretty typical [physical therapy] exam: looking at muscle strength and . . . force control and joint mobility and muscle length, posture, [and] gait. . . . The next step is to make some hypotheses about how those exam findings correlate with the stated problems . . . and then tagging certain ones . . . "Well, I think it's this or this and that, and so I'm going to do that," . . . and then track on the functional goal. . . . Then I take data on a small selection of things that I think are important about the child, reflecting which little subsystems I think are the control parameters. . . . Then I want to see that change, and I want to see the function change. . . . That's my sort of hypothesis: that if I push on this one hard enough, the system will reorganize, and I'll get a different function. I like a system that makes sense, and I don't like dogma. . . . I like big ideas that encompass all of the things—all of the aspects of life and not just one little part of it—and things that help give an explanation or a suggestion or a helpful thing, no matter what the problem is.

The only thing that can get you through is a system for looking at whatever comes up because the things that come up are totally unpredictable, and you just have to have a way of just putting things into perspective and considering where the parents are coming from and where the child is coming from and what is it that needs to happen right now in order to kind of unstick the system and unstick their system and keep their family moving and keep their life moving. And to me, that's the essential thing. . . . It's a compilation of all those different pieces that were picked up along the way: the teaching thing and the systems thing and the whole family thing and that tension between, you know, what you can actually do with that child's body and what the whole life of the family is about and how that plays out. And you don't get to separate them. . . . You can pretend that you are separating them and that you're just working on the child's body, but I think you're really fooling yourself and doing a disservice to the family.

Janis also frequently discussed a systems approach to patient management decisions and indicated that this influences her clinical decisions, such as who in the family to involve, when to treat, and when to teach. She identifies external systems affecting children, including family and caregivers, as well as physiologic systems.

4

> **JANIS:** When you are working with people, everyone is an individual and there are so many systems involved and you are really trying to figure out what enables them. . . . One of the things I've learned is that I take the systems approach and I look at all the systems and I realize how important the autonomic system is to the motor system, you know, (laughs) . . . and I feel like if I lose the baby autonomically, I lose the baby. I mean, sometimes I let babies cry because I think that . . . babies *should* cry. That's what they do. It's one of the ways they learn. But I know how much the autonomic system is going to affect their state system and the motor system so what I'm trying to do is sort of help control all those systems so that we have them working together rather than sort of pulling the child apart. Yeah, that's what I've learned. Nobody ever told me that, and I wished they did now, when I was a student. Really looking at those kinds of behavioral changes . . . I didn't learn that for a long time and that really has made a difference in my treatment, and not only looking at the behavioral changes in the baby but looking at the behavioral changes in the family.

When asked how her clinical decision-making process has changed over her career, Janis again emphasized the importance of taking a broad approach to each patient's problem:

> **JANIS:** Probably in looking at assessing a child, getting broader and broader in terms of my assessment, [and] starting out with the child but also figuring out what is going on with the family. What the family's needs are and also what the family's needs are within their home and the child's within the home and within the community. I think that as I have sort of taken it more like a general approach to what's going on, not just with the child but the whole system. I now use that whole system approach, and that's really affected my ability to do a better job with the child.

Expanded Roles with Patients and Families

Expansion of clinical judgments made by these experts creates different relationships between the therapists and patients' families than might be found in other physical therapy specialties. Pediatric physical therapists become significant individuals in the lives of their patients' families. Each expert recounted stories of parents with whom they have stayed in touch, regardless of whether the child was in treatment. Therapists are often asked to solve family problems concerning children. Lucy gives the example of a particularly complicated client who was receiving care from several providers. A child who was dyspraxic and nonverbal, treated by Lucy from 12 months to 3 years of age for motor deficits, has a mother who has difficulty dealing with her child's needs. Lucy has not seen the child for 8 months, and she receives a call from the mother, who requests a consultation. Several aspects of the child's progress and care with other professionals concern the mother, who needs some guidance.

> **LUCY:** She called me because I'm the one who stuck by her since the baby was a baby, and she trusts me. She trusts my advice. So I came in and . . . I guess previously I would have . . . I would have thought . . . I would have been real kind of frantic about it, like, "Well, what does she want from me?" you know? I mean, I'm the [physical therapist] here . . . You can tell me about the bicycle problem, but I'm not a potty trainer, and I don't know what these people are doing. And I wouldn't have been able to cope with all of her requests, except to refer her to my friends and then bug out of there as quickly as possible. But today I felt like, okay, this is a real-life situation. Parents don't divide their children up according to what discipline their problems belong to, and she is coming to me as someone to really help her. . . . And so I had a process, you know . . . identifying issues, prioritizing them first, and then deciding what the options were for each one and then assigning each of us the next step and making a plan for what we were going to do next. . . .
> I was able to conceptualize what was going on as, okay, here's a frantic mother who's got all these situations, and how can I sort it out, simmer it down, and do something productive in 1 hour . . . and be, you know, be efficient about it . . . and think about, okay, what's the best way to allocate county resources here, and personal family resources, and how does that relate to insurance company resources and health care reform?

Team Player and Patient Advocate

The multidisciplinary nature of pediatrics means that making decisions usually involves negotiating care of children with other pediatric team members. As the therapists' confidence in their own clinical judgments grew through continued study and, in particular, clinical experience, their ability to disagree with a team consensus strengthened. Each expert described the ability to intervene as a critically important skill for a pediatric physical therapist. Each therapist had a story that helped cement this concept for her. Lucy's story of a successful intervention on behalf of her patient Hansie, recounted earlier in the chapter, is similar to Janis's story, which occurred early in her career and involved a disagreement with a physician about the care of a child with a brain injury.

> **JANIS:** I had been seeing this child. [The disagreement] was about how long this child should be in the hospital and where this child should be

referred after hospitalization, and he had only seen this child once, and I had been working with this child. So it was that kind of issue. I felt like I knew the child, knew the family. I knew the progression of this child in terms of the head injury, and I also knew the outside in terms of what is out there and whether it would be better for him to be an outpatient or whether it would be better for him to be in a pediatric rehab facility. That was a big issue.

Elizabeth recounts a story of a child who had an unsuccessful outcome from muscle-lengthening surgery. She says she regrets not fighting enough on behalf of the child.

> **ELIZABETH:** I feel as though I didn't do a good job defending that child, even though it wasn't my mistake.

Diagnosis through Patient Observation: What is Normal?

Perhaps some of the most difficult clinical decisions pediatric therapists make involve diagnosis and prognosis of neurologic disabilities in infants. Janis, who works in a busy clinic environment, must consult with 8–10 complex patients in each session. Her clinical judgments must be efficient, accurate, and delivered with appropriate care for the clients she sees. Janis summarizes what her clients want from her in the following way:

> **JANIS:** People come in here and they want to know what is wrong with their baby and why, and how they can be fixed, and how fast can this be fixed.

Equipped only with medical information that can vary from brief referral letters from pediatricians to extensive hospital charts, Janis enters each examination room with a few hunches about what she might find with a child.

> **JANIS:** Before I go in, I have certain ideas, but they are just ideas. When I go in there, then I can build on them, and then they go off in different directions or they may go off in different directions. I certainly cannot make a diagnosis by looking at a chart that does not tell me anything except that the baby is small and [health care team member] Melissa says that she doesn't move too much.

The decision about what type of data to gather on the patient is based on her hunches from the medical record and on the family's description of the child's condition. This allows her to focus and prioritize her evaluation.

> **JANIS:** If they tell me [the baby] cannot calm [itself], the biggest thing that I think of first of all is autonomic instability, and then I think about all the things that I need to consider to build on, like what's going on with the autonomic nervous system, when is it that they are crying, is it all the time or only at certain times, what happens when they cry and do they get real stiff? It's like if they give me a presenting problem, then I have this idea. So I go along with some systems approach to it.

4

When pediatric physical therapists make diagnoses and prognoses, they struggle with the often intangible question, "Is this child normal?" To answer this question, they often structure evaluations that allow them to compare activity of the child with normal infant activity across numerous physiologic and behavioral systems. Their evaluations then rely on significant amounts of observation and analysis of the child's problems and compensations.

> JANIS: I really feel like we don't sit back and watch enough. . . . We know something is wrong, so we just go in there and start using our hands, and I think that what I have learned from being a therapist for a long period of time is that I am using my hands less and less and that I am sort of really trying to key into what's the movement pattern. . . . Why are they doing whatever they are doing and how can I intervene or work through the parents to intervene?
>
> I prioritize, too, so that it's like I watch a movement or watch somebody move around, and then I might try to figure out what's missing or what the problems are. I sort of go through something in my mind in terms of things like "How old are they? What should I be seeing?" and then "How should it look?" So I'm looking at restrictions in movement, whether I should be looking for symmetrical patterns or asymmetrical patterns. What kind of [range of motion] activities they should be able to do and what's not there, or how much restriction do they have, and whether they're limited by even a soft-tissue problem.
>
> ELIZABETH: The other thing I'm seeing as I see her walk is that her ability to reciprocally move her legs at the hip and knee are really good. So the problem is more isolated in her foot and ankle. So there is a discrepancy. The other reason I'm worried about her ankles is there is a discrepancy between the amount of problem she has at the subtalar joint in her ankle and the amount of difficulty she has moving her hips and knees. If you just looked at her hips and knees you would expect her feet to look better, so that's not a very good sign.

Eventually, these experts must come to a decision about the child. They are very sensitive to the impact such a decision may have on a family. Also affecting these diagnostic clinical decisions are their personal experiences of being wrong. Janis believes that earlier in her career she would have jumped more easily than she does now to diagnostic categories for children with abnormal movement patterns.

> JANIS: Yeah, definitely, because I think what I've learned over time is the more you know, the more you don't know. Everything's gray. I used to put children in categories and think, "Yeah, this is it." There are certain things that you can look at. I mean, there are ways of predicting ambulation, and I do look at those things too, but I also have seen some people doing so much in terms of variation that I don't buy into stereotypical thinking anymore.

What has happened with me is, the more I see children, the more I feel like I'm less likely . . . less able to predict because there are so many variables that occur between the first time you see them and as they go along. It's hard. I thought Samantha had CP in January. I thought that was what was happening. I was worried. I was trying to figure out if she was going to be in the mild range or if she was going to be in the moderate range. I didn't think she was in the severe range, and what I'm seeing now is that she's able to break out of a lot of things like the stereotypical motor patterns, so that I feel like she is going to be more functional than I had initially thought she was going to be. You know time will tell. You know CP is not a progressive lesion, but the manifestations of CP change overtime. You know a lot of things affect motor behavior, including things like growth, and so you keep seeing that the motor pattern doesn't exactly stay the same, and so I don't know what's going to happen exactly. For me it's kind of fun. It's exciting to see her make the changes that she's making.

These experts have evolved extensively to expand the scope, efficiency, and accuracy of their clinical judgments. Underlying this professional development is significant self-learning and reflection. Perhaps close personal relationships with patients and patients' families facilitate the storage and retrieval of rich and useful clinical knowledge, which is put to good use every day they practice.

SKILLED MOVEMENT

The treatment settings observed during this study included noisy, cluttered pediatric treatment gymnasiums, private examination rooms, and intensive care nurseries. Each practitioner required space to sit with or hold the child and (for older patients) a selection of toys, balls, and games. Very little treatment equipment was used, other than the floor, mats, treatment benches, walkers, mirrors, and steps. Each therapist had the necessary flexibility to conduct repeated hour-long treatment sessions on the floor or mat and to assume often contorted positions while working with the patient. Therapists must effectively gain their patients' trust because they often are required to move patients into potentially frightening, unstable, or painful postures.

While handling a child, expert therapists simultaneously assess with the "eyes in their hands" and communicate caring toward the child. Elizabeth comments that young therapists can be too focused on assessments, preventing their touch from communicating the comfort needed by children. Expert therapists' handling techniques achieved results quickly and efficiently. Often, just the tap of a finger could regain or shift a child's focus or cause an extremity to be repositioned. Elizabeth and Lucy both mentioned the fine-tuned kinesthetic awareness they believe has developed throughout their bodies that allows them to sense changes in a patient's muscle tone or emotional state.

These skilled movements have been developed over years of practice by, as Elizabeth puts it, "paying attention to what is in front of you and what your hands tell you." Again, the process of reflection allows these therapists to increase their skilled movements by analyzing motor performance cognitively and kinesthetically.

**PERSONAL
ATTRIBUTES**

Undoubtedly, these practitioners' concepts of who they are as pediatric physical therapists are influenced heavily by personal values and beliefs. In several personal aspects, these experts are very similar; in others, they differ quite a bit. The experts are uniformly highly intelligent, acknowledged by the numerous awards each has won during her formal educational experience. Are they intellectually curious? These three therapists could be described as driven to know, understand, and be able to solve their patients' problems. They each have completed self-directed formal and informal educational experiences and are constantly using educational resources and consultation with colleagues to solve patient problems. They have chosen to practice in environments where their access to intellectual stimulation is higher than average, and they seek opportunities to teach within their specialty area. Despite this drive to remain up to date with research and practice in pediatrics, they are dissatisfied with the state of their knowledge and performance.

> **JANIS:** I don't know how any of these other [experts] feel, but I still have that feeling . . . you never feel like you totally know what you're doing. That's why I keep trying to learn as much as I can.

> **LUCY:** I don't consider myself an expert clinician. . . . I always feel a struggle. . . . Every once in a while I have some kind of a breakthrough, or, you know, every once in a while something will come together just right, but mostly I feel like I'm just struggling. So I think it's hilarious that they think of us as . . . expert clinician[s].

Observing these pediatric practitioners always brings about the following conclusion: These people love their work! The care and joy observed in their interactions with children and their families is undeniably genuine. The time they are associated with the patients is unique in physical therapy and can actually present a problem, as one therapist found she had formed strong bonds that were difficult to break.

> **LUCY:** I'm not doing enough of a good job of preparing them to leave me. And I'm realizing it now because some of my children are transitioning into school, and the parents don't want to let me go. I mean, it's like I'm part of the family now. . . . To a smaller degree, it's like losing a child. I hate to see them walk out of the door for the very last time or being carried out the door for the last time, but it's like breaking a bond. You have to break a bond, which is not comfortable for me.

The therapists also seem truly devoted to their patients, and their patients are intensely involved with them. During one session, a child showed adoring focus toward her therapist. As the therapist moved the child from exercise to dance step to role play, the child rarely took her eyes off her therapist. This activity seemed to be a very important hour in the child's day. The children observed in this study could not have had more passionate advocates than their physical therapists. These physical therapists accept no boundaries when dealing with their patients, and they move outside their traditional roles with knowledge and skill.

How did these therapists develop their high level of commitment to children who are disabled? Although one of the subjects recalls feeling strongly about children from an early age, two of the expert therapists credit families with teaching them about the preciousness of these children—one child at a time. Expert pediatric physical therapists believe in children, just as parents do; this creates the bond of hope between therapists and parents that is desperately needed by the families. The therapists' triumphant celebrations of even the smallest gain in function becomes a shared occasion of joy. All three subjects laugh in self-deprecation as they call pediatric therapists "bleeding hearts." They believe that pediatric practitioners are self-selected, persistent optimists.

The three expert therapists each had different personalities and various individual traits, suggesting that no one personality type is required to become a successful pediatric physical therapist. Janis is intelligent, is focused on family needs, and is a small size, which seemed helpful in not overwhelming babies. Elizabeth is enthusiastic, intelligent, caring, and efficient, moving with the flexibility and grace of a dancer to juggle activities. She works as smoothly with the distraught child as with the happy one, combining creativity and extraordinary patience. Lucy might be (by a slim margin) the most extroverted practitioner, with one creative play idea up her sleeve after another. Whether the patient or Lucy laughs more during therapy is hard to determine. Lucy exhibits childlike joy during much of the therapy sessions.

Each of these pediatric therapists engages in much reflection and has no difficulty posing and answering her own questions about her professional development, use of knowledge, or decision-making processes. Most questions posed during the study generated thoughts that had been already considered by the therapist, as evidenced by the swift responses and frequency of comments such as, "Oh yes, I've wondered about that . . . and, I used to think . . . but now I know."

CONCLUSIONS

The path to excellence for the three pediatric practitioners has been an exciting and rewarding journey for each (Figure 4-1). In a profession that cannot expect 40 years of continuous practice from each entrant, these three experts have followed career paths that have provided the necessary challenges to remain engaged in the practice of physical therapy. Their paths have wound through formal education, continuing education, encounters with clinical experts, practice with intellectually challenging teams of providers, and periods of self-directed

Figure **4–1** ■ Path to expertise in pediatric physical therapy.

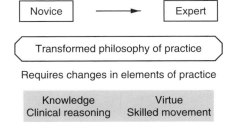

learning. They quickly redefined their roles with their patients and then broadened the scope of knowledge they needed to perform those roles. They deepened their physical therapy content knowledge, transforming it into meaningful clinical knowledge through constant analysis. They began their practices in single-disciplinary roles with limited and prescriptive clinical decisions and progressed into interdisciplinary and multidisciplinary roles that required significantly more sophisticated clinical judgments. Very little has gone unnoticed during their years of practice: They have effectively learned from each patient encounter. They are admirable individuals and virtuous clinicians who care for children who have unlucky starts to life. Their stories are models of clinical practice that can guide all pediatric practitioners.

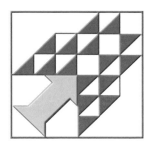

Tree of Life — A traditional pattern showing growth and longevity.

5 Expert Practice in Geriatrics: You're Never Too Old

Laurita M. Hack

CHAPTER OVERVIEW

BACKGROUND

CLINICAL PRACTICE THEMES
    Philosophy of Geriatric Physical Therapy
      Practice

Types and Sources of Knowledge
Clinical Reasoning
Personal Attributes and Professional
    Development
CONCLUSIONS

TRACY: Well, if I'm treating a whole patient, then anything that concerns her is a concern to me. . . . If it's important enough for the patient to complain about it, then it's important enough for somebody to address the problem.

BEN: In rehabilitation, it's better to fail by trying than fail without trying.

PHYLLIS: People sometimes say, "Why don't you become a doctor?"
There's enough in [physical therapy] to keep me busy until the day I die.

Caring for patients as people, needing to challenge and be challenged, and having an excitement for practice are typical qualities of the clinicians we interviewed as experts of geriatric physical therapy.

BACKGROUND

Tracy is a 59-year-old black woman. She grew up in a large city and did her undergraduate work in biology at a small women's liberal arts college near her home. She became a physical therapist in 1960 after completing a certificate program and began her career at a large city hospital in her hometown. After 2 years she left that facility for a nearby university hospital but returned 1 year later to the city hospital, where she remained for 14 more years until the hospital closed. At the hospital, she gradually assumed more responsibility and became coordinator of the clinical education program. She next worked for 6 years at the city's long-term care facility, where she was director of the physical therapy department. For more than 13 years, she has worked for a large geriatric facility with a strong religious commitment. The facility has several levels of care, including wellness programs, home care, outpatient care, acute care, rehabilitation, and a nursing home. She is director of physical medicine and rehabilitation and coordinator of clinical education. The department includes physical therapy, occupational therapy, and speech pathology. Tracy is the mother of five and grandmother of three. For many years, she was essentially a single mother because her husband traveled for long periods. She has shared her home with her mother and has been the primary caregiver for all three of her grandchildren.

Ben is a 48-year-old white man. He grew up in a rural county near a large metropolitan area and did his undergraduate work in political science at a small, but select, college near his home. He became a physical therapist in 1971 after completing a certificate program. He had planned to enter the Army's physical therapy program after a successful Army Reserve Officers Training Corps career in college, but he was rejected because of his gender (at the time, the army program was only for women). He joined the army after completing his certificate, however, and was stationed in the western United States and abroad as a physical therapist. After his army service, he earned a postprofessional master's degree. He had entered the program intending to specialize in pediatrics but switched to geriatrics after working in several nursing homes to support himself while in school. On completion of his academic program, he decided to return to his hometown to be closer to his family. He joined an existing practice but determined that he preferred working individually. Several years later Ben invited a relative who had become a physical therapist under his guidance to become a partner in his practice. The practice constructed an outpatient office in a suburb of a fairly large city that includes a large gait and functional activity area, an aquatic exercise pool, and a large area for the therapists' offices. In addition to an outpatient practice, the partnership maintains a contract in a nursing home, where Ben has practiced for more than 13 years, and a home care practice. Ben is also an active member of the Section on Geriatrics, an adjunct professor at two educational programs, and a frequent contributor to the geriatric literature. Ben is married, the father of two children, and an active member of his community.

Phyllis, a 47-year-old white woman, did her undergraduate work in physical education at a college near her home in a rural area. She became a physical therapist in 1973 after completing a master's program. She worked in the Army for 3 years and then spent 3 years in Asia working as a physical therapist and fulfilling a religious commitment as a missionary. After deciding to return to her hometown, she accepted a job at a prestigious specialty center but left shortly after starting because of ethical conflicts. She then worked as a reviewer for her state's department of health and subsequently as director of physical therapy at a community hospital, during which she completed a master's degree in public administration. She helped start a rehabilitation department at a local nursing home, using a connection through her church, and subsequently opened her own practice, continuing a contract with the nursing home and adding an outpatient practice and other nursing home and home care contracts. She is certified in the clinical specialties of geriatrics and neurology and continues to practice each summer in the Army Reserve program. Phyllis is single but plays an active role in the lives of her parents, siblings, nieces, and nephews (Table 5-1).

Table 5–1. Professional Profiles of Expert Geriatric Physical Therapists

	Phyllis	Ben	Tracy
Years of clinical experience	23	25	36
Practice settings (past and present)	All, including international, Army, outpatient practice (owner), home health care, nursing homes	All, including international, Army, outpatient practice (owner), home health care, nursing homes	Inpatient (chronic adult), nursing home, geriatrics center with all levels of care; has had only three employers in 36 years
Education	Bachelor of science Master of science in physical therapy Master of public administration	Bachelor of science Certificate Master of science (PT)	Bachelor of science Certificate
Advanced clinical education	Geriatric-certified specialist Neurology-certified specialist Continuing education	Continuing education	Continuing education
Teaching experience	Instructor Clinical instructor	Instructor Clinical instructor	Clinical instructor
Professional associations	APTA (active; held office)	APTA (active; held office)	None

PT = physical therapy; APTA = American Physical Therapy Association.

CLINICAL PRACTICE THEMES

PHILOSOPHY OF GERIATRIC PHYSICAL THERAPY PRACTICE

The three therapists' stories help illuminate the philosophies each brings to his or her clinical practice. These therapists have a clear perspective on the rules that guide practice, whether the rules apply to individual patient care or their practices in general. They understand that touch and physical interaction with patients is extremely important, which was proved by the videotaped sessions. All three strongly identified being rooted in their communities as part of their ability to strive toward excellence, and they identified education of patients as essential to their practice of therapy.

Clinical Practice Decisions

These expert clinicians demonstrate many common features in the choices they make: They chose their practice settings to meet the needs of their patients; they see their patients as vital members of society; they hold high standards for themselves, their patients, and others; they recognize the importance of risk-taking to achieve these high standards; and they strongly espouse their own roles as advocates for their patients. The kinds of decisions they make follow directly from the first sort of decision listed—to choose the practice of physical therapy and to focus that practice on the care of older people.

Focus of Practice. Tracy, Ben, and Phyllis became physical therapists because physical therapy appeared to be a way to develop their interests in learning and people.

> **PHYLLIS:** I was very strong in science in high school, and that was kind of a draw for me. But I also wanted to work with people. This is sort of a real good blend.

> **BEN:** That's when I thought I want to go to physical therapy school. And it was just putting all of my likes together. . . . It's a value on thinking.

All were educated in postbaccalaureate programs. They discussed the options they had available when they completed their college educations. Phyllis rejected two occupations (athletic training and medicine) that had been suggested to her. At the time the therapists were making career decisions, physical therapy was not well known, and the decision to pursue physical therapy was not always supported by others.

> **TRACY:** When I said I wanted to be a physical therapist, they looked at me like I was crazy. I knew I wanted to be a physical therapist. . . . I was going to help people walk again.

These were not passive choices made by teenagers influenced by other people. They were active choices made by people with many options.

None of these therapists sought geriatric care as his or her first career specialty. Instead, they all began with generalist work. Ben and Tracy had even developed skills in other specialties before choosing geriatrics. Even now, they have quite varied practices and see patients of all ages with many different types of diagnoses. They have a special focus, however, on the older patients in their practices. Their choosing geriatric care as a specialization seems rooted in a concern for patients who have special needs and their beliefs that they have skills to meet these needs.

> **TRACY:** I thought I was a good therapist, and most therapists didn't want to work with those patients. But they're entitled to as good care as everybody else.... They needed me.

> **PHYLLIS:** I knew that I could affect people, that I had talent in the area, and that I felt I should be out there using it to help people, when there maybe weren't people who were as qualified, so I thought that's where I should do things.

> **BEN:** I just didn't like my older patients falling through the cracks in the health care system.

They all have a high regard for the value of the work they do. Tracy began her career at the city hospital, where she worked with all kinds of patients, many of whom had few options for health care. She volunteered at a university hospital that was next to the city hospital while she prepared to enter a physical therapy program. After she started working, the therapists with whom she had volunteered kept encouraging her to return to the university hospital.

> **TRACY:** They always said to me, "Why don't you come back [to the university hospital]?" And they would say things like, "They give you time to go shopping and to leave early." Isn't that ridiculous? It just seemed stupid to me to take the job just for the prestige of saying I worked at [the university hospital]. Somebody advised me that only the best worked at [the university hospital].... But money was never the reason why I took a job. I planned to work at [the city hospital] from the time I finished school because that's where I could do the most and where I could learn the most.

Vitality. These therapists certainly did not choose geriatrics out of pity for geriatric patients. They have genuine regard for their patients, with a strong belief that older patients, even the very old, remain valuable, autonomous members of society. Frequently, Ben talks to patients about life expectancy:

> **BEN:** Often people come [to physical therapy] after they've had injuries and they're fearful, depressed, thinking "This is the end for me." And I say, "Wait a second: You've got this life expectancy ahead of you. Now, how are you going to live? Are you going to succumb to this injury or are you going to try to rehabilitate to the highest potential?"

The therapists also believe that each patient should reach his or her maximum potential, regardless of the patient's age or level of disability. This is an interesting perspective for clinicians who have chosen to work with geriatric and neurologic patients.

> **PHYLLIS:** I look at every patient as if I am going to make them an Olympic athlete, and then I pare that down a little bit for each one.... I kind of look for the maximum for that individual.

This belief is perhaps best revealed by two incidents that reflect the sternness of expert clinicians attempting to push their patients to maximum function. These might be considered negative episodes, but they also reflect the intense value these therapists placed on maximum function. On one tape, Tracy was working with a patient in a nursing home who had multiple neurologic trauma of unknown origin and behavioral problems. He was not happy with his therapy and began talking rapidly and loudly, disturbing the other patients. Tracy firmly informed him that his behavior was inappropriate and consistently redirected him to the task. She was displaying little tolerance for his distracting behavior. On a subsequent tape, however, she gently teased him and displayed a very different type of relationship. When asked about the approach on the first tape, she acknowledged that someone watching might easily think she was scolding the patient, but she explained that she knew that he was capable of making progress and that he had established a goal of being able to get to the dining room independently. She knew that he needed to be able to perform certain tasks to reach his goal, and she thought it was important to hold him accountable for these tasks. He and his family had asked her to persist in helping him meet his functional goals, even in light of his occasional inappropriate responses. Tracy therefore changed her approach with the patient to match his behavioral needs. She was willing to risk being seen as too tough to help the patient reach his potential.

This view was reinforced when Phyllis was working with one of her patients who did not perform to Phyllis's expectation. Phyllis was trying to encourage the patient to come from standing from a mat table to ambulating with increased weightbearing on her legs, rather than being dependent on her arms for bearing weight. The woman reached out to Phyllis in panic several times, and Phyllis assisted her to stand. Each time Phyllis removed the patient's hands from herself and placed them at the patient's side. Finally, Phyllis had to discontinue intervention because the patient would not cooperate. Phyllis was visibly disappointed and reflected this disappointment in her tone of voice.

> **PHYLLIS:** It is just a characteristic throughout the rest of my life, too . . . when people don't produce to their potential and have the ability and just don't do it . . . I get unhappy.

She also expressed disappointment with herself for not being better able to match her goals to the patient's goals, but she stated that she could not easily give up on helping the patient achieve a goal that she knew the patient was capable of physically.

Phyllis extends these standards for physical performance to her fellow therapists, who, she believes, should understand the feeling of being physically challenged because that is what physical therapists do to patients.

> **PHYLLIS:** The physical aspects of . . . not that we can experience everything ourselves . . . but knowing what it is like being pushed out of breath yourself, I think you are able to identify. And I think that a

[physical therapist] who is not much more than a couch potato cannot be a good [physical therapist].

Risk-Taking. The therapists demonstrated a willingness to take risks with their patients. Phyllis said she had learned to take risks from a mentor, who encouraged her to push patients, never asking more than they could physically do but always getting them to do as much as possible. During the study, she encouraged one patient to work through pain after a surgical procedure and tried to get another patient to come to standing although the patient was clearly afraid. When asked about each of these instances, she said that she "looks for the maximum for each individual."

> **BEN:** On our mug [given to patients], it says something to the effect that in rehabilitation it's better to fail by trying than fail without trying. . . . That is a foundation here.

> **TRACY:** Sometimes I watch the [other] therapist and I think, "Well maybe you're not progressing this patient quick enough." And it's not because what they're doing isn't right. But because looking at the patient and how they're responding to the therapist, for some reason I can see that that patient could be pushed a little harder than what they are being pushed. And you could get more out of them.

Advocacy. Advocacy was identified as a serious responsibility. The therapists believed that they had the obligation to insist on not just adequate care but the best possible care for their patients. Each was willing to adjust his or her clinical practice to gain control over the ability to give good care.

> **TRACY (on discussing the encroachment of managed care–type standards into nursing home care):** Well, getting me to be an efficient machine may be getting me to be something that I don't think is being a physical therapist. Then I'd have to make decisions about whether my own personal philosophy would allow me to behave like that. You could be efficient, but you are not doing anything for the patient. I really think I am not a crusader, but I think at some point in time, I would just have to say, "Look, if you don't like the way I do things, I'll just do it someplace else because I think what you are doing is wrong."

The therapists all talked about instances in which they had to challenge reimbursers about coverage of care for patients. A patient of Ben's was denied Medicare coverage by an intermediary (an insurance company under contract to manage Medicare claims in a particular geographic region) because Ben had used a diagnosis of gait dysfunction in documenting the patient's care. This diagnosis is included, however, in the *International Classification of Diseases, Ninth Revision (ICD-9)* used by health care providers in describing patient conditions. He contacted the publishers of the *ICD-9*, who provided documentation that this was a recognized diagnosis, and forwarded the documents to his U.S. Representative, who in turn contacted the Health Care Financing

Administration (HCFA). HCFA then issued a directive to all of the intermediaries that gait dysfunction is an acceptable diagnosis.

Physicality

The therapists all understood the role of their bodies and their patients' bodies in the practice of therapy. They used their own bodies very effectively in working with patients and had an exquisite sense of what their patients were communicating through their bodies. The therapists valued touch as a means of evaluation, treatment, and communication. Phyllis demonstrated a masterful touch when performing a neck massage in preparation to do cervical traction with one outpatient. As she carried out the soft-tissue work, her voice softened, her conversation turned to items of personal interest to the patient (rather than discussion related to the patient's health care problem), and she beamed with joy as the patient responded to this personal intervention by relaxing and allowing Phyllis to complete the soft-tissue mobilization. When asked about this episode, she talked about the importance of helping patients to relax and of using touch to help patients remember how to use their own bodies appropriately.

Ben describes his use of touch as a way "to lend a sense of security":

> **BEN:** I try to use touch a lot. It's one of the first things that attracted me to physical therapy as opposed to medical school. And that is how we get to know our patients. We handle our patients.... I remember working with a woman who was pleasantly confused and had bilateral amputations. I remember sitting on the mat hugging her. Trying to check her balance but at the same time to extend a sense of security to her....
> I want her to see what she can do without me, but at the same time I'm trying to give her support. So I think I've done that—I think it's been part of what I perceive is physical therapy, as a hands-on profession.
> I have a lot of concern about the dependence on machines.

All three commented that technology or equipment is not as important as using their heads and hands. None of them were ever observed using modalities, and sometimes they even indicated that they did not support increased use of modalities.

Community

The therapists have a strong sense of community, whether in urban, suburban, or rural environments. This sense of community not only linked them to their families and friends, but also to their patients, even when their patients were different from themselves. Phyllis talked about working at a number of different bases in the Army and then overseas on missionary activity. She described looking forward to returning to a community where she could connect with her patients. In the videotaped sessions, she frequently discussed community events and mutual friends with patients as a way to help them relax.

During the study, Ben introduced one of his patients to the researchers. He proudly explained this woman's role in the community as one of its leading editorial commentators. Her letters to the local paper were a community institution. She beamed at his knowledge of her role in the community. Ben identified this as not just building a personal connection to a patient; he also believed this interaction was important for a professional sense of community.

> **BEN:** I have this attitude that when people come to my office, they become part of my medical family.... I like the community. That's why, while it's been over a year since I had rehabilitated [a patient], I would stop to see her once in a while just simply to say, "Keep up your exercises." It helps them to know that I'm around and if something happens I'm going to try to get them back [to functional levels].... They have transcribed their affections, their concerns, and their respect to me and my colleagues and my students.... I view them as part of my medical family.... We're going to stay [in this town], and 15 years from now if she has problems, we're going to know where she was today.

Teaching

Teaching is another important aspect of physical therapy for the therapists. They place a high value on explaining everything to patients, including medical status and what the therapist is and will be doing. Phyllis noted that if a patient does not understand what is happening, the patient cannot make necessary changes in behavior, nor can the patient comply fully with the therapist's activities. Ben continually provided his patients with information, especially in his outpatient practice. He comments, "I like my patients to know what I'm thinking." His reception area had patient handouts and a book on osteoporosis.

In one videotaped session, Phyllis spent extensive time with a patient explaining a medical procedure and a typical course of recovery from surgery. She saw value in talking to the patient about all aspects of care, not just issues related directly to physical therapy. She also spent a lot of time teaching specific exercises and activities with the three patients whose treatment sessions were videotaped. She incorporated the patient's specific interests into the program, spontaneously taking advantage of items in the patient's room to provide functionally related teaching. She also used this technique in her office when she worked with two patients with head trauma.

> **PHYLLIS:** As a [physical therapist], you teach, and knowing how to teach is so important and enables you to be more successful.

In addition to considering teaching patients as essential to practice, the therapists also value teaching colleagues. All three participated in clinical education, and Tracy commented that she would sooner give up attending continuing education courses than give up students. Ben and Phyllis participated in academic didactic courses in physical therapy education programs and continuing education.

TYPES AND SOURCES OF KNOWLEDGE

The therapists were not immediately able to make sophisticated and complex decisions. They all described sources of knowledge that helped them become better therapists. *Knowledge* usually implies information gained, but it can also refer to the processes of acquiring information and using that information in complex decision making. Each therapist identified mentors that had inspired them by example to assess the methods by which they acquired knowledge. They all noted that patients are excellent sources of information and that knowledge obtained through patients comes not only from information patients provide but also from interactive processes involved in providing care. They also identified students as an important source of knowledge. Each of them talked about various levels of reliance on more traditional sources of knowledge, including entry-level education, postgraduate education, continuing education, and current literature.

Mentors

Mentors who made a significant contribution to development were readily identified by each therapist. They all talked enthusiastically and in detail about the significant role mentors played in their lives. Although they identified mentors who had been in the faculties of their physical therapy educational programs, they also identified other college faculty, clinical colleagues, and family members who had served as role models and mentors.

Ben particularly focused on his family as a source of knowledge. During his résumé sort, he designated his family as the most important influence in his life. He spoke of the direct information he learned from his family.

> **BEN:** My family obviously teaches me. I have used my father as a research subject, and I may write an article about my daughter because of [a health problem] she had last year.... I kept a daily diary on my son's development. I observed him very, very closely.... When my son wanted to learn scuba diving, I learned with him.... And my wife is a special educator, so we share a lot of information.

Ben also talked about the values he learned from his parents. He describes his parents as vitally important in his life.

> **BEN:** My father...he's 86...he's maintained a very sharp mind. He's probably more open-minded than 50% of the college students today.... My mother taught us a love of literature, and we went to the theater, music, fine arts a lot. I think that gives you an appreciation for differences.

When asked if she could identify people who had an important influence on her career, Tracy talked of professional mentors. She first described a college teacher.

> **TRACY:** In college, there was [a professor] who was in charge of the biology department. I wasn't exactly an "A" student, but she was looking for students who knew how to learn, not just how to take tests well. When I told her I was interested in physical therapy, she set up a class where she and I were the only two people in the class. In her own quiet way she encouraged me to keep going when others didn't think I could do it.

In addition, Tracy mentioned the importance of one of her physical therapy professors.

> **TRACY:** She inspires everybody to do anything. She was a great professor. She just had a way about her that when she taught you something you

just learned. She knew herself and she knew how to get people involved, so she basically had a lot of influence.

Tracy also mentioned several therapists with whom she worked in the early years of her career. She identifies them as the source for her comfort with taking risks and giving her the recognition of the need for developing a strong patient–therapist relationship despite cultural differences.

When asked about mentors, Phyllis very quickly identified four clinical colleagues who had made vital contributions to her development. Only two are physical therapists. One of these was her first clinical supervisor, with whom she has maintained contact for more than 20 years. Phyllis still turns to this person to discuss professional issues and patient care.

> **PHYLLIS:** She was very good at throwing articles at you and discussing things and figuring things out. She was very good with sharing with everybody, but she soon realized that not everyone wanted to know these things, so we would cooperate and share.

Another therapist Phyllis identified as influential worked with her during her missionary years and when she returned home. This mentor had died not long before the interview, and discussing his role as her mentor often brought Phyllis close to tears. Whereas the first mentor identified had been a source of intellectual challenge, the second was a source of values and personal example.

The other two people Phyllis identified included an orthopedic surgeon and a dentist. From the dentist, she learned to use conversation and connection to help patients tolerate pain. Of the orthopedic surgeon, she said:

> **PHYLLIS:** I always marveled at his perceptiveness, that he realized where [his patients] were coming from—their purposes—and could stay a step ahead of them. He would allow them to experiment and try things, but he would never do anything detrimental to the patient. . . . We had some tough cases together. Just the way he tried to conduct himself . . . I tried to model after him. . . . That was an excellent start. You can't ask for better than that.

Patients

Ben, Tracy, and Phyllis eagerly discussed how much they had learned from their patients. This knowledge seemed to develop in a variety of ways. These therapists clearly valued the information they received from their patients. They saw this information as being as important as—if not more important than—information gathered from sources such as charts, referrals, or colleagues.

> **TRACY:** If I'm treating a whole patient, then anything that concerns her is a concern to me. . . . If it's important enough for the patient to complain about it, then it's important enough for somebody to address the problem.

They learned from and about patients by interacting with patients. Ben has a very clear systems review that he uses with patients, much of which involves gathering data by touch. He also repeats this data gathering frequently during the course of care.

BEN: Every evaluation is a treatment; every treatment is an evaluation.

TRACY: I just watch people. . . . Actually I'm getting a little slow at it. I used to be better at it. There are just things that don't seem—this is very scientific!—that just don't seem right to me. Because looking at the patient and how they're responding, I can see that the patient could be pushed a little harder. . . . We have to learn how to listen to what they're saying, what they're saying behind what they're saying. You can get them to participate better if you just take the time to listen to them.

They also use knowledge gained from each patient to enhance the care they provide to the next patient. They have a "patient database" in their minds to help guide clinical decisions. Ben said that he has developed his precise systems review through clinical practice. He also uses his clinical experience to informally adjust the norms on various tests for the geriatric population because formal geriatric norms are not available. He has conducted research to help develop geriatric norms for procedures such as spirometry testing and dynamometer testing.

When I asked Phyllis abut her "clinical eye," she described a skill to recognize rapid or severe changes in physical status without using objective measures. She learned this skill "with the patients teaching me." When asked if she used continuing education to develop the skill, she said, "No, I think it is experience."

Students

Each therapist enjoys teaching, views teaching as an integral part of practice, and sees teaching as one of the important ways to acquire new knowledge. All three are involved in clinical education for physical therapy students. Ben frequently teaches continuing education courses across the country, Phyllis leads discussion groups of colleagues seeking to improve geriatric care, and Tracy is involved in the education of a number of health care practitioners. For these therapists, *student* has a broad connotation. They learn from students in a number of ways. Certainly transfer of new knowledge occurs, because students often report the latest information from current literature.

TRACY: I think students are good for my department because basically it makes you rethink what you are doing, and it makes you throw out some of the things you were doing because the reason you were doing them may not be as sound as you thought it was. It keeps me aware of what the schools are teaching and how thinking is changing. [If asked to choose one source of new information,] I'd take the students, because it's not just me they bring a lot to. They bring a lot to the department.

The therapists also learn when they organize information to transfer knowledge to students. This is particularly true for knowledge related to decision-making processes, such as the organization of patient examinations, diagnosis, or prognosis. Ben described the process of explicating his detailed systems review to students developing their own methods for caring for patients. He and Phyllis described methods of transferring information from practice to the classroom and clinical teaching.

PHYLLIS: I think it reinforces your clinical skills when you have to teach it to anybody.

Other Sources

Ben and Phyllis talked about their need to read as a means to stay current with new findings and views. They read widely and continually. Tracy has a much more focused approach, reading specific material as she finds a need for it in her practice. She seems to use discussion with others as her primary method of acquiring new knowledge. They all mentioned specific articles and texts that had influenced their clinical decisions. Ben cited clinical data from his readings in the course of treatment.

The therapists all participated in continuing education, but in different ways, at this point in their careers: They chose programs that had specific information they identified as important. Each cited specific courses over the years that had given him or her specific examination or intervention skills. They also mentioned courses as a means of meeting and understanding other clinicians. Phyllis looked at a list of courses taken over her career and talked about the importance of the ideas generated by several of the teachers.

PHYLLIS: I think that everybody has something to offer, and you have to look at what they can offer you and what you can take from that.

Phyllis and Ben have pursued postgraduate work. Ben has a degree from a program specifically designed for physical therapists, and Phyllis has a degree in advanced management education. Both commented on the contribution these programs had made, but each saw his or her program as part of a progression of learning, not a conclusion.

Consistent with all of the therapists in the study, none of these therapists identified entry-level education as significantly important at this point in his or her life. They acknowledge it as the foundation of their careers, but they all saw that they had moved beyond it. They also valued their entry-level education for the teachers they had encountered, but none saw it as a source of his or her current ability to practice well.

PHYLLIS: Of course, to be a [physical therapist] you have to go to [physical therapy] school.

CLINICAL REASONING

The therapists understand their responsibility as diagnosticians working within a disability framework, which includes focusing on patient function, setting mutual goals with their patients, recognizing the importance of motivation, and managing many tasks simultaneously.

Diagnosis and Prognosis within a Disability Framework

These therapists had a very good understanding of their priorities in clinical decision making. Although they all believe that understanding traditional medical diagnosis is important, understanding function and appropriate classification of patients related to their functional levels is more important to them. Each talked about the importance of knowing the patent's prior functional status.

> BEN: The diagnosis itself is not as important as "Functionally, what am I seeing that's happening?"...Yeah, I like to know the diagnosis, especially when it comes to fractures and other conditions. But I think that, at least in my experience, maybe it's misleading, especially here.... The diagnosis is important, but often the medical diagnosis that comes on a transfer sheet is not the functional reason for a physical therapy diagnosis, and so often that's completely ignored as far as the reason for physical therapy at the hospital. So, yeah, I pay attention to it but it's...I don't really perseverate right there.... To get to a definitive *ICD-9* code is not as important, because, for example, many of these people have mobility problems. Now, what's the reason that their mobility is jeopardized or having rise in their immobility? Is it a little bit of arthritis? Is it a little bit of neurological problems? Is it a little bit of spinal stenosis? Is it a little old history of lumbar disk disease? Is it a little of this and a little of that? So it fits into a gait disturbance—a gait abnormality. However, that's not a very clean diagnosis, but it fits probably a large percentage of people that we see.

The therapists also recognize that patients often require more than a simple analysis of a single system or problem.

> BEN: I think I see the musculoskeletal folks having a neurological organization to that musculoskeletal performance or that biomechanical performance. Whether you think it's a Feldenkrais concept about the organization of the system...or you want to call it a pattern of Bobath, I don't think that the neuromusculoskeletal systems are separable.... To learn something, you've got to start to categorize or discriminate or set—put in certain blocks. But I don't think our patients are that way. They haven't read the book to say that this is all muscular or this is all neurological.

The therapists demonstrated confidence in their abilities to make appropriate clinical decisions about patients. They expressed little hesitation about their ability to predict prognosis, although they were willing to give the patient the benefit of the doubt, and they all reported stories of persisting with physicians to have issues more fully evaluated. They were willing to go to colleagues, including physicians and insurers, to defend plans and goals for the patient. They approached this not only because of their perspectives on advocacy, but also because of confidence in themselves as good decision makers.

> BEN: I understand systems. I understand the Medicare system. But, for example, the question about gait disturbance came up in my previous office. We suddenly started to get hammered about the diagnosis of gait disturbance. Well, what other diagnosis are we going to list on the billing form? Well, it's not necessarily just arthritis because there hasn't been an acute flare-up of the arthritis and there hasn't been a stroke that's listed. But why is this person not walking well compared to 6 months ago? Well,

if there's not any other condition, then it fits the *ICD-9* description of those conditions listed in that section. The Medicare folks said, "Hey, forget it. Our intermediary wrote and said the gait disturbance is what happens when someone drinks too much." Well, clearly that does happen when you drink too much but that's intoxication and not a gait disturbance, due to these ill-defined conditions that we see in geriatric patients. So I wrote to my representative in Washington, D.C., and said, "Hey, why is this getting denied because it's a proper diagnosis?" And he wrote up through HCFA, and it comes back and says, "Well, the intermediary has determined that this is an ill-defined condition and you've got to come up with a better diagnosis." So I called the people who wrote the *ICD-9*, and I said, "Wait a second. Why do you even put this in the book if we're not supposed to use it?" He said—the guy that I spoke to—"You're supposed to use this." So I said, "You write me a letter about that, please," which he did. And I then sent this back to my representative, who then sent this on through Health and Human Services in HCFA, and they then wrote back and said indeed there is a gait disturbance. So they stopped making that denial. And I think probably there was something that came down through the system that was said throughout the country: To get all your papers together for a review takes time and energy, which means you're not treating patients. So I guess what I'm saying is don't tell me this is the way it's going to be when you can't substantiate it.

PHYLLIS: I know what to do, so I do it.

Because Ben has practiced in a particular nursing home and its affiliated life care community for more than 13 years, he has come to know many of his patients personally and is able to follow the changes in their conditions. He often is called on by the facility staff to help make decisions about the need for further testing or hospitalization.

BEN: I try to take a more aggressive stance here because I knew where she was. And always when something happens and there's a precipitous decline, can it be corrected if we figure out what it is? . . . I'm the only one out there who's trying to say "Let's see what we can do." Of course, I'm the only one who knew her when she was completely independent.

Maximum Function as a Mutual Goal

These therapists share common definitions of *success* in physical therapy: the absolute maximum function of which a patient is capable. They are able to articulate in detailed and accurate ways the specific goals and matching interventions that help a patient reach maximum function.

PHYLLIS: I look for the maximum for that individual, you know? I tell my patients that they have to do their exercises because the muscles are weak and you have to strengthen them. You have to work just as hard as an Olympic athlete, not just do them when you want to. . . . What I don't like is taking patients down to [physical therapy] and doing nothing but walking. I'm sorry, but you can't violate the hip musculature and go through muscles [with fracture surgery] without having them weakened. There's nothing like specific exercises to make muscles better.

Although these therapists frequently offer comfort, especially to patients in pain, they have high standards for their patients. These standards are set to help give patients options. They frequently commented on the need to give people a chance. If the patients were not able to perform, the therapists were willing to discontinue care. This view also pervades their clinical decision-making processes.

> **BEN:** I'm usually right in my assessment with this person as good or excellent rehabilitation potential, but in the years I've practiced, I've seen some people that I've felt initially had excellent potential and they died within a week or two. And I've seen some that I thought had poor potential and they were the ones that went home. So that's why it's better to fail by trying.

> **PHYLLIS (discussing progressing patients from walkers to canes):** It's the patient's choice. Sometimes I leave both articles there, so they can play around with them, and let them decide. That's a more mature way to provide therapy.

Motivation

Ben, Tracy, and Phyllis recognize the importance of incorporating motivation for the patient into their plans of care.

> **TRACY:** As much as you do for a patient, if they don't do anything, except you doing for them, there's no point in doing it, because it's a wasted effort. If the patient doesn't at some point say, "Hey, I can do this," and take that step ahead, then you're [only] doing it to the person. I mean, anybody can manipulate a body and get something, but you're going to lose it all if the patient isn't invested in what you are doing and take the initiative in what you are doing.

Whether dealing with a mobile outpatient needing treatment for a musculoskeletal problem or with a patient in a nursing home who is very ill with multiple comorbidities including dementia, the therapists work with patients to develop mutual goals.

> **PHYLLIS:** [Home health care] has made me let go of a lot of my goals.... I've got to pay attention to what the patient wants and be satisfied.

Management of Multiple Tasks

Each of the therapists manages multiple clinical tasks. They have the ability to scan the environment and recognize changes.

> **BEN:** I watch.... I think I often will take a gestalt perspective. That is, I'm working with someone. I will remove myself and stand behind the scene of me treating, thinking, "What is happening here? What am I seeing?" ... My senses are all open. They tease a lot because, I may be

out in the hallway, but I hear someone's breathing change as they're working in the parallel bars. I'll hear that. Usually my hearing is terrible, but when I'm working with my patients, I try to keep all of my senses open.

TRACY: Basically I keep an eye on everybody that comes through. I basically watch what everybody's doing and ask questions about why they're doing what they're doing. I see things that I think need to be attended to. . . . I was the person keeping track of things. It was very easy for me to remember who went with what. Even in my family, I was the person who took care of things.

PHYLLIS: I guess we can attribute [being able to manage many tasks] to my mother. There was so much going on in my home, with seven brothers and sisters. And then I guess I learned it in the Army. You had to know everybody else's cases to do rounds, so you trained yourself to pick up on things. You never knew who was going to ask you what.

Personal Attributes and Professional Development

Hunger for Knowledge

These individuals exhibit many characteristics that can be identified in any expert, particularly expert health care practitioners. Although they all have a high regard of knowledge, the therapists acquire knowledge from different sources. Two are very well read, are able to cite references, and use research materials to design care for patients. The third focuses on learning from the many students she taught. Regardless of the source, they all have the need to keep learning.

BEN: I get nourishment from my teaching and my writing and my research. . . . It helps in my thinking with my patients.

Do the Right Thing

All three exhibited a strong need to do the right thing. They did not try to maximize their incomes or make their lives less stressful; instead they made choices based on what their patients needed. Ben discussed leaving a thriving practice because he wanted to spend more time on his teaching and research. Tracy chose facilities where the patients were neglected by others. Phyllis reported challenging a prestigious center because she perceived unethical behavior on the part of the staff. Each had clearly reflected on these episodes or decisions and saw them as essential parts of their personal and professional lives.

BEN: I tried to do some work [with some other therapists]. It kind of unraveled, partially from seeing students and from writing. They saw these things as costs to the practice and they didn't want that to happen. That's one of the issues they talked about at [college]. Money is not the most important issue. Balance comes from all aspects. Physical therapy is so multidimensional. You teach, you do lots of professional activities, you do some writing. You're a parent. See, you're enriching yourself in the whole—all those dimensions.

TRACY: Money was never a reason why I took a job specifically. I planned to work at [the city hospital] when I finished school because I felt that was the place where I could do the most...I owed something to the people. They were people just like all other people who needed medical care. And here [her current place of employment—a long-term care facility], they need me more than other people did...I've always been interested in helping a person who I knew might not get help because they were not necessarily going to get everything back.

PHYLLIS (discussing her response to testifying against a colleague in a licensure investigation): I just couldn't live with myself without reporting it. It's just something within you. It's something that gives you power that you survived it. It was something that affected patient care quality.

The therapists have considered and chosen career paths that relate to their personal values. Tracy speculated at some length about her response to the increased pressures of managed care and administration.

TRACY: I guess some people would say that I build up some type of empathy with the patient. Sometimes when you build up that relationship, you shouldn't just snatch it away because it's the end of their treatment period, because what you do is something added to their life and they may not be ready in 3 weeks to have it removed, until you're able to replace it with something. . . . You could be efficient, but you're not doing anything for the patient. I really think I am not a crusader, but I think at some point in time, I would have to say, "Look, if you don't like the way I am doing things, I'll just do it someplace else, because I think that what you are doing is wrong."

Phyllis commented on the same issue from the perspective of independent practice:

PHYLLIS: That's total clinical work. That's using all your guns to get whatever is necessary accomplished with your patients. It gives you the freedom to do as you want to design and create, so it's like your nirvana of [physical therapy].

However, the therapists do not make unrealistic decisions. Although Phyllis commented on the joy of working in a practice that allowed a great deal of freedom, she mentioned the value of input from others.

PHYLLIS: Even though you have agencies like Medicare telling you what to do . . . But sometimes there are good aspects to that as we get more efficient and productive than we have been in the past.

It was interesting to note the role that participation in organized religion played in each of their lives. All three spontaneously talked about their church activities. Ben included his church-related responsibilities in his discussion of the important activities in his life. Tracy and Phyllis talked about the role religion had played in shaping their values and choices. Phyllis spent several years in a church-based health care program in Asia and has continued a religious affiliation in her nursing home work. Tracy identified mentors with religious careers and discussed the inspiration religion provided for her in her work.

> **TRACY:** Basically, the thing that has gotten me through everything has been my religion and my beliefs.

Energy

As might be expected, all three demonstrated a very high level of energy. Although they manage busy lives that involve many different things (e.g., family, community, profession, church, sports), all approach their activities with gusto.

> **BEN:** I don't sleep a lot. . . . Well, I think it's because there's a lot of life, so I'm going to do these things that all excite me, then I sleep.

> **TRACY:** I don't think I've ever reached a point where I was what you'd call "burned out." My family is very close . . . so that part of it relieves a certain amount of tension that a lot of people have in my work day. I've always had a big capacity to like people.

> **PHYLLIS:** [Lots of activity] just helps me to keep growing. Sometimes people reach plateaus or stagnate. I don't think I have ever been in stagnation. It just helps me to keep the wheels going, to get more interested in topics and ideas.

CONCLUSIONS   Each of these therapists was educated at a time when physical therapy was still being developed as a profession. Physical therapy has advanced to its current state, however, because of therapists like Tracy, Ben, and Phyllis (Figure 5-1). Each has a desire to learn, a high standard of professional conduct for themselves and their colleagues, and a zest for life. Their personal characteristics, intimate knowledge of physical therapy, and extreme respect for patients has helped create their excellent decision-making skills.

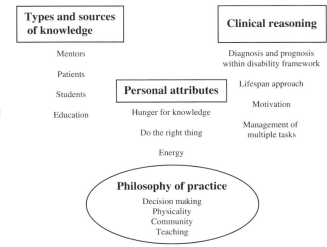

Figure **5–1** ■ Conceptual model for geriatric physical therapists.

Although they are extremely skilled and focused therapists, they should not only be regarded as serious and committed individuals. They each displayed humor, enthusiasm, and compassion when interacting with patients and being interviewed. As the population of older people in the United States grows, the field of physical therapy can only hope that more therapists assume the characteristics of these expert geriatric clinicians. Ben, Tracy, and Phyllis set a high standard, but they are examples of what can be achieved when the focus is high-quality care.

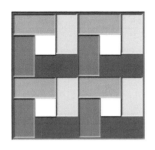

Bright Hopes — A variation of the classic log cabin pattern, with light center squares rising from the dark background.

6

Experienced Practice in Neurologic Rehabilitation: Experts in the Making

Katherine F. Shepard

LEE: In my first job, I found I liked the neuro patient because, unlike the orthopedic patient, it wasn't cookbook. No matter how many patients you see that have a stroke or head injury, they all have different backgrounds and their infarcts or head injury or whatever would affect them differently. Even though you may have some common characteristics of, for example, a right CVA [cerebrovascular accident] versus a left CVA, there was always something a little different, and I thought that was interesting.

The three physical therapists studied in neurologic rehabilitation had no more than 12 years of clinical experience each, but all were identified as experts by their peers. The therapists identified themselves as experienced but not necessarily expert, as they continued to pursue more formal and informal knowledge regarding the care of a diverse patient population with neurologic disorders.

Finding very experienced therapists working in neurologic rehabilitation patient care at least 50% of the time was difficult. Most clinicians who work in traditional neurologic rehabilitation settings move into administration by the time they have been working for approximately 10 years. The move to administration appears to be partly because of experience—that is, they are needed to oversee departments and supervise less-experienced staff. They also move to administration because their bodies give out from the heavy physical work involved in this type of clinical practice. Although all three had less clinical experience compared with most experts in the other clinical areas studied and each worked in different clinical sites, they exhibited similarities in their professional development and approach to clinical practice. They have many characteristics of experts in the making.

BACKGROUND

Lee is a certified clinical specialist in neurology who has been in the field almost 10 years. She works part time in the outpatient department of a major rehabilitation hospital and part time in home care.

Kellum was one of the first physical therapists in the country to become a certified clinical specialist in neurology. She has practiced for approximately 7 years in a variety of clinical settings and for 8 years in a research setting. At the time of the study, she was the only physical therapist in an otolaryngology outpatient clinic at an internationally recognized medical center.

Kate, who recently became a certified clinical specialist in neurology, has been in the field almost 12 years. She practices in a hospital-based rehabilitation department and is the clinical education coordinator. All three hold master's degrees in areas related to treatment of patients receiving neurologic rehabilitation. In addition, all are married, and two (Lee and Kate) have young children. Table 6-1 provides additional demographic information.

The clinicians report they enjoy neurologic rehabilitation practice because of the complex physical and often concomitant psychoemotional dysfunctions presented and because of the opportunity to work with many people in the health care of patients.

Table 6–1. Professional Profiles of Experienced Neurologic Physical Therapists

	Lee	Kellum	Kate
Years of clinical experience	10	7 clinic, 8 research	12
Practice settings (past and present)	Home care Outpatient rehabilitation Inpatient rehabilitation	Acute care Rehabilitation research department in children's hospital Otolaryngology clinic	Neuroscience unit in rehabilitation hospital Inpatient rehabilitation
Education	Bachelor of science Master of science	Bachelor of science Master of science	Bachelor of science Master of science
Advanced clinical education	Continuing education NCS pending (delay due to pregnancy)	Continuing education NCS	Continuing education NCS Neurodevelopmental treatment certification
Teaching experience	Continuing education instructor University classroom Clinical education instructor	Continuing education instructor University classroom Clinical education instructor	Continuing education instructor University classroom Clinical education instructor
Professional associations	APTA	APTA (active; held office)	APTA (active; held office) National Stroke Association

NCS = neurologic clinical specialist; APTA = American Physical Therapy Association.

6

> **KELLUM:** I think in some ways it is more complicated, more multifaceted. It's not that orthopedic problems are singular—there are some really complicated orthopedic problems—it's just that people have so many issues—paralysis, cognitive problems, language problems....I found it challenging, interesting, and that those people really needed help. I liked working with them and their families.

All three have been influenced by several role models who were physical therapists in the field. None described a single mentor. Instead, they were influenced by people they observed and worked with for relatively short periods during their careers.

> **LEE:** One of my role models was a therapist in her 60s who I observed practicing rural home care when I was a high school student. She was very influential now that I think about it...how she thought and how she carried out her evaluation and treatments....Given a home environment, you have a variety of diagnoses and you have to know a little about everything. She was very thorough.

KELLUM: Jean Ayers was a powerful role model for me. She was thinking in ways that other people weren't. She was very criticized for her research but definitely was a hard thinker and would talk about it in class. I just thought it was wonderful the way she was constantly reading, constantly evaluating her theoretical framework for treatment and evaluation for the kids she worked with. She was far ahead of her time in terms of her thinking.

KATE: The role model who made a big difference was my clinical instructor at Harmarville [Pennsylvania]. I did have a penchant for neuro and why and how does the brain work and what does that mean, but at that point in time I knew nothing. It was very hard for me to apply what I'd learned. I had a wonderful [clinical instructor] who was just amazing with patients. She gave me a sense for seeing what the patient is doing, analyzing it, and figuring out how you can help them. She put a little extra time into working with patients. She also put extra time in with me as a student teaching those skills. And she was so excited about what she did! You know, before I went to Harmarville as a student, I thought I was going to be an [orthopedic therapist].

PHILOSOPHY AND PRACTICE

GATHERING INFORMATION TO RETURN PATIENTS TO THEIR PRIOR LEVEL OF FUNCTION

Similar to the other expert clinicians studied, the three neurologic rehabilitation clinicians carefully observe and listen to patients. In particular, they listen closely to the patients' descriptions of their lives before any neurologic insult occurred. Their focus is to return patients to previous levels of function as closely as possible. They are not satisfied by minimal improvement; they want to provide a return to a way of life.

LEE: You see here I am allowing her to move the way she wants to move. (The patient is going down steep stairs by leaning forward using both handrails and descending step over step.) I also have had patients who have *never* gone up or down their stairs step over step with alternating legs. So, I am not going to teach them something new. This is something I talk with students about both in the labs I teach and in the clinic. They need to be open-minded as to where the patient is coming from. Your expectations have to be similar to the patient's expectations. You can't have them do something they've never done before or have no interest in.

Kate also expressed a desire to provide patients with the best opportunity to recover function:

INTERVIEWER (summarizing information Kate has provided): So that is the image you have in your head: home, the function, what's going to be happening. Is that what guides you in how far you push or don't push a patient?

KATE: It does to some degree. Even if I know the patient is going to go home with 24-hour nursing care, I will still try and push them as far as I feel they can go just to make them as independent as possible.

FOCUS ON FUNCTION

In conjunction with knowing the functional status and interests of a patient before a neurologic insult, the clinicians think constantly about their patients' return to their own settings and the activities in which they will be involved. Teaching and preparing patients—even putting them in positions that look to be physically difficult and sometimes risky—is in concert with what they anticipate the patients want to do and will do in their home environments.

> **INTERVIEWER:** I am impressed with how much you are pushing this patient [67-year-old woman recovering from an aneurysm]. She has had a good workout—endurance, balance, cognition—all within multiple functional tasks within nearly every room in the house. For an hour and a half, you are just steadfast with her.

> **LEE:** Yes, I think you have to be given she was a very active woman before, very bright. You only have so many treatments and you want to get the most you can out of every treatment.

> **INTERVIEWER:** Having this 380-pound man with right CVA and extensive sensory loss bend over and pick something small up off the floor looks very precarious.

> **KATE:** Yes, I was a bit nervous about that. It was a bit nerve-wracking. But knowing he was going to go home and take these risks, it was appropriate for him to be able to practice so he learns how to do it, feel comfortable doing it, and be safer.

> **KATE (3 weeks later):** The OT [occupational therapist] went to see that patient after discharge. He told her he was getting into his car and dropped his car keys on the ground. Someone was going to stop and pick up his keys but he picked them up before he could be helped. And he said, "Well, I was cursing Kate when she was making me pick things up off the floor. But when I dropped those car keys I was saying, 'Thank you, thank you, thank you'" (laughs).

COLLECTING QUANTITATIVE DATA IN A QUALITATIVE CONTEXT

When the neurologic therapists are involved with treatment, they constantly evaluate and collect quantitative data related to function and continually monitor cognitive and psychoemotional states. When they watched videotapes of themselves working with patients, they inevitably noted the patient's cognitive, affective, and motor status and level of competence in the present task and described what they were going to do next.

> **NOTES MADE DURING OBSERVATION:** Lee's calm, gentle, and friendly demeanor is undergirded by the constant collection of objective data in the outpatient rehab clinic. During Lee's work with four patients, she collected the following data: flexibility (range of motion), weakness (manual muscle test), endurance (number of repetitions), cardiac status

(blood pressure, pulse), functional ambulation status (distance, steps, curbs), pain (description and location during specific activities), falling (when, under what circumstances, which way, how many times), joint stability (knee ligaments), and cognitive assessment.

OBSERVATION RATHER THAN WRITING

These clinicians do very little writing while they are working with patients, an indication of how carefully they listen to their patients and how much they are actively thinking about what is happening.

> **KELLUM:** I have this short amount of time to figure out what the problem is and to figure out what I need to do to get them started with exercises. Sometimes I need to hook them up with people in their community. All that has to take place quickly. . . . The reason I don't write anything down is because I just want to pay attention to the person's movement, the look on their face and all that. If I write it down, it distracts me. I actually miss information if I write it down. I like to be in tune with what is happening to people. Like when people are real dizzy they get a look on their face. They may not say anything but you can just see they don't feel well. It tells you something about how they are tolerating the evaluation. I don't write for that reason: I don't want to miss anything.

Riolo noted that a survey of neurologic clinical specialists and a random sample of the neurology section membership identified that experts differed from entry-level practitioners by the efficiency and proficiency of skill performance (1).

CLINICAL REASONING

The therapists' clinical reasoning was based on constantly thinking about (reflecting) how patients presented themselves (motorically, cognitively, and psychoemotionally) when performing a task. Tasks were set specifically for patients based on prior function, present dysfunction, and long-term goals. The therapists' decision-making processes have been honed by experience and influenced by an understanding of the benefits of motivating patients to be intimately involved in their treatment and to achieve their highest levels of function.

> **LEE (asked to describe what guides her treatment program):** I think always making the task challenging to the patient but at the same time enabling them to carry out the activity. I am always thinking about the long-term goal and working in that direction, trying to simulate the context, the environment as much as possible even if I am in the clinic.

During one observation Lee was working with a patient in the clinic alongside a newly hired novice therapist. The following is an excerpt from the investigator's field notes of that observation:

> **NOTES MADE DURING OBSERVATION:** I note that patients and Lee engage each other in conversation. Lee says to [the patient], "How far have you been walking? Any problems?" She continues checking out which leg

is easier to move first and continues discussing this with the patient while they walk. Lee is safety guarding and watching the patient's face for fatigue/discomfort as she continues a constant conversation about upright activities (function, weakness, and fatigue) in the patient's day.

By contrast, the novice therapist in the treatment area gives short, curt commands (e.g., "Sit there," "Roll up your sleeves. I'm going to take your blood pressure") and admonishments (e.g., "You're not still smoking are you? I smell it on your clothes.") This is the *only* conversation this young physical therapist has with his patients. There are long minutes of silence between these directions and admonishments and further directions and admonishments.

Kellum described her clinical reasoning style as intuitive and noted that pattern recognition was the basis for her intuition. She also describes checking out this inductive approach by returning to a deductive method, especially if her intuition failed.

> **KELLUM:** I feel that I form opinions pretty quickly about certain patterns. I get an intuitive feeling about problems after I have observed them for a while—that is, people's problems and how well they will typically do and what to expect. . . . I do trust myself, because I think I am a pretty good observer, and I am certainly willing to change my mind if something convinces me otherwise.

PATIENTS AND FAMILIES PARTICIPATE IN CLINICAL DECISION MAKING

Patients and their families, if available, were important to the clinical decision-making processes of the therapists. Patients were consulted about their past and their present motor problems, and priority was given to teaching functional tasks the patient was most interested in learning. Long-term goals were consistently part of the therapist's conversations with patients. Trusting and working through collaboration and cooperation was also integral to the work of the neurologic rehabilitation clinicians.

> **KELLUM:** I feel I spend the majority of time explaining to people what the problem is and then teaching them the ideas behind the therapy and then getting them to help me design their exercise program. They do all the work. When they come back, I check on their progress. The more I explain the idea behind the intervention, the more they buy into it and the more accurate they are in what they tell me when they come back.

In another example of this kind of collaboration, Lee engages her patients in reflecting on task performance, assessing what went well, and discussing what they might do next time.

> **LEE (discussing a video of her with a patient):** Here I am trying to get the patient's insight into what she just did and how difficult it was. I think it is always good to get the patient's feedback before going on to a new activity, especially one that is as challenging as the stairs. I want to see what she thought was challenging and how comfortable she felt.

INTERVIEWER: What kind of specific questions do you ask?

LEE: I asked this patient how she felt and what she thought was difficult or easy. I asked if she felt comfortable going up and down with alternating legs. The questions are pretty specific to the task. I think new grads may not give the patient a chance to speak, give them a chance to give feedback. They are more in the mode of we will do this, this, and this, and that's it.

TEACHING PATIENTS AND FAMILIES

The clinicians constantly teach patients about the pathologies underlying their dysfunctions and how they can take responsibility for their own health. For example, all of Lee's outpatients were on home programs. These programs were reviewed and updated at each patient visit. Much of Lee's teaching is accomplished by asking patients questions that require them to think about and make decisions regarding daily activities.

NOTES MADE DURING OBSERVATION: Lee pursues with the patient why he is pushing so hard on the exercise bike at home when he has just injured his knees. She brings the patient around to deciding to lay off his new bike by a series of questions in a conversational tone of voice. For example, "Do you think you need to get this injury cleared up before you get on the bike again?"

Family members are also taught about techniques for returning function. When family members were present, they were included in learning about the patient's activities and how they can best participate.

KATE: This patient's husband came to therapy every day and he lifted her all the time. He couldn't wait for her to initiate. I mean, it took probably a minute or two for her to process anything. And I kept saying to him, "You know, try and let her do as much as possible. It's important for her recovery to let her do that." So, part of it was training him. Regardless of the setting they go home to, I still try to make them as independent as possible. I try to get them where they can be and try to train the family.

BELIEVING PATIENTS

The clinicians accepted and responded to what patients said about their physical disabilities. Labeling or blaming patients was not part of their clinical reasoning processes.

KELLUM: I have heard some therapists say, "That person is not very impaired." But you hear the patient say, "This gets in the way of everything I do." You have to really learn to hear what they are telling you and look at what they do. Although subtle, it's significant. Subtle but significant! For some people it's very validating because they are so happy that someone else saw their problem. The problem has been so significant to them, it gets in their way, but nobody has noticed it.

LEE: It is a challenge working with a long-term disability. This patient is convincing me about his pain because he is a worker's compensation case, and he probably had to convince people in the past. He has low self-esteem, depression, and weight problems. You need to be aware of these things and attend to him. It will take work to prevent further injury and increase strength and endurance.

ADVOCACY

The therapists often assume advocacy roles for patients under their care. They encourage patients and family members to call them if they have questions and make an additional effort to ensure that patients are taken care of properly.

KATE: I think part of the reason that I got more time for this patient, to be perfectly honest, is that the head of the rehabilitation unit rotated off in December. We had an attending come on that was not familiar with a rehab unit, and he left us to our own decisions. So I said, "We need to work on this and this and this." Usually, the utilization review nurse gives us a lot of hassle, but she didn't seem to give us as much when the head of the rehab unit wasn't there. So, we were able to get more time for him—6 weeks instead of 4 or 5 weeks. And he deserved it.

6

NOTES MADE DURING OBSERVATION (Lee in outpatient rehabilitation): The patient's knee brace is broken, and the orthotist has finally arrived with a temporary knee brace. The orthotist doesn't appear interested in following through with this patient. (He is halfway out the door even though the temporary knee brace he brought wasn't big enough to fit over the patient's knee.) Lee persists, calling to the orthotist across the room. "He needs this now. How should we fix it?" The orthotist suggests using tape around the broken brace. Lee turns to the patient and says, "The tape didn't work last time, did it?" The patient suggests a heavier tape might work, and Lee and the orthotist agree. The orthotist leaves and Lee goes off, gets the heavier tape, and fixes the brace. During the next visit, the patient says he needs a new brace. Lee agrees and says she will talk with the orthotist and will also "see what other braces are available on the market." When I talk with Lee later that evening, she reports she has already found another source for a better, new brace.

PHYSICAL THERAPY SKILLS

KATE: I use my hips, my hands, my neck, my shoulder. Sometimes I think it looks easier than it is. I may even have to stop and think, "Did I use my hip to help them keep their hip in extension when they went into stance?" I guess there's a negative to that, too. When they go home, no matter how much you train a family, they're not going to know how to use their bodies like that. So, I may start out that way but then I always work on getting hands-off.

All three experienced clinicians practiced without modalities and with little equipment, except for instruments needed to take measurements (e.g., a goniometer or blood pressure unit). The major tools they used in their work with patients were their own eyes, ears, hands, bodies, and minds. In fact, all three clinicians reported that observational and listening skills were more important than hands-on skills in evaluating and treating patients.

> **KELLUM (when asked about the most important skills for working with neurologic rehabilitation patients):** I think you need to have good observation skills. You need to be good at listening to what people are telling you because I think that people pretty much tell you what the problem is. They tell you a lot—more than you can learn from evaluating them.... You can always learn the manual skills; learning to listen and observe accurately [is] much harder.

The therapists' physical contact with patients and specific uses of touch were fascinating to watch. The four kinds of physical contact or touch documented by Helm et al. (2) were clearly demonstrated by the clinicians: 1) touch to gain information (e.g., tension, pain, balance), 2) touch to guide or stabilize a patient during an activity, 3) touch to reassure or praise the patient, and 4) touch related to a specific technique.

TOUCH TO GAIN INFORMATION

> **KATE:** I have to feel what the patient is doing. Somebody will say, "Well, what do you think is wrong?" or "What can I do to make his gait better?" And I say, "Well, I don't know. Let me feel." And then I can say, "There's not enough weight shift" or "you need to facilitate this aspect of movement" or so on.

TOUCH TO GUIDE OR STABILIZE

Touch to guide or stabilize was used sparingly by all three clinicians, especially in home and outpatient environments. The therapists realized that patients were moving within their homes and in public constantly without their guiding or safety guarding. Much of the guarding was done without contact.

> **NOTES MADE FROM OBSERVATION:** Kellum is working with an outpatient who has been experiencing sudden balance loss. The patient is walking rapidly down a long hall, turning her head from side to side to see if the balance loss can be simulated. Kellum is walking on the patient's right side. She has her right hand cupped over the patient's shoulder (not touching) and her left hand at the patient's low back (not touching). She is matching the patient's pace stride for stride. When the patient starts to loose her balance, Kellum restrains her touch until absolutely necessary to prevent a fall. As Kellum noted, "Well, she is going to walk out of here and I am not going to be with her."

TOUCH TO REASSURE OR PRAISE

Touch to reassure or praise often included a quick, firm pat on the patient's arm or shoulder if standing or on the patient's knee if sitting. These therapists were also quick to offer more body contact in the form of a prolonged steadying hand or a hug if the patient appeared upset. Hugs were also freely given in response to patient initiation or on a special occasion, such as discharge.

TOUCH TO PERFORM A SPECIFIC TASK

Many instances of touch for performing specific tasks were used during evaluation and treatment. Touch during evaluation included taking measurements, such as strength or range of motion, or performing a specific neurologic function test, such as vestibular testing. During treatment, touch was used for specific interventions, such as gentle mobilizations, to help with the patient's hand or foot placement during transfer or ambulation activities, or for adjusting patient clothing or assistive devices.

TYPES AND SOURCES OF KNOWLEDGE

> **KATE:** I feel very comfortable calling and talking and asking questions. Who do I call? I talk to nursing. If that doesn't help, I talk to the resident. Then I go up to the attending [physician]. I think there are some people that aren't as comfortable, or afraid to ask because they think they may look stupid. And maybe I do look stupid, but at least I get my answer.

The therapists studied appeared to have five types of knowledge. The first type is a detailed understanding of a patient's current physical, cognitive, and psychomotor status. This knowledge was collected primarily from observations and evaluations, but it also was collected from medical records and whoever could provide current information (e.g., family members, physicians, psychologists, nurses, other therapists). For example, to determine an accurate diagnosis, Kellum repeats tests physicians have done and recorded in the chart.

> **KELLUM:** I want to see for myself, both for me to learn and in case I see something they didn't happen to see, and then I would talk with them about it.

> **KATE:** I try to gather as much information as I can. For this particular patient, I would go and talk to the OT and the neuropsychologist. I would say, "Well, what do you think? How should we handle this patient?" We come up with different approaches on what might work or what might not work.

The second type of knowledge comes from understanding the patient's life before the disability and is gathered mainly from patients and their families.

> **KATE:** Premorbidly, this patient [with a severe CVA] sounded like a real card. He is in his 80s, but he went dancing probably three or four nights a week. He had a lot of lady friends. He walked a lot. So premorbidly, he was very active. Then, my guess is there was the start of dementia—that is, some cognitive problems that were not very apparent in his own environment. . . . In treatment when he hears something, he's distractible. I figure if I'm ever a stroke patient, I'll be one of these highly distractible people that can't concentrate on what they need to do because I am used to doing so many things all at once like this patient apparently was.

The third type of knowledge includes knowing about a patient's family, family interactions, and living context. This knowledge came from patients, families, home visits, and observations of the family interacting.

> **KATE (after a home visit):** This patient did not have a safe living situation. I was trying to let him know, trying to talk about safety with him, but that was something he didn't see as a problem. Of course if you saw his house, you would agree that, for him, safety was never an issue because he was a very large man and the amount of clutter he had throughout his house was not safe, even for a normal-sized person.

The fourth type of knowledge involves being aware of what it is like to have a disability. This comes from empathy (crossing over to experience what the patient is experiencing) that the therapists try to gain through experiences with patients, patients' stories about returning to function with a disability in society, and their personal experiences with disability.

> **INTERVIEWER:** You have figured out how tough it is for a patient with sensory loss. You've said that three or four times. But how do you know what that feels like?

> **KATE:** I know how I would feel if I had no idea or sensation that my leg was underneath me and you ask me to shift some weight onto it. I mean, think about the times when you've had your mouth numb and you have no control over one side of your mouth from a dentist. . . . Now think about the whole side of your body being that way.

Lee attributes much of her awareness and sensitivity to patients to her husband having a visual disability. Together, they have many friends who also have disabilities.

> **LEE:** My husband is very resistant to using too many assistive devices which would make him look disabled. Certainly, that is very typical in the neuro population. You want to give them a brace, but they say, "I don't want to wear a brace. It will make me look disabled." . . . I have also had the opportunity to go with my husband to employment situations where we fill out an application and go through the whole employment process. Seeing discrimination certainly gives me a different perspective on disability. I know how it is for him to have to worry about a ride to wherever he needs to go. This is the kind of problem that our patients have.

The fifth type of knowledge is knowledge of the impairment, functional limitation and resultant disability of the patient, and the currently espoused physical therapy theories and techniques that can be applied to those conditions. Some of this knowledge came from advanced academic study, continuing education courses, and colleagues.

> **LEE (discussing why obtaining her master's degree in physical therapy was the most influential factor in her professional growth):** The dynamical action system theory: That was an update. My whole treatment approach changed, definitely. That wasn't in my curriculum in

my bachelor's program. I used to be more of an NDT [neurodevelopmental treatment] traditionalist. I think my outlook and my actual carry-through of treatment has changed. What I do today, I wouldn't have done when I first started.

> **KATE:** One of the things I like best about annual conference and combined sections meetings is the poster and platform presentations. I purposefully seek out those things that might affect the patient types I am working with, so I can see what's new information and think about how that can help me, like, "Oh, that's a really good idea!" Sometimes I look at posters and say, "We already did that. How come I didn't think about doing a poster on that?" (laughs).

The greatest source of knowledge for these clinicians, however, appeared to come from reading and, particularly, reflection during clinical encounters (thinking in action) that resulted in effective pacing of patients and the discovery of new treatment strategies—that is, the creation of craft knowledge. These clinicians were constantly thinking and questioning what was going on during treatment.

> **KELLUM:** You learn to teach yourself. You need to ask questions, to think about what you are doing. I can see two people with a vestibular injury: All their test results look the same, and these two people are completely different in terms of how they're doing with treatment. Why is that? How can I explain it? What is it? By trying to figure it out, it helps you to begin to identify the problem, and that makes for good scientific inquiry.

> **KATE:** Sometimes I'll stop and be thinking about something, and I've had patients tell me, "Oh gosh, she's thinking. I don't like that. That means she's going to come up with some other diabolical scheme that she'll make me do." It's true. I think about how to make something more functionally oriented or how to come to simulate something that might be a little more meaningful for the patient.

> **LEE (asked about what she was thinking during a review of one of her videotaped sessions):** I am analyzing not only why she is having difficulty but also trying to see what she is doing different this time as compared to the last. I am also looking for any facial or arm gestures that would give me signals about fatigue or discomfort, seeing if she is getting to the breaking point of getting frustrated ... seeing if she is about to give up.

PERSONAL ATTRIBUTES

CARE, COMPASSION, AND PATIENCE

All three clinicians exhibited compassion and patience while working with patients. Voice tone, touch, and how they talked about and worked with their patients demonstrated that these clinicians care deeply about their patients. This compassion drives their practical work rather than interfering with it.

> **KATE:** I often take patients to bathrooms if they have to go. I mean, you have to do that at home. We need to learn to do it anyway. Might as well do it.... I put people back to bed. I'll clean them up and change their

clothes. I have done that on numerous occasions. Seems like that's how it should be.

INTERVIEWER: If you were to choose a young therapist who is graduating from school to come work with you, what would you look for?

KELLUM: Someone who is patient—that's an important quality. Someone who is sensitive to the problems these people have because you can't always see the problem. They don't look like other people who have neurological disorders. But as we have discussed before, it is a very significant program for these people and their frustration is that other people don't see what the problem is.

The care and concern demonstrated by these therapists was consistent and quietly done. Patients and their families may sometimes be unaware of the thought, concern, and feeling of responsibility that the therapists bring to their work.

LEE: I was concerned when the second attendant had just started. [The patient's husband] said they were trying to get away from using an attendant because [the patient] didn't always feel comfortable having someone with her all the time. I was very shaken because I thought maybe he wasn't seeing what I was seeing. I was concerned at that moment. But then I think he was just trying to see how much assistance she needed without the attendant there.

KELLUM: My main role at the research center in my prior job was to get kids with thoracic and lumbar spinal cord injuries standing and walking with these devices. Well, these devices are at the feasibility stage but far and away from being practical.... The best thing I could do for the kids who were participating in the research was to be there for them when they needed me. I would work often late at night in the lab and they would come down and we would shoot the breeze.... I felt they gave a lot more in terms of their involvement in the research than they were getting—a lot more. I had parents say to me, "Take care of my kid while he is there." That's a huge responsibility, which I took seriously.

PERSISTENCE RELATED TO PATIENT ADVOCACY

The care and compassion the therapists demonstrate is the basis for the persistence they show in finding resources for and following through with patients. In their assumption of advocacy roles, they are well known for "bugging" people to get patients taken care of properly.

LEE: I have spoken with the MD [physician] at the rehab center who is following the patient and told her about the discharge from home care and my anticipation that she would be followed by outpatient therapy. The MD said she would write the prescription. Then I made a follow-up call to the secretary to see if the patient could be scheduled for outpatient therapy soon. She did not have a prescription yet from the MD.

So a week and a half later I made another contact with the physician. She apologized that she did not get a chance to write the prescription. She wrote it then while I was with her. Then I checked with the secretary again and she still didn't have the prescription. I wish I had just taken the prescription from the MD when I was there. Now I am going to have to call her again.

KATE: A week or two ago, I got into hot water with nursing because there was a stroke patient who came down who had basically no balance whatsoever. He needed to be in a wheelchair. I called upstairs and said, "I can't find any contraindications for this patient not to be in a wheelchair. I would like you to put him in one." The nurse said, "We would rather you didn't. He's so big we would break our backs transferring him from bed to wheelchair." I said, "Actually, he's not that bad." I got kind of worked up about this one. I spent a lot of time on the phone trying to find out this information, going through the chart, making sure there wasn't a problem. I said to the nurse, "Well, you know it is really in his best interest to be up instead of lying flat all this time. I'd be willing to come up and show you what I have done and how to do it. How to make it easier." The nurse said to me, "You called and asked me my opinion. If you didn't want it, why did you call?" I went up right before lunchtime and waited for this specific nurse to come on. When she saw me with this guy in the wheelchair she said, "Can you come help me with him and bring about 100 other people with you [to help with the transfer]?" And they had four different nursing staff plus me to get this guy into bed. And it only took me. So, she was not happy. I mean, I could tell by the demeanor on her face that she just thought this was completely ridiculous to have even tried this. And then when she saw me do the transfer, she said, "Oh, maybe it wasn't so bad." And that took up part of my lunchtime.

EMBRACING NEW KNOWLEDGE

KATE: I think a lot of where our practice is going in neuro [physical therapy] may depend upon technological advancement and basic science research in terms of the brain and how it functions. You know when [magnetic resonance imaging] first came out they talked about how wonderful it was, because you could see structures so much more clearly. But it still doesn't tell you a lot. Like, you have this tiny little infarct here and look at this patient has a complete dense hemiplegia, whereas this other person has this huge area of the brain that's affected and, look, all they don't have is isolated finger movements. Why is that?

The clinicians all enjoy encountering new knowledge. They are committed to learning and seek information from all viable sources, including patients, colleagues, research findings, professional presentations, and other health care professionals. Lee recalls being shocked at her first job to find that another therapist was reading a popular magazine at work rather than a physical therapy journal. They love working with patients receiving neurologic rehabilitation because of the challenge of complex dysfunctions.

> **KELLUM:** This patient has been seen by physicians who know as much about vestibular testing as there is to know. She does not have a clear vestibular disorder that we are able to test. And then they send her to me (laughs), which is not atypical! They say, "This person has a problem, and we can't quite figure out what to do. See what you can do." That happens a lot! (laughs)

> **KATE:** I'm on the education committee. It's partly selfish because there are things that I want to know about and hear about. Striving and learning has always been important for me. I can count the number of days I missed school in high school. There were three or four missed days, and two of them were because I was looking at colleges. I used to go into school throwing up sick....Since early on I've been a member of the orthopedic and neurological sections. Friends have said to me "Ortho and neuro?" Well they are related, you know.

Commitment to learning is the foundation of their high levels of responsibility to the patients and their obvious joy in becoming increasingly effective in evaluation and treatment of patients receiving neurologic rehabilitation.

> **LEE:** I can think back to working with amputee patients in Michigan. One gentleman in his mid-60s was involved in a motor-vehicle accident and had a resulting unilateral below-knee amputation. I was working with another patient on the other side of a really big gym—maybe 300 feet, wall to wall. He didn't have his prosthesis, and he hopped over on his intact leg. All the way over to the other side of the gym! If that doesn't change your impression of a 65 year old! Not only him but I can think of people in their 80s who have jobs—they are still employed! It gives you a different perspective on people and what goals to set for them.

MORAL RESPONSIBILITY

Moral responsibility to patients includes an unquestionable honesty. Kellum reports that she, along with physicians working with her, has misdiagnosed patients. She related that the first diagnosis was an easily correctable problem: benign paroxysmal positional vertigo. The actual condition turned out to be a degenerative cerebellar problem.

> **KELLUM:** Absolutely I will tell them. I made a mistake. I told the patient I had treated him assuming that [benign paroxysmal positional vertigo] was the diagnosis. I knew something was wrong the second treatment when the patient didn't respond as predicted. They have a right to understand what happened. And people don't seem to get mad at you. They're certainly upset. They're unhappy that the problem wasn't a simple one, but they don't seem to get upset with you.

The clinicians also assume a moral responsibility for their colleagues, which manifests itself through rectifying inappropriate patient treatment or billing.

LEE: I saw a patient in the outpatient clinic who I felt had received a brief, inadequate treatment from a physical therapist in home care, and I was aggravated by it. I didn't want to know the name of the therapist, but I certainly made sure the [Visiting Nurse Association] followed up with the therapist just to make sure it didn't happen again.

INTERVIEWER: Why does that aggravate you?

LEE: Two reasons: One, ethically the physical therapist has no right to be providing inadequate treatment. They need to be there for the time they are supposed to be there. Secondly, the therapist is shortchanging the patient. The patient is deserving of the best treatment they can get. They shouldn't be shortchanged either by a short 10- or 15-minute treatment or by a therapist who [describing another example] was just watching the patient walk with a walker when the patient walked independently!

INTERVIEWER: I see you feel strongly about this. You appear angry.

LEE: Oh yeah, very angry. I am calm now because I went to the office and reported the incident and they followed up on it. If I hadn't taken any action, I would have more anger stored in me.

CONCLUSIONS

The most powerful theme in this cross-case analysis is concerned, committed, and persistent focus on return of patients to the functional status they experienced before disability. Functional status includes motor, cognitive, and affective components of recovery that are relevant for the patient and his or her family members in the patient's home environment (Figure 6-1). The basis of this focus is a patient–therapist partnership that allows the therapist to teach patients about dysfunction and disability to permit patients to understand and take as much initiative as possible in their own recovery. The work of the clinicians included assessing current status (motor, cognitive, and affective), planning the next

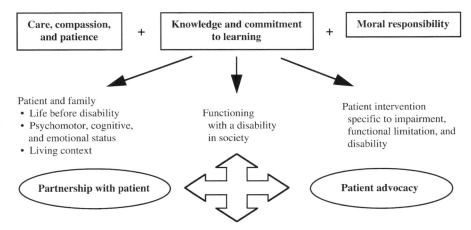

Figure 6–1 ■ The work of expert neurologic rehabilitation clinicians in the making.

treatment intervention, and moving swiftly to identify and involve other people in the health care system who could play a role in the patient's recovery. They are driven to find information about neurologic disorders and their treatments. Their skills are powerful but subtle: intently observing, questioning, and listening; quickly discovering the uniqueness of each patient and treating within this uniqueness; and carefully and skillfully using their hands and bodies. They love working with patients and are dedicated to being exceptional in the complex and sometimes confounding work of neurologic rehabilitation.

REFERENCES

1. Riolo L. Skill differences in novice and expert clinicians in neurologic physical therapy. *Neurol Rep.* 1996;20:60–63.
2. Helm JS, Kinfu D, Kline D, et al. Acquisition of a touching style and the clinician's use of touch in physical therapy. *J Phys Ther Educ.* 1997;11:17–25.

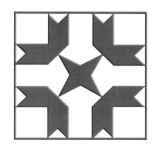

Hands All Around — A stylized pattern showing hands joined together to create.

7

Expert Practice in Orthopedics: Competence, Collaboration, and Compassion

Gail M. Jensen

ANNA: I look at the patient as being a mystery. I love to get a new patient because it is a new problem to solve. It is exciting, and if it wasn't, I wouldn't be practicing today.

PEDER: I think you need impeccable methodical evaluation skills, which include your ability to screen and prioritize your examination, to get to the core problem—problems and concerns and needs of that patient—quickly. You have to interpret the data you collect and communicate to the patient in a succinct, easily understood framework. The physical therapist is accountable to the patient for the success of the program, and it must make sense to the patient.

ISAAC: Therapists should answer questions until it does make sense, and patients must consider themselves as a patient and therapist who is responsible for the outcome of their program. The patient is both the patient and therapist. The need for the patient to become their own therapist means I am as much a coach and guide as a therapist. Patients must be in control in the treatment process and be willing to make changes in both behavior and lifestyle that are often necessary to achieve maximum recovery.

This chapter describes three physical therapists who practice in orthopedic outpatient settings. Each therapist was the subject of a qualitative case report. This chapter is a qualitative case study that provides examples of expert practice in orthopedic physical therapy.

BACKGROUND

The clinicians studied have substantial clinical experience: two of them have been practicing for more than 30 years, and the other has been practicing for almost 20 years (Table 7-1). They all described their entry-level educations as good, but none of them spoke of either professional education or physical therapy faculty as making significant impressions on their careers in orthopedics.

ANNA (discussing her Army preparation): I always felt good about it. When I came out and matched myself against other physical therapists coming out, I had an extremely good education. What was good about it was I was trained by people who had come out of the profession to teach for 2 years. We were in the clinic from the beginning. We started with little things and then gradually built on that foundation.

Continuing education courses in orthopedics did not give them sufficient or significant training because it did not address their needs. All of them sought additional, long-term training and education in manual therapy programs. All these experts have a drive to do well, a desire to be the best they can be, and a passion to seek more knowledge about what they are doing with patients. The therapists studied were all highly motivated.

PEDER (discussing continuing education courses): You never talk about integration, the total treatment regimen....I would take something in a continuing education course, and it just wasn't good enough for me. I found that I was exposed to numerous evaluative and treatment procedures but

Table 7–1. Professional Profiles of Expert Orthopedic Physical Therapists

	Isaac	Peder	Anna
Years of clinical experience	31	19	31
Practice settings (past and present)	Rehabilitation center HMO Acute-care hospital Private practice Corporately owned practice	Rehabilitation center HMO Private practice	Acute-care hospital Rehabilitation center Private practice HMO
Education	Bachelor of science Master of science	Bachelor of science Master of science	Bachelor of science
Advanced clinical education	Continuing education Long-term course	Continuing education Long-term course	Continuing education Long-term course
Teaching expertise	Clinical faculty long-term manual therapy courses Continuing education	Clinical faculty long-term manual therapy courses Clinical faculty for clinical residency Continuing education	Clinical faculty long-term manual therapy courses Clinical faculty for clinical residency Continuing education Academic faculty
Professional associations	APTA IMTA (active; held office)	APTA IMTA (active; held office)	APTA IMTA

HMO = health maintenance organization; APTA = American Physical Therapy Association; IMTA = International Manual Therapy Organization.

7

that no one ever talked about how you use them beyond the first day. There was no talk of integration or the total treatment regime. I saw how I grew with an ongoing continuing education program with a mentor at Mass General [Massachusetts General Hospital] where I was.

Isaac is committed to becoming the best therapist he can be and pursuing challenging and important experiences. After finishing his physical therapy education, he decided to develop additional clinical skills by enrolling in a long-term course that focused on therapeutic exercises. After the course, he became the physical therapy director at a medical center in an urban area. Again, he found himself wanting to learn more so that he could help all of his patients.

In addition to speaking about developing their clinical skills after entry-level education, all of the experts mentioned clinical mentors who had influenced their thinking and practice techniques at key points in their careers. They identified long-term manual therapy training as an opportunity to learn how to solve clinical problems, attributing much of this understanding to working with mentors who facilitated their clinical thinking and reasoning processes.

> **ANNA:** I did this course at a clinical facility that was part of an HMO [Health Maintenance Organization]. We went all day long for 1 month and also had access to treating patients. This was a real turning point in my career. It was the first time I realized that I can do something and make change and make change up front. So after that I went and worked at another clinical facility in that same HMO.

> **PEDER:** You were asked to take it all in and synthesize information, and then you would get a live patient. You were forced to make decisions and you made a lot of mistakes, but you learned. I think the clinical supervision is what helped me learn light years faster. I was forced to put knowledge to work on a patient and had close evaluation of applied clinical skills. I had to test and retest and assess and prioritize my interventions.

The therapists also identified clinical mentors whom they admired for their skill and ability to help patients with tough clinical presentations. The clinical mentors inspired these developing experts to reach an exceptional level of practice.

> **ISAAC:** I was in the clinic now doing what I had learned from the mentor in the therapeutic exercise course. What I would find is that a patient I would treat and could not help...well, I would see them in 2 or 3 months in the hallway at our clinic. I would say, "How are you doing?" They would say they went to see this therapist who helped them in one visit. I said to myself, "Oh my gosh. I have to find out what he is doing."

These clinicians have practiced in a variety of settings, including rehabilitation centers, hospitals, outpatient clinics, and private practices. For all of them, motivation continues to come from meeting patients and being challenged by difficult cases. Consequently, they sought practice settings that provided them access to patients with challenging cases.

> **PEDER:** Every patient becomes a competition and a little mini research project. I think part of it is my competitive nature. I don't enjoy treating easy patients. I get satisfaction out of improving the tough patients.... I don't get everyone better, but improving someone's quality of life is part of helping someone. I might not get them back to work, but I might improve the quality of their life, so there is that competitive drive to take someone, especially if they have been somewhere else, and do that. And then there is the pressure from the medical community,...and I happen to be lucky. I get a lot of referrals from the best spine doctors around, and they send you their wife. You know the pressure is on.

Although they enjoy the challenge of patient care, the expert clinicians also welcome opportunities to teach. In addition to teaching students, they teach their peers in long-term courses and other professional activities. All of these therapists also have made contributions to the physical therapy literature. Most of these contributions are in the form of book chapters, specialty articles, and other educational materials. Although all three have had some experience with clinical research, writing papers or book chapters and gaining publication does not appear to be a priority. Two of the three experts also have had significant involvement in professional activities with the American Physical Therapy Association and the International Manual Therapy Association.

<table>
<tr><td>

CLINICAL PRACTICE THEMES

</td><td></td></tr>
</table>

PHILOSOPHY OF PHYSICAL THERAPY PRACTICE

This section discusses major clinical practice themes (e.g., philosophy of practice, types and sources of knowledge, and clinical reasoning), beginning with an overview of each therapist's philosophy of physical therapy practice. A therapist's approach or philosophy of practice was used as a key to understanding how that therapist did his or her work. Each of the three experts is described by metaphors intended to be conceptual descriptions of that therapist's approach.

Although many similarities exist among these three expert practitioners, each had his or her own identity as a practitioner. All of the therapists shared similar beliefs and values about their roles as therapists (e.g., facilitating patient independence and movement), but how each practiced and performed varied.

Isaac: Healer and Teacher

Isaac, who describes himself as a healer and teacher, focuses on withholding any judgment about patients and tries to find ways to stimulate healing. His views about health are based on a foundation of integration of mind and body. He always works to empower patients.

> **ISAAC:** I think that as physical therapists, a more generic term for us is healers. . . . What does it take to be a healer? That is a question that is incredibly important to me. How can I be the best healer I can? . . . My answer is in order for me to be the best healer I have got to be able to stimulate the healing in the person that I am healing. It isn't in me but in my ability to stimulate the other or the patient. The healer is within us all.

Peder: Competitor and Craftsman

Peder came from a strong athletic background and took tremendous pride in working hard and finding success. His work with patients is a blend of constant dialogue and substantial hands-on intervention for identifying and treating soft-tissue and joint problems. His evaluative approach to patients is disciplined, yet highly interactive.

> **PEDER:** You have to get to the core problem—the concerns and needs of the patient. You have to have impeccable methodical evaluation skills, which include your ability to screen and prioritize your examination, to get to the core problems—problems and concerns and needs of that patient—quickly.

Anna: Detective and Listener

Anna loves "listening to the patient's story and solving the mystery." She uses a strong evaluative framework and has mental discipline but also has an admiration of how much patients know, if therapists allow them the opportunity to speak.

7

ANNA: You have to know what you need to know to solve the problem. You are following a line of questions. The more you do it, the more you can let the patient do it. You don't have to ask them. If you just go in and listen to them, they will tell you. You can compartmentalize after you have heard enough stories, but while you are learning, you have to keep control over it so you can sort through it.

Anna also stays in practice because of the challenge of patients. She enjoys treating new patients and helping make a difference in their lives.

ANNA: I try to put the pieces together throughout, and if I was not, I would not still be doing this. I think throughout my whole career I have always done a little something to add to it so it is not just plain patient care. I needed something else.

Although each practitioner has a unique identity, the therapists share two strong similarities in how they conduct practice. First, they set consistently high standards for themselves. They all discussed how their patient loads have become more difficult over time because other practitioners send them tougher patients with more complex problems. All of them identify a professional responsibility to solve tough patient cases. They also withhold judgment about patients and do not readily categorize patients with labels such as "noncompliant," "poor historian," or "malingerer." The second similarity is an intense focus on patients that involves making patients' needs and goals a central aspect of evaluation and intervention processes. They try to understand who the patients are, what brings them to physical therapy, and how they can return to activities important in their lives.

TYPES AND SOURCES OF KNOWLEDGE

Physical Therapy Knowledge and Skills

All three experts have strong foundations of general practice knowledge that concentrates on assessing movement problems, facilitating movement through manual procedures, and teaching specific exercise to improve patient function. The aim of their work with patients is to facilitate the return to valued activities.

PEDER: Our goal here is to get you back to golf. [Peder shows the patient a floor exercise]. Now let's try that again. You are not strong enough yet to go low. You have to be able to stabilize that back on your own.

ANNA: I try to remember that she is 59 years old and still working in a cannery. That is important, and that is pretty tough work.

The experts used a consistent evaluative framework that has similar core elements yet is dynamic and can change during the evaluation process. Evaluation begins immediately and is interactive, occurring between practitioner and patient.

PEDER: The evaluation process should begin when a patient walks into the treatment room. An interview process occurs in which the manual therapist guides the patient's description of his or her symptoms by defining the location and behavior of those symptoms, obtaining the patient history, and determining any precautions that may preclude treatment.

ANNA: That concept of collecting relevant information and making change on the spot is essential. Making change where the patient feels better means that that you could do something. That approach was a whole new light and made treating exciting to find a problem and change it.

The therapists considered listening to the patient a critical component of their work—a skill that helped guide their selective data-gathering process.

ISAAC: Not only do you have to understand the presenting problem, but in the process of understanding the problem, you have to understand the cause of the cause to understand just where this thing came from. I think that the way you help a patient to get better is your ability to observe and understand them as a human being, a total human being.

ANNA: You have to know what you need to know to solve the problem. You are following a line of questions. The more you do it, the more you can let the patient do it. You don't have to ask them. If you just go in and listen to them, they will tell you. You can compartmentalize after you have heard enough stories, but while you are learning, you have to keep control over it so you can sort through it.

Additional elements of their clinical practices include clinical skills of observation, palpation, and hands-on manual therapy procedures. The manual skills of palpation and manual therapy, at times, appeared to be unconsciously used, applied often as they were talking and interacting with the patient. Their eyes and hands are important tools for doing their work. All three of the experts had long-term education in manual therapy and spoke of the importance of working with patients to help solidify these important skills.

The abilities demonstrated by these experts consistently illustrated that each possesses superb manual skills and strong observational skills. The therapists differ, however, in how much they rely on each of these skills. For example, Peder attended more to manual skills than the other two, whereas Isaac spent intense periods listening and teaching patients, and Anna used a mix of skills as she investigated problems. The strongest skills of each therapist were governed by the guiding philosophy of that therapist, whether that was teaching and healing, being skilled in manual techniques, or solving mysteries.

Equipment usually was avoided during treatment sessions, although hot packs and ultrasound occasionally were used. Patients were treated with the therapists' hands and given instructions for home exercise. The exercises prescribed were always few, simple, and specific to the movement problems. Any equipment recommended was usually easily available, such as exercise bikes, soup cans, and exercise balls. One therapist had designed exercise tools for patients to do specific mobilizations at home.

Knowledge of Patients

Knowledge gained from and about patients was important in the practices of all three therapists. Knowledge of patients came from listening to patients and then shaping evaluations and interventions to fit the patients' needs. Although one expert, Isaac, was the most holistic and humanistic of the three, all of the experts acknowledged the importance of understanding the patient and what he or she wants and needs. Patients should be understood in the context of who they are and how they live.

> **ISAAC:** You have to get to the core problem—the concerns and needs of the patient.

> **ANNA (responding to a question about the importance of listening):** I think that is one of the things about our work—that is, how you modify. You get a lot of good information if you just let [patients] give it to you as it wants to come out. I am experimenting, and I have recently changed my first question to patients to "How can I help you?" rather than "What is your problem?" because sometimes they will tell you, "All I want is advice on this activity," and that is a very simple thing.

Patients were also valuable because they allowed the therapists to learn through their own thinking processes.

> **PEDER:** Don't allow yourself to treat the same diagnosis the same way. They all react differently. You know, it's like thinking out loud. Don't be afraid to not know the right answer right now, but prove your answer through your process.

> **ANNA:** When I came back from Australia and taught part time, what I really needed to do was see a lot of patients so I could consolidate all the knowledge and skills I gained. You need that intensity of patients, and perhaps that is why I really enjoy this end of the work now.

> **ISAAC:** In order to involve them in what I am doing I just talk out loud. Okay, I am trying to figure out whether your injury was here and is affecting this or is it in both places and each is feeding on the other. So I get the patient involved intellectually in a problem-solving process without feeling like they don't have control. In fact, the control comes from involving them in the thinking and proving to themselves that we are on the right track. It demands a degree of accuracy so that you don't look like a fool. You want the patient to appreciate the process and not see it as a lack of knowledge on your part.

Knowledge of Teaching

Each of the therapists was strongly committed to teaching patients about their bodies and how to care for themselves. The exercise programs given to patients were tailored specifically for individual patients.

> **ISAAC:** With all patients, you can see them as unique human beings trying to deal with life just as you are. What they are here for is to understand their

problem and become their own therapist. The patient must be involved in their own therapy and must understand what I am doing and become part of what I am doing.

When Anna was asked how she effects change with patients, she quickly replied, "I do more teaching....I explain to people more so they have a better understanding of their condition."

Isaac used several methods to teach patients. His routine for teaching exercises involves demonstrating exercises to patients, then having the patients perform the exercises as he guides them. In addition, many patients received patient education materials (e.g., booklets or videos). These materials were designed by Isaac for individuals with chronic upper quarter pain problems.

> **ISAAC:** I demonstrate because I want them to see. I am thinking of all of the ways that people access knowledge. Some people are auditory, some are visual, some are kinesthetic, and I will use all of those to communicate with my patient. I don't know that they are predominantly auditory, visual, or kinesthetic, so in my teaching, I will combine all of those methods. I will want them to visually see me, I will want them to hear me express it, and I will want them to kinesthetically feel it as they are doing it.

Teaching adaptations for home, work, and exercise continued as the treatment progressed. A patient's valued activities, whether work or play, were usually considered within the exercise regimen.

> **PEDER:** I think that health and wellness is an individual thing. I've had patients that get up in the morning and make sure the kids are fed and clean, lunches made, dropped off at school, and 9 hours of work was [the thing that provided happiness]. They survived the day, and that is health and well-being to them. Or you have a person that is a daredevil—driving a mountain bike 55 miles per hour and not crashing. That is happiness to them, so you have to change your treatment program and be more aggressive.

In teaching patients exercise, care was taken to break down the steps and explain the movements in the exercise.

> **ISAAC (guiding a patient through the actual exercise):** Go back to the segment below, and now that is the area causing your problems. We can make a difference there. Now just try rolling and just slide yourself down [patient is doing exercise; Isaac guides the patient through the exercise with his hand on the patient's pelvis]. Now, as you roll up, this is for the upper part of the spine [Isaac corrects patient's hand position], and then roll back and forth. Now again.

> **PATIENT:** Do you think I should have an MRI [magnetic resonance imaging]?

> **ISAAC:** No—even if it could be done at no cost—because you don't have a back problem that would ever require surgery the way it is right now.

7

PATIENT: Do you think I have a slipped disk?

ISAAC: I think it matters as far as you having a handle on what it is.... The body is the best healer, and it knows what is going on at the cellular level. What if I told you had a disk [problem], and someone else said you had a facet [problem], and someone else a muscle problem, and each one of us gave you the right thing to do? I suggest you have an injury to a mobile segment and that injury went through a repair process and the repair led to some stiffness and some problems with coordination and endurance and strength or flexibility. The solution is to get through all of them. The physical stress of doing all of that is the body needs to repair itself, and you are using the roller to address flexibility and the pelvic exercise for coordination and the walking for endurance. Then we work through getting you better, and you will be guided by your own body rather than knowledge that we don't know for sure anyway.

In addition to teaching patients, all of the experts continue to be engaged in teaching colleagues through workshops, seminars, and long-term courses. They taught early in their careers, beginning with supervising students. All have been involved with educational programs and have been faculty members of long-term manual therapy programs.

The therapists' knowledge about teaching generally came from clinical experiences, learning from patients what worked and did not work, and being involved in mentor activities. Only one of the experts has had formal course work in education.

ISAAC: You have to prove your worth to the patient, and that's the most humbling experience of all.

Knowledge of the Health Care Environment (Context)

Because the experts made it their business to know patients beyond musculoskeletal problems, they also were involved in managing patients within the health care system by assuming roles of patient advocates. For two of these experts, being advocates meant spending additional time trying to get the best for patients—calling case managers, writing evaluations quickly, and in some cases doing pro bono work for patients who did not have additional insurance coverage. For the third expert, who worked within a large health care organization, advocacy work involved "going the extra mile for the patient," which could include following up by referring services, providing recommendations for other interventions if physical therapy is unsuccessful, or speaking directly to physicians. Two of the therapists also periodically consulted with patients over the phone about their conditions and exercise programs.

ISAAC: I expect the patient to be better within this period of time, and I give an expectation level to him: "If this doesn't happen, you call me." This call method has evolved over time, and it is this ability and need for the patient to become their own therapist that means that I must give them a process for thinking, and I have got to be able to reinforce it. Otherwise, I am doing nothing more than anyone else who just hands out a sheet of paper and says, "Go home and do your exercises."

All of the experts had good interactions with other health care professionals, including physicians. Physicians and other colleagues often referred patients with difficult cases to them. The experts also confidently provided professional opinions and treatment recommendations to physicians.

The experts had a sense of responsibility to their communities. Peder is active in several community organizations, Isaac makes a point of personally knowing and treating members of his local community, and Anna is focused on being an instrumental part of the health care organization where she works.

Clinical Practice Knowledge

Thus far, no mention has been made of expert discussion and application of content knowledge often associated with physical therapy education (e.g., anatomy, kinesiology, pathology). This might be owing to how data were gathered—that is, through observational and interview methods of clinical practice. Another factor might be the central importance of clinical knowledge in professional practice settings. Strong evidence exists that knowledge used by professionals in practice is not traditional knowledge found in textbooks but is the knowledge that clinicians adapt and shape as they integrate their understanding of signs, symptoms, and responses to treatment into their clinical knowledge bases. The adaptation and shaping of their clinical knowledge comes from thinking and reflecting as they practice. Figure 7-1 shows a working conceptual model of expert orthopedic practice. The types and sources of knowledge and skills described in this section are part of an integrated whole seen in clinical practice knowledge.

In the three case reports, the clinicians did comment about aspects of biomechanics and anatomy as they reviewed videotapes of patients, but this was

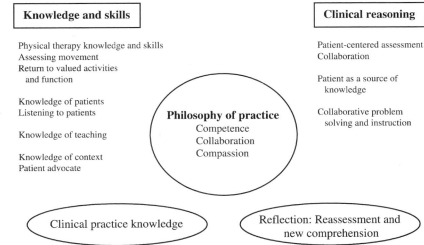

Figure 7–1 ■ Conceptual model for orthopedic experts.

always done in the context of the patient's story. It appears as if these collective stories or "patient scripts" develop significant meaning for the experts over time, as illustrated by the following examples:

> **ANNA:** I constantly try to make everything make sense to see how certain clinical pictures behave. If you go in and listen to [patients], they will tell you. You can begin to compartmentalize after you have heard enough stories.

> **PEDER:** I want to get a picture of where she hurts on her whole body, and I want to know how those areas relate to her problem. She might hurt at T12 [thoracic level] or L1 [lumbar level]. She could have a pelvic problem or a hip problem. I have to find that out. I am also looking for clusters of signs and symptoms that fit certain pathologies. You see me here finding out . . . the symptoms, their behavior and their descriptors, their relationships—that helps me decide on a working hypothesis. Now, there is a functional test. You can look at her spine. I counted three times that she went off to the side, so I did unilateral movements L4/5 [lumbar level], and that is the involved side. You see this is a tough thing to teach. You have to go back and think laterally. You have to accept some uncertainty—that is, you trust yourself, your own judgment—because what happens is the student wants a diagnosis, but the system that you are using is a continuum of going this way, and you make decisions that initially may be quite uncertain. I'm proving to myself, and I have to prove to the patient, that if I treat them at L3/4 [lumbar level] or whatever that I have changed her symptoms, and that is critical. You see, so many people that think you have to treat the specific region of symptoms to make it better.

CLINICAL REASONING

Clinical practice is a collaborative venture between the therapist and patient. Therapists' reasoning and decision-making processes were guided by their philosophies of practice, patient needs, and application of knowledge to particular cases. The reasoning strategies used by the experts were multiple and involved not only using problem-solving sequences but also gathering evidence from multiple sources (e.g., knowledge of specialty, patients, or teaching; patient cues; hypotheses generating; reassessment techniques). The descriptions of the orthopedic experts' clinical practice and reasoning methods come from a number of data sources, including observations, interviews, and examination of materials.

Patient-Centered Assessment

The clinical reasoning process with patients began with gathering patient data that were selective and specific to that patient's experience. This specific focus on the patient was done with a definite and consistent evaluative structure, adapted to the particular patient.

NOTES MADE DURING OBSERVATION: [Peder] is carefully observing and recording what he sees and hears. He is intent on comprehending the patient's problem—that is, what do they want or need?

ISAAC: A lot of therapists cut the patient off, and they want to get to the physical exam. What brought this patient to me? Not only do you have to understand the presenting problem, but in the process of understanding it, you have to understand the patient as a person and a human being.

NOTES MADE DURING OBSERVATION: [Anna] starts a new session by asking why the patient has come. What is the patient's understanding of his symptoms? This helps in targeting her data gathering with the patient.

In the interview process, the experts were all eager to gather essential information pertinent to the patient and the patient's problem.

Collaboration: The Patient as a Source of Knowledge

Patients were trusted and respected sources of information and knowledge for the clinicians. The clinical practice and reasoning processes became a collaborative effort between therapists and patients. The therapists wanted to know about patients as people, which included understanding what was important to them, what kind of work they did, and what other factors influenced their movement problems.

ISAAC: I am trying to get inside of his head and understand what brings him to me. I say I think that he is in his middle 40s and beginning to have problems with his low back and neck, and he is concerned. His concern is as much to know that it is not serious and to know that he is going to get better, that he can control the symptoms, and that the problems won't affect his job or marital relationship. Understanding him as a person and where he comes from will allow me to better direct my care and meet that need of his.

NOTES MADE DURING OBSERVATION: In working with a new patient who has experienced a neck injury in a car accident, Anna asks, "What is the worst part now?" [She puts her hands on the patient's to identify the area.] "Which is the part that interferes with your life the most?" She uses this information to decide which problem is most bothersome to the patient and where she will start with her treatment intervention.

The therapists work quickly to understand the patient as a person as a central aspect of their evaluation and intervention process.

PEDER: You have to learn what the patient wants within the first 5 minutes because then you can focus your patient and say, "Look, if we can change this and this, we might be able to get you back to horseback riding, or we might be able to get you back to weight lifting." If you don't know what they want or need, well then, you're going to waste your time. You need a patient profile. What are your hobbies? Are you doing them now? Can you work? . . . What do you expect from me? What is your problem? What do you do? Where would you like to go after therapy? What is your goal? These kinds of questions help you focus everything to what is meaningful to them.

Collaborative Problem Solving and Instruction

The therapists were challenged by patients' problems and saw the development of solutions as opportunities for collaborative problem solving. Problem-solving processes occurred at multiple levels. They investigated movement problems and determined primary sources of problems (e.g., posture, joint dysfunction) in conjunction with patient function and need. This collaborative process involved teaching patients more about their musculoskeletal problems and how their daily activities affect the musculoskeletal system.

> PEDER [reviewing a videotape of his interactions with a patient]: I want to clarify with her right now, to make sure about our contract. They need to know that I really care and I hear them, so here we are talking about sitting. I want to try to get at what makes it better or worse and make it as objective as I can. The patient comes back and says, "Oh, it is a little better." And you say, "Well last time, you could only sit 30 minutes, and now it is an hour." Well, then they perk up. I asked her that question, and then I put it in my notes. I told her, "I'm going to hold you accountable because it will help with our decisions." Now I am formulating a working hypothesis and I am trying to figure out if in or out of the car is what bothers her, because it flexes her back, hip, neck, or what? I'm trying to relate that functional motion to my evaluative findings.

> ISAAC: The physical therapist is accountable to the patient for the success of this program. It must make sense to the patient, or the physical therapist should answer questions until it does make sense. Patients must consider themselves as a patient/therapist who is responsible for the outcome of the program. The success of the treatment depends upon the effectiveness of the patient's role as a patient/therapist. This statement is a keystone to effective treatment. The patient is both the patient and the therapist! Patients must be in a position of control in the treatment process and must be willing to make the changes in both behavior and lifestyle that are often necessary to achieve maximum recovery.

Patients were also active collaborators in diagnostic processes. Frequently, initial exercises given to patients were specific to movement problems and part of the diagnostic processes.

> ANNA: I am of the belief that the majority of people will not do a lot of exercises. Part of the diagnosis is with exercise. Exercise also helps me decide what is wrong with the patient. When I am not really clear, I will give them one thing to do at home, and then I will get more information. Like the lady I saw today. She had the really sharp pain, but after she did the exercise a few times, it went away. If I had given

her a couple of other things to do, then I would not have learned the full value of that and she would have not been as much better as she was.

Isaac also discussed how patients should be instructed when the therapist makes a clinical diagnosis.

> **ISAAC:** My clinical diagnosis is that we need to increase extension. I want to involve [the patient] in that thought process. While I haven't proved myself right, my experience tells me that I am going to prove it right or at least involve him in that process. If we prove it right, then I am reinforcing intellectually what he needs to know. I want them to intellectually understand what is going on because I want their belief system and their visualization to strengthen the process. So I empower their intellect to give them a reason for why they are doing the story. I want my story to be valid, although I am willing to change my story if there are not any facts. The ultimate lesson I want them to learn is that the story is only an intellectual hook. The real hook is the response of the body and tissue to what they are doing. But if they say something is wrong, then give them the hook, but emphasize the assessment. They must assess and prove the value of everything they do in their functional movements.

Ongoing Process of Reflection: Reassessment and New Comprehensions

The clinical reasoning processes of the therapists are driven by continual assessment based on successes and mistakes. This process demonstrates the experts' dependence on reflection while practicing. Reflective practice contributes to the development of clinical practice knowledge (see Figure 7-1).

Peder emphasizes that therapists should have evaluation frameworks that are flexible: "You have to continue to assess and treat, assess and treat, and it is the mental discipline that enables you to know when to add or delete something to the program. You continually rerank your hypothesis."

> **PEDER:** Here is a functional test I am doing. She said she felt weak in her legs. I'm looking at her spine. See how it changes. . . . Now you will see after I treat her how that changes. . . . You see, you collect your data, relate that to your hypothesis, and reproduce the symptoms in a certain movement. Is it hip movements versus back movements? I've got to treat an area and reassess those movements. This is a laborious process. Now look at this, a positive [sacroiliac (SI)] test. I did something to the lumbar spine that affected that test but I did not change her SI problem. I can't just look at one test but have to think laterally. I have to prove to myself, and I've got to prove to the patient, that what I treat is changing them.

Evaluations also included checking to see if the patient understood and realized what was happening to his or her body and determining how he or she adjusted to the intervention.

> **ISAAC:** I get the patient involved intellectually in a problem-solving process without feeling like they don't have control. In fact, the control

comes by involving them in the thinking and proving to them and having them prove to themselves that we are on the right track. I want people to trust me. "When I know I am right, I'll tell you and you can trust that. But until I know that I am right, I am going to give you a hypothesis that we are going to test." I use those words. With this patient, I want her to realize that she is getting better because she is doing the right things, not because of any other reason.

These experts were challenged by tough patients and made mistakes. They were not afraid to acknowledge and learn from mistakes. One of the experts commented, "Remember, if you can make a patient worse, you can also make them better." The therapists consistently devoted rigorous thought to tough problems, trying to sort out what was going on or what should have been done differently. Peder continues to be challenged by patients—tough patients. In one of his "failures," he was unable to communicate adequately with the patient.

PEDER: I had this 37-year-old weight lifter with a basic C7 [cervical] nerve root problem that is chronic. His goal is to weight lift, and he has a 3/5 strength in his triceps muscle. He has had three treatments, and he is no better and says, "Why am I not better?" Well, it is going to take time. So, I go through the progression of healing in my head, and I think about him. I'm already thinking, "I don't think I did a good job the first day in explaining things, setting things up." It wasn't that I was technically incorrect in what I did or [was] not competent . . . but somehow I did not communicate to him.

Peder considers risk and learning as part of a lifelong education.

PEDER: You know I have done things to people and their symptoms have become worse and then gotten better. That is the risk you take. You see, I think that what we do with our patients does not come without risk. You just minimize the risk. I look at risk as not knowing the outcome. If you are careful, you can predict the outcome. Sometimes you are wrong.

Anna's reflective process was constant. She was not worried about making mistakes and having to solve problems along the way. She integrated her own creative techniques with her problem-solving processes.

ANNA: Oh, I did something the other day. The only objective sign— I had a lady with trochanteric bursitis—was really her low back. The only objective sign was hip lateral rotation not medial. All hip movements are fine, but lateral rotation in 90 degrees of flexion reproduces the pain. If you palpate, you can find soft-tissues changes at L4/5 [lumbar] and S1 [sacral]. I could make it better but not clear it. So I thought, "Oh well, I'll rotate in flexion," which means you are really side bending away and that is what happens to the pelvis. I will put her in side bending and rotation prone. Well, that got at it better, but it still didn't get it. So I finally had to put her in flexion and dropped the other leg over the side of the table so I could externally rotate her and hold it with my thigh while I did my mobilization. Now, retrospectively, I can think of three other patients if I had done that it might have helped.

Experts also learn by thinking about what their patients do.

ISAAC: I had this patient who was coming to me for thoracic outlet syndrome, but it was very clear that she had a very debilitating back problem that had progressed to the point she was looking for a nursing home. So I go through my evaluation and start mobilizing her spine. I gave her a home program to start moving herself and breathing and relaxation exercises. That is all I did. . . . She comes back 2 weeks later and she is doing great! She is better than she has been in years. I am thinking to myself, "What is she doing to make all this change?" Well, she had taken everything I said on face value and added common sense to it. The face value was this may hurt, but we are trying to remodel things, so do it for a few minutes every hour, then over time it will start to make a change. In the meantime, she starts doing the breathing and listening to music and starts doing more and more exercise. She learns how to twist her own body over the roller. She comes in and says all of this, and I say, "Wow! Have I ever learned something from you." What I am saying is that you give someone a process to work with, and then they will adapt that process to their experience to everything. They will be able to take it and score a touchdown before you even know what it is they did to score that touchdown.

All three of the experts had similar postgraduate education experiences in manual therapy, but their clinical practices did not center on one particular philosophy. Each of them had his or her particular approach to practice that was consistent with his or her philosophy of practice. For example, Isaac routinely works with mind and body issues with patients and teaches his patients about their problems.

ISAAC: We look at the problem and say, "What is it that is keeping this patient from moving? Is it physical? Is it psychological? Is it emotional? Is it intellectual?" Then look at the person and try to determine what factor that is stopping them from moving. Sometimes it is emotional, and by that I mean they have a belief system that if they move they will get worse. A belief system that says they must not move. You have to access that belief system to make a change in that person and give them a choice. It is not that you are saying they are wrong and this is how they should do it, because they will be worse. You cannot judge them.

Peder used manual techniques with most of his patients and then moved them to exercise programs.

PEDER: Every patient becomes a competition and a little mini research project. . . . I don't enjoy treating easy patients. . . . So there is that competitive drive to take someone, especially if they have been somewhere else, and do that.

Anna is motivated by the challenge of solving a puzzle.

ANNA: I try to put the pieces together throughout, and if I was not, I would not still be doing this. I think throughout my whole career I have always done a little something to add to it so it is not just plain patient care. My stimulus now is just enjoying the patients and being able to work with the patients here and share what I know.

| PERSONAL ATTRIBUTES | ### INTENSE FOCUS AND INNER DRIVE: COMPETENCE |

All of the experts are hard working and able to focus on work, whether it is treating patients or preparing paperwork. They are highly motivated to develop and maintain their professional competence and enjoy people and are challenged by patient care.

Isaac is patient, dedicated, and respectful and loves people. His philosophy is the foundation for the beliefs and values evident in his practice. He knows himself well and uses his understanding of his limitations as the basis for choosing activities that keep him challenged. He could be described as a healer and teacher. Isaac's beliefs and values about health and wellness are central to his practice. He considers himself a facilitator and a coach. The central aspects of his practice demonstrate processes of reasoning and action that are similar to those found in teaching. He works in collaboration with patients to help them understand their bodies, their musculoskeletal problems, and the techniques used to address their problems.

Peder has a wonderful sense of humor combined with a strong focus on all of his senses (particularly his hands, eyes, and ears) for gathering and making sense of data. His mental discipline and competitive spirit are central aspects of his character. He relishes challenges and is constantly engaged in learning from those challenges. Peder has a tremendous sense of fairness and equity.

PEDER: I think you should have an idea [something you believe in] that is good for your teaching or your profession or your family or whatever, and then you must carry it out in an equitable manner. You reach that goal you have set. You do it in a way that is not arrogant.

Peder demonstrates excellent manual skills and astute communication skills. He is determined to remain in his private practice despite a rapidly changing environment because he believes in the quality of patient care his clinic provides. He works collaboratively with his patients toward their goals. His advice for new graduates is as follows:

PEDER: I think you need to teach them an evaluative framework that is open-minded. They need to know the psychomotor skills in terms of a physical exam. They need to perform the same tests the same way and then they have to have the skill to adapt the test to the patient. They have to understand how to retest and have excellent communication skills. They have to know how to phrase questions, and they need to know that this is a lifelong learning process. It takes a long time.

Anna is a focused, energetic, and respected therapist who loves her work and her life. She enjoys the challenge of working with patients and trying to solve problems. Asked about ways to help students think, she recommends that they read mysteries to sharpen their analytic skills. "While they are interviewing, they need to listen and think so that the data they collect flows."

> **ANNA:** You have to know what you need to know to solve the problem. You are following a line of questions. The more you do it, the more you can let the patient do it. You don't have to ask them. If you just go in and listen to them, they will tell you. You can compartmentalize after you have heard enough stories, but while you are learning you have to keep control over it so you can sort through it.

Anna enjoys coming to work, getting ready for the day, reading the patient charts, and reviewing radiographs to prepare her for identifying and solving problems. Although Anna would be the first to suggest that she is not particularly good and empathetic with patients with long-term problems, one of her most memorable patients is a woman with chronic pain who could not tolerate any touch at all. Anna described how she helped the patient realize her limitations, control her pain, and manage her medications. This case represents a success story in which both the patient and the therapist learned.

PROBLEM SOLVING: REFLECTION AND COLLABORATION

All of the experts are secure in their own problem-solving processes, although they sometimes do not arrive at the correct answer. Their methods of gathering data, understanding patients, identifying movements that cause symptoms, and experimenting with treatment techniques are used consistently.

> **ANNA:** When you talk about a car, there are certain signs and symptoms when it is not working right. That never occurred to me in my own practice until I went to Australia. My biggest evaluation skills were [manual muscle tests], goniometry, and gait analysis. I realized that I could do something and do something that could make change. . . . You can collect relevant information and make change with a patient on the spot.

> **ISAAC:** What I am doing now is not a lot different than 10 years ago; it is just more sure. I think I make decisions faster and progress the patient faster when my decision is the right one, but I change quicker when the decision doesn't produce the change I expect. This whole issue of expecting or making a prognostic decision in your own head and then applying treatment to make that come true—when it doesn't confirm your hypothesis, you rethink it with the expectation of being able to create another hypothesis.

The therapists also continue to stay engaged in clinical work because of the challenges presented by patients. These challenges are driven by their reflective processes.

PEDER: I do this thousands of times. I've done it thousands of times. I figure I have had about 23,000 patient visits in my career . . . but what keeps me in practice is I am challenged. Every patient is a mystery. It is me against that patient, constantly analyzing and rethinking.

RESPECT FOR PATIENTS: COMPASSION

Respect for patients was evident during interview sessions and observation. Knowing what brings patients to physical therapy and understanding the patient's needs were considered very important.

ISAAC: From the patient's perspective, what is their problem?

NOTES MADE DURING OBSERVATION: Anna has been working with a woman with severe osteoarthritis of the knee and made little progress in changing her symptoms. During this visit, she brings the radiographs in to show the patient why her joint is so painful. Anna then moves closer to the patient and takes her hand as the patient relays her fears about surgery for her knee. Anna reassures the patient by telling her about other patients she has worked with and how much she respects the orthopedic surgeon. She then calls the orthopedic clinic to set up an appointment for her patient.

The therapists consider patients as human beings and not just problems to be fixed. These therapists frequently work with patients as advocates to help them negotiate the health care system.

CONCLUSIONS

These expert orthopedic therapists have advanced skills in manual therapy and share similar beliefs and values. They each are strongly motivated to develop competence at the highest levels. Their evaluative work is patient centered and is intended to allow them to understand patients and movement problems in the context of the patient's life. The skills of listening to patients are coupled with the skillful use of observation and palpation. Their intervention processes are collaborative ventures between patient and therapist. Although these experts differed in the ways that they practiced, they all consistently engaged in processes of reflection leading to new understandings. Helping patients understand their movement problems and teaching them specific exercises were common intervention strategies. They shared a focus on clarity of reasoning based on clinical evidence and patient need. Reflection in action was the critical skill used for competent, collaborative, and compassionate practice.

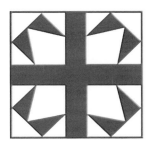

Cross and Stars — A pattern built from the combination of the traditional cross block with the star block to create a new view.

8 Expert Practice in Physical Therapy

On the most general level, the study of expertise seeks to understand and account for what distinguishes outstanding individuals in a domain from less outstanding individuals in that domain....In nearly all human endeavors there always appear to be some people who perform at a higher level than others, people who for some reason stand out from the majority. Depending on the historical period and the particular activity involved, such individuals have been labeled exceptional, superior, gifted, talented, specialist, expert, or even lucky (1).

A premise of our argument is that there exists no well-defined standard that all experts meet and that no nonexperts meet. Rather, experts bear a family resemblance to one another and it is their resemblance to one another that structures the category "expert" (2).

What does expert practice look like in physical therapy? What dimensions may account for those practitioners who handle complex patient cases and are known as *expert clinicians*? Do expert physical therapists resemble one another in what they know, what they do, and how they think? As detailed in Chapters 4–7, clinical expertise can be described through examination of the nature of knowledge used in practice, clinical reasoning and judgment, and the developmental journey of practitioners. This chapter is intended to recontextualize and develop an emerging theory of expert practice in physical therapy that should help demonstrate the usefulness and implications of our study's findings.

A key directive in our study was exploration of everyday practice in its natural setting—the clinic. This is consistent with the argument that a professional's skill level is adapted to the context of practice. Learning from clinical practice is a legitimate source of knowledge (3–5). The challenge for us was to understand the methods of reasoning experts use to think about, construct, and solve clinical problems in practice (5). Rothstein (6) states this idea well in the following passage:

I have come to the personal conclusion based on observation of outstanding clinicians. Good clinicians may not always be aware of reliability coefficients, but during their practice they have gleaned some insights into the errors associated with their measurements. They appear to almost intuitively take into account the possibility that their measurements may be error-ridden. They know when to second-guess their measurements and when to take other measurements. I do not believe that they are actually doing this intuitively, but rather because of their experience.

Each of the specialty areas of pediatrics, geriatrics, neurology, and orthopedics has different expectations of its practitioners and requires significantly different types of clinical decisions and actions. For example, orthopedic physical therapists are frequently confronted with patients in good health who are experiencing temporary episodes of impairment or loss of function. The mechanism of the injury must be identified, and the best course of action to relieve the symptoms and restore function must be pursued. The clinical decisions of neurologic, geriatric, and pediatric physical therapists more commonly focus, however, on diagnosing movement disorders and planning an appropriate treatment strategy that allows the most complete restoration of function in the face of permanent disability. Despite the different demands placed on each specialty area, considerable overlap exists in certain dimensions of practice.

COLLECTIVE SAMPLE

CLINICIAN PROFILES

Professional profiles were compiled for each of the 12 clinicians and are detailed in Chapters 4–7. All 12 therapists have practiced in a number of facilities, and 11 have practiced in a minimum of three different clinical settings (Table 8-1). The therapists also have extensive clinical experience, ranging from 10 to 31 years of practice. Of the 12 therapists in the sample, 11 are active members of the American Physical Therapy Association, and several have participated in other professional groups related to their clinical specialty areas. The majority hold master's degrees. Most acquired clinical specialty education through a combination of short- and long-term continuing education courses and graduate education. All of the clinicians were actively involved in teaching in a variety of settings, including continuing education, clinical education, and academic education.

PROFESSIONAL JOURNEYS

How did these therapists get where they are today? Although their specific paths have varied, the group does share some core characteristics. These therapists appeared to be highly motivated and driven to continue to learn and work toward excellence through lifelong learning.

8

> **JANIS (pediatric clinician):** I don't know how any of these other [experts] feel, but I still have that feeling...you never feel like you totally know what you're doing. That's why I keep trying to learn as much as I can.

> **ISAAC (orthopedic clinician):** Be the best you can be, be self-directed, and seek knowledge. Even if you are going to be a bank robber, be the best you can be.

> **BEN (geriatric clinician):** I get nourishment from my teaching and my writing and my research....It helps in my thinking with my patients.

> **KELLUM (neurologic clinician):** When I first graduated [from an undergraduate program], I never questioned what I did. I mean, not in the way I do now. I think if you get really good at critical thinking, it really helps you learn because you keep asking yourself questions that others would ask you. You learn how to teach yourself. I learned that in my master's program. You need to ask questions, to think about what you are doing. And now I ask myself all the time. I can see two people with the same condition, and all the test results look the same, and these two people are completely different in terms of how they're doing with treatment. What is that? How can I explain it? What is it?

Table 8–1. Professional Profiles of Expert Therapists

Clinician	Years of Clinical Experience	Education	Practice Settings	Advanced Specialty Education	Teaching Experience	Professional Involvement
Orthopedic clinician 1	31	BS MS	Rehabilitation Acute care HMO PP (owner)	CE LTC	CE Clinical faculty (LTC)	APTA IFOMT
Orthopedic clinician 2	19	BS MS	Acute care HMO PP (owner)	CE LTC	CE Clinical faculty (LTC)	APTA IFOMT
Orthopedic clinician 3	31	BS	Rehabilitation Acute care HMO PP (owner) Military	CE LTC	CE Clinical faculty (LTC) AC	APTA IFOMT
Pediatric clinician 1	15	BS MS	Pediatric clinic and school Acute care	CE NDT	CE CI AC	APTA NDTA
Pediatric clinician 2	30	BS MS PhD candidate	Rehabilitation Acute care UAPP PP (owner)	CE PNF	CE CI AC	APTA

Pediatric clinician 3	24	BS
		MS
		PhD
			Adult long-term
			  care
			Acute care
			UAPP
			Consultant for a
			  state board of
			  education
				CE
				NDT
					CE
					CI
						APTA
						NDTA

Geriatric clinician 1	23	BS MS MPA	Rehabilitation Acute care Home care Nursing home Military	CE NCS GCS	CE CI	APTA
Geriatric clinician 2	25	BS Certificate	Outpatient practice Home care Nursing home Military	CE	CE CI	APTA
Geriatric clinician 3	36	BS	Acute care Nursing home Geriatric center	CE	CE CI	—

(Continued)

Table 8–1. Professional Profiles of Expert Therapists—Cont'd

Clinician	Years of Clinical Experience	Education	Practice Settings	Advanced Specialty Education	Teaching Experience	Professional Involvement
Neurologic clinician 1	10	BS MS	Rehabilitation Outpatient practice Home care	CE NCS (pending)	CE CI AC	APTA
Neurologic clinician 2	15	BS MS	Rehabilitation Acute care Research laboratory	CE NCS	CE AC	APTA
Neurologic clinician 3	13	BS MS Certificate	Rehabilitation	CE NCS (pending) NDT	CE CI AC	APTA

BS = bachelor of science; MS = master of science; PhD = doctor of philosophy; MPA = master of public administration; HMO = health maintenance organization; PP = private practice; UAPP = university-affiliated pediatric program; CE = continuing education; LTC = long-term course; NDT = certified in neruodevelopmental treatment; PNF = certified in proprioceptive neuromuscular facilitation; NCS = neurology-certified specialist; GCS = geriatric-certified specialist; CI = clinical instructor; AC = teaching in academic classroom; APTA = American Physical Therapy Association; IFOMT = International Federation of Manipulative Therapists; NDTA = Neurodevelopment Teachers Association.

These therapists sought mentors to assist them with their development. Their mentors were frequently clinicians that they admired and respected for their work.

8

KELLUM: Jean Ayers was a powerful role model for me. She was thinking in ways that other people weren't. She was very criticized for her research but definitely was a hard thinker and would talk about it in class. I just thought it was wonderful the way she was constantly reading, constantly evaluating her theoretical framework for treatment and evaluation for the kids she worked with. She was far ahead of her time in terms of her thinking.

PEDER (orthopedic clinician): I also saw how I grew with a mentor in my first job, and he influenced me to go to Australia and seek additional training.

LUCY (pediatric clinician): I became very enamored of [teacher Margaret Rood's] ideas...and really started reading journals—doing things that I had never done before, like reading journals, starting to read books. She was the person who got me back to studying. I had not cracked a book since I had gotten out of [physical therapy] school because I thought I knew everything and I could just kind of fly by the seat of my pants in any problem that I ran into.

For some of the clinicians, mentors also included faculty or family members. They often sought more than one mentor depending on where they were focusing their energies.

TRACY (geriatric clinician): She inspires everybody to do anything. She was a great professor. She just had a way about her that when she taught you something you just learned. She knew herself and she knew how to get people involved, so she basically had a lot of influence.

BEN: My family obviously teaches me. I have used my father as a research subject, and I may write an article about my daughter because of [a health problem] she had last year....I kept a daily diary on my son's development. I observed him very, very closely....When my son wanted to learn scuba diving, I learned with him....And my wife is a special educator, so we share a lot of information.

Other personal attributes shared by the clinicians studied are discussed as part of the core dimensions of our theoretical model of expert practice in physical therapy.

THEORETICAL MODEL OF EXPERT PRACTICE

PHILOSOPHY OF PHYSICAL THERAPY

What does philosophy have to do with the practice of physical therapy? *Philosophy* can be defined as the love of or search for wisdom (7). John Dewey, a well-known American philosopher and educator, defined *philosophic reflection* as the need to identify the modes of thought and action that prevail in a given culture (8). Both of these definitions provide insight into our naturalistic study of physical therapists. We were immersed in the culture of physical therapy practice, trying to understand more about the thoughts and actions of our colleagues in actual practice settings. As we shared our cases and discussed the thoughts and actions of the therapists, a concept called *philosophy of practice* emerged. The theoretical model in Figure 8-1 shows four major

Figure 8–1 ■ Expert practice model developed for physical therapy.

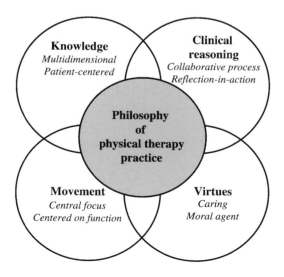

dimensions of expert practice in physical therapy: 1) knowledge, 2) clinical reasoning, 3) movement, and 4) virtues. Each therapist's philosophy of practice, comprised of components from each of the four dimensions, is at the center of our expert practice model. This philosophy of practice represents a therapist's vision of practice—that is, what it means to practice physical therapy, including the therapist's beliefs about the purpose of physical therapy and his or her goals for patients. As we spent time with our therapists and gained more insight into how they did their work, we found that each of them held his or her own identity as a practitioner. The experts' beliefs about what being a therapist means, their goals for patients, and their beliefs about the role of physical therapy in health care were central to their practices.

The experts had a relatively common understanding of their roles as physical therapists, regardless of clinical specialty area. They all emphasized that practice begins and ends with patients. This translated into listening intently to a patient's story, understanding the context of the patient's life in designing and implementing treatment, and collaborating and teaching patients and families to regain function and enhance quality of life. These therapists did not judge patients or label them *difficult, noncompliant,* or *malingering.* Instead, they assumed responsibility for trying to solve complex clinical cases. Discussing and analyzing these four dimensions of expert practice helped reveal how this philosophy of physical therapy is constructed.

MULTIDIMENSIONAL KNOWLEDGE BASE

The types and sources of knowledge used by the therapists are integral components of the model of expertise in physical therapy. These clinicians hold a deep understanding of their clinical specialty and continually work toward enlarging the scope of knowledge pertinent to their practices. They are engaged in learning when they transform their knowledge base through reflection—that is, thinking critically about practice. They tend to ask themselves questions such as, "Why didn't this intervention work with this patient?" "What am I doing wrong?" and "How can I work to solve this problem?"

The experts' specialty knowledge is multidimensional but centered on the patient. Although professional education was an initial source of knowledge, it was not enough and did not help them solve their clinical problems.

> **ELIZABETH (pediatric clinician):** The first year I was out of school, I immediately felt like I had to go back to the things I learned in physical therapy school and refile everything because I felt like everything I learned was from one perspective and I needed to immediately pull it out by diagnosis. When I started doing that—from my notes, say—I went back to my kinesiology course, and they mentioned a couple of things for one diagnosis or another, I pulled that stuff out, and I realized when I did that, the net total of the packages I had for any given diagnosis were really incomplete to me. So I went to the library and just started looking up spina bifida or muscular dystrophy or any of the diagnoses and just [started] pouring through articles. Now, that time period I loved, because I had never done anything like that before in terms of being completely self-initiated, completely for myself.

KATE (neurologic clinician): I tell students this all the time: The actual skills you learn in [physical therapy] school—like transfers and bed mobility—these things I don't think are as important as being able to look at a situation and problem solve to find your answer to best help the patient.

ISAAC: I was in the clinic now doing what I had learned from the mentor in the therapeutic exercise course. What I would find is that a patient I would treat and could not help...well, I would see them in 2 or 3 months in the hallway at our clinic. I would say, "How are you doing?" They would say they went to see this therapist who helped them in one visit. I said to myself, "Oh my gosh. I have to find out what he is doing."

As mentioned, clinical mentors were instrumental in the professional development of these expert clinicians. They admired mentors for their skills and ability to help patients, particularly in tough cases. A number of mentors usually were present at different points in each therapist's development. These mentors stimulated their thinking and helped them understand and solve clinical problems and often encouraged them to return to school and learn more.

PEDER: I basically worked 7 days a week....You were asked to take it all in and synthesize information, and then you would get a live patient. You were forced to make decisions, and you made a lot of mistakes, but you learned. I think the clinical supervision is what helped me learn light years faster.

An important source of their knowledge comes from patients. Listening to patients was identified as an essential evaluation skill.

ANNA (orthopedic clinician): You get a lot of good information if you just let your patients talk and give it to you as they want it to come out.

LUCY: One thing that I think I've really improved on with practice, and because of specific course work I've had with specific people, is shutting up and listening, and that was real hard for me to do. I just always want to jump in there with a solution no matter what it is....I've gotten much more information from listening than I ever did from structuring my questions....It really isn't a problem getting the parents to tell you about the child....It's mostly just giving them the permission to tell you...and acknowledging—honoring—what they say.

TRACY: We have to learn how to listen to what they're saying, what they're saying behind what they're saying. You can get them to participate better if you just take the time to listen to them.

Use of knowledge goes beyond understanding a patient's movement problem or mechanism of injury; it requires understanding the patient's life and social systems at work and home. For expert clinicians in pediatrics, neurology, and geriatrics, breadth of knowledge included dimensions such as normal and abnormal physical, psychological, and social development of individuals. This was in addition to their understanding of multidimensional movement problems.

LUCY: Today, I was doing a consultation with a much richer background of knowledge, not just about child development, but about family issues, about adulthood interactions, about early intervention policy at the national level...a general theoretical base about seeing the child as an integrated whole.

DESCRIPTION OF ONE TYPE OF KNOWLEDGE USED BY NEURO-LOGIC CLINICIANS: An in-depth knowledge of patients' current physical, cognitive, and psychomotor status. This knowledge was gleaned not only from observations and evaluations but also from the patient's medical record and whoever could give current information (primarily the patient's family members, physicians, psychologists, nurses, and other therapists).

BEN: Often people come [to physical therapy] after they've had injuries and they're fearful, depressed, thinking "This is the end for me." And I say, "Wait a second: You've got this life expectancy ahead of you. Now, how are you going to live? Are you going to succumb to this injury or are you going to try to rehabilitate to the highest potential?"

The experts in orthopedics demonstrated more focus on understanding patients' movement problems and teaching patients to care for and manage their problems at work and home.

ISSAC: With all patients, you can see them as unique human beings trying to deal with life just as you are. What they are here for is to understand their problem and become their own therapist. The patient must be involved in their own therapy and must understand what I am doing and become part of what I am doing.

None of the experts mentioned specific areas of traditional content knowledge in physical therapy, such as functional anatomy, biomechanics, or pathophysiology. They were much more focused on knowledge they had gained from reflecting on practice (i.e., thinking about and learning from patients). The experts compiled breadth and depth of clinical knowledge that evolved not only from experience with patients but also through their reflective processes. This clinical knowledge involves knowing how to interpret and do things in practice. For example, clinical knowledge comes from linking patient signs and symptoms with the pathophysiology of disease processes. It is also knowing how to best manage a patient and his or her family. Clinical knowledge comes from listening carefully to a patient and sorting out the patient's expectations and integrating that with knowledge about the patient's movement problem.

BEN: I try to see the musculoskeletal folks having some neurological organization to that musculoskeletal performance or their biomechanical performance....I don't think the neurological system and musculoskeletal system are separable....To learn something, you've got to start to categorize or discriminate, but understand the whole....Our patients are that way.

KELLUM: I feel sometimes I form opinions pretty quickly about certain patterns. I get an intuitive feeling about problems after I have observed them for a while, people's problems and how well they will typically do and what to expect.

ELIZABETH: The importance is to have a continual building, and because my heart is in the clinic, everything I would hear...struck some connection to what I knew to be true of children in the clinic, that stuff really caught my attention, and when I hear stuff that conflicts with what I feel I've known to be true when I actually have watched a child, then I do question it....I do want to explore it further before I just take it. I can't take it on the assumption of someone...if it really conflicts with what I've experienced in the clinic.

ANNA: I constantly try to make everything make sense to see how certain clinical pictures behave. If you go in and listen to [patients], they will tell you.

CLINICAL REASONING: CONTEXTUAL COLLABORATION

The clinical reasoning and decision-making methods used by the experts were collaborative processes between therapists and patients or patients and their families. The patient as a valued and trusted source of knowledge was the center of the assessment process. The therapists focused on a patient first as a person. For example, they were interested to know what valued activities or goals the patient had and to understand how movement problems interfered with those activities. They also wanted to know about the kinds of support the patient received at home and work. Patient and family data were selectively gathered and specific to each patient.

PEDER: You have to learn what the patient wants within the first 5 minutes because then you can focus your patient and say, "If we can change this and this we might be able to get you back to horseback riding."...What are your hobbies? Are you doing them now? Can you work? What do you expect from me? What do you do? These are the kinds of questions that help you focus on what is meaningful to the patient.

ISSAC: What brought the patient to me? Not only do I have to understand the presenting problem but in the process of understanding it, you have to understand the patient as a person and a human being.

JANIS: Part of what I feel like I do is try to work towards whatever independence the child could have. So it is important for me to help the family deal with what is going on with the child all the time, not just the end results of [the condition].

LEE (neurologic clinician): I think about making the task challenging to the patient but at the same time enabling them to carry out the activity. I am always thinking about the long-term goal and working in that direction, trying to stimulate context, the environment, as much as possible, even if I am in the clinic.

For these expert clinicians, the medical diagnosis is a supplemental, additional piece of data but is not the focus of their intervention strategies; the patient's function and family needs are central.

TRACY: The diagnosis itself is not as important as, functionally, what am I seeing that is happening. I like to know the diagnosis, especially when it comes to fractures and other conditions...but what is the reason their mobility is jeopardized? Is it a little bit of arthritis? A little bit of neurological problems? Is it a little bit of stenosis?

PEDER: Don't allow yourself to treat the same diagnosis the same way. They all react differently. You know, it is like thinking out loud. Don't be afraid to not know the right answer right now, but prove your answer through your process.

KELLUM: I can see the two people with a vestibular injury. All their results look the same. And these two people are completely different in terms of how they're doing with treatment. Why is that? How can I explain it? What is it? By trying to figure it out helps you begin to identify the problem, and that makes for good scientific inquiry.

After the problem is identified and the context is understood, the therapist engages collaborative problem solving with the patient and family, teaching them about movement and function as the intervention proceeds.

KELLUM: I feel I spend the majority of time explaining to people what the problem is and then teaching them the ideas behind the therapy and then getting them to help me design their exercise program. They do all the work. When they come back, I check their progress. The more I explain to them the idea behind the intervention, the more they buy into it.

LUCY: I'm trying to influence the dad's behavior because...it's kind of a conflict, because a parent knows a child better than anybody who sees the child once or twice a week, and I really have to respect their instinctive ways of interacting with their children.

ISSAC: The physical therapist is accountable to the patient for the success of this program. It must make sense to the patient, or the physical therapist should answer questions until it does make sense. Patients must consider themselves as a patient/therapist who is responsible for the outcome of the program. The success of the treatment depends upon the effectiveness of the patient's role as a patient/therapist. This statement is a keystone to effective treatment. The patient is both the patient and the therapist! Patients must be in a position of control in the treatment process and must be willing to make the changes in both behavior and lifestyle that are often necessary to achieve maximum recovery.

PHYLLIS (geriatric clinician): Knowing how to teach is so important and enables you to be more successful....If the patient does not understand what is happening to them, then the patient cannot make the necessary changes in behavior, nor can the patient fully comply with the therapist's activities.

In their clinical reasoning processes, the experts were not afraid to take risks and learn from mistakes through reflection. Patients were not blamed if the therapist could not figure out solutions. The therapists were challenged by tough cases and welcomed opportunities to learn from patients.

> **PEDER:** You know, I have done things to people and their symptoms have become worse and then gotten better. That is the risk you take. You see, I think that what we do with our patients does not come without risk. You just minimize the risk. I look at risk as not knowing the outcome. If you are careful, you can predict the outcome. Sometimes you are wrong.

> **LUCY:** I'm real up front with the parents about what's possible and what isn't. And I give them articles to read, or, you know, whatever they want; if it's research articles, I give them research articles or books or whatever.... They tell me what their goals are.... I'm there to consult with them on their goals, and I will share whatever information I have, but I certainly don't know everything, and I'm open to any other information. It puts you into different waters with respect to the families, and it makes it a lot easier in some ways.

> **KELLUM:** I have heard some therapists say, "That person is not very impaired." But you hear the patient say, "This gets in the way of everything I do." You have to really learn to hear what they are telling you and look at what they do. Although subtle, it's significant. Subtle but significant! For some people it's very validating because they are so happy that someone else saw their problem. The problem has been so significant to them, it gets in their way, but nobody has noticed it.

> **BEN:** On our mug [given out to patients], it says something to the effect that in rehabilitation it's better to fail by trying than fail without trying.... That is a foundation here.

MOVEMENT: A CENTRAL FOCUS AND SKILL

Skilled facilitation of movement is a central focus for all of the experts. In the data-gathering processes, hands-on skills and assessment of movement are accomplished through palpation and touch.

> **JANIS:** I have a tremendous memory for how a child feels in my hands, and I often don't see these children for 6 months. I make notes after an examination. I'm glad to have my notes, but I trust my memory.

> **BEN:** I try to use touch a lot. It's one of the first things that attracted me to physical therapy as opposed to medical school. And that is how we get to know our patients: We handle our patients.

> **PEDER (explaining the evaluation procedure he is using):** I want to get a picture of where she hurts, the quality of the movement, and I want to know how those movements relate to her area of symptoms.

KATE: I have to feel what the patient is doing. Somebody will say, "Well, what do you think is wrong?" or "What can I do to make his gait better?" And I say, "Well, I don't know, let me feel." And then I can say, "There's not enough weight shift" or "You need to facilitate this aspect of movement" or so on.

In pediatrics, play is the movement medium used for evaluation and treatment:

ELIZABETH: See, now he's starting to play with me. He's starting to play with my face. He wants me to, you know, puff air into my cheeks—you know that silly game children do. See, I feel that level of trust is just worth a million dollars. And now we are getting all the physical stuff we need.

Function was consistently the underlying reason for movement. Returning a patient to a prior level of function or designing exercises to fit with the patient's work or home environment was an important outcome.

LEE: You see here I am allowing her to move the way she wants to move. [The patient is going down steep stairs by leaning forward using both handrails and descending step over step.] I also have had patients who have *never* gone up or down their stairs step over step with alternating legs. So, I am not going to teach them something new.

ISSAC: I demonstrate the exercise to them because I want them to see. I want them to hear me, and I want them to kinesthetically feel the exercise as they are doing it.

Use of equipment either in the clinic setting or for home programs was limited. Treatment settings included patients' homes, treatment gyms, private examination rooms, and intensive care nurseries. Standard equipment consisted of treatment plinth, therapeutic mats, mirrors, steps, and basic assistive devices. Exercise programs used readily available items in the home environment and often were a vehicle for collaborative problem solving for the patient and therapist. Patient movement was facilitated and guided by the therapist's hands as instructed in exercise programs. Exercise programs were usually composed of simple exercises that were directly linked to functional movement or, in the case of pediatrics, were related to function and fun.

KATE: [A former patient] was getting into his car and dropped his car keys on the ground. Someone was going to stop and pick up his keys but he picked them up before he could be helped. And he said, "Well, I was cursing Kate when she was making me pick things up off the floor. But when I dropped those car keys I was saying, 'Thank you, thank you, thank you.'"

ANNA: I am of the belief that the majority of people will not do a lot of exercises. Part of the diagnosis is with exercise. Exercise helps me decide what is wrong with the patient. When I am not really clear, I give them one thing to do at home and then I will get more information. I tell them, "You learn and I will learn from this exercise."

JANIS: What I'm trying to do is help people learn how their baby moves and ways that they can help their baby move easily, more easily, and prevent certain problems and, hopefully, sort of incorporate what I'm showing them into whatever they're doing so that it doesn't become such a burden. I try to say that this shouldn't be something that's really going to stress you. This should be something that you can do when you're playing, when you're diapering.... So I teach people to do a little bit of light stretching because it can just be incorporated into play.

VIRTUES: CARING COMMITMENT

The moral commitment these therapists demonstrated in practice was consistently strong. They all set high standards aimed at doing the best for patients and maintaining professional competence. Clinical practice for these therapists is exciting and provides them with the opportunity to continue learning through reflection. They are constantly intrigued by patients' problems and the challenge of trying to solve them.

ANNA: I look at the patient as being a mystery. I love to get a new patient because it is a new problem to solve. It is exciting, and if it wasn't, I wouldn't be practicing today.

JANIS: I still have that feeling... you never feel like you totally know what you're doing. That's why I keep trying to learn as much as I can.

PHYLLIS: I don't think I've ever reached a point where I was what you'd call "burned out."

KELLUM: The only part I can't tolerate is feeling that I'm not doing a good job for the patients. That's the part I can't tolerate.

The experts were all able to communicate a sense of commitment and caring about patients. These therapists were confident yet humble and morally committed to patients. These characteristics often translated into advocacy roles that meant spending additional time trying to get the best treatment for patients by having conversations with case managers, writing additional letters or documentation, or serving local and professional communities.

ISAAC: I expect the patient to be better within this period of time, and I give an expectation level to him: "If this doesn't happen, you call me." This call method has evolved over time, and this ability and need for the patient to become their own therapist means that I must give them a process for thinking, and I have got to be able to reinforce it. Otherwise, I am doing nothing more than anyone else who just hands out a sheet of paper and says, "Go home and do your exercises."

LEE: I have spoken with the MD [physician] at the rehab center who is following the patient and told her about the discharge from home care and my anticipation that she would be followed by outpatient therapy. The MD said she would write the prescription. Then I made a follow-up call to the secretary to see if the patient could be scheduled for outpatient therapy soon. She did not have a prescription yet from the MD. So a week and a half later I made another contact with the physician. She apologized that she did not get a chance to write the prescription. She wrote it then while I was with her. Then I checked with the secretary again and she still didn't have the prescription. I wish I had just taken the prescription from the MD when I was there. Now I am going to have to call her again.

BEN: We have been in this community 15 years, and I know this patient. I have this attitude that when people come to my office, they become part of my family.

Our information about experts has been merged and a theoretical framework that represents a comprehensive yet simple model for our data has been presented. This framework includes four dimensions of expert practice: 1) knowledge, 2) clinical reasoning, 3) movement, and 4) virtues. A shared component, the therapist's *philosophy of practice*, is central to the framework. What does this theory mean? What is the role of prior knowledge and literature, particularly when one is developing his or her own grounded theory? When students begin their first qualitative projects, they often struggle with how the literature fits with the perspective of gathering and interpreting data from the participants in the field. This focus on understanding human behavior from the perspective of the subjects does not mean that research should be done in isolation from the literature. As one of our mentors pointed out, "One should go into the field to collect data with an open mind, not an empty head." Morse (9) argues that the process of recontextualization is the real power of qualitative research. In the process of recontextualization, the work of other researchers and established theory is used to link new findings with established work. The final section of this chapter recontextualizes our theories of expert practice for physical therapists by discussing our theory in light of established theory and research on expert practice.

BUILDING A THEORY OF PRACTICE: KEY ELEMENTS

This chapter has proposed a theoretical model of expert practice in physical therapy. The model builds on concepts from theoretical work on expertise from cognitive psychology (1,2,10–13); grounded theory work on clinical reasoning; and expertise from several professions, including nursing (3,14), occupational therapy (15), physical therapy (16–22), medicine (12,23,24), and teaching (2,11). The key elements of our theory of expert practice are summarized in the following sections; Chapter 14 discusses implications for physical therapy clinical practice and education.

KNOWLEDGE AND CLINICAL REASONING

Knowledge and clinical reasoning are key components of expertise. One of the fundamental differences between experts and novices is the knowledge brought to solving problems (1,2). For the expert physical therapists, the primary component for the use of knowledge and clinical reasoning is the patient (Box 8-1). Although knowledge used in practice is multidimensional, patients are key sources of knowledge. Specialty knowledge in an area of clinical practice is visible in evaluation processes and intervention and appears to be closely linked with the patient and the patient's presentation. Focusing on patients helps these therapists tailor their assessment process to the needs of the patient and family. In turn, the patient continues to be a primary source of knowledge for the therapists as they learn from their experiences or reflect in action. They are not afraid to take risks, and they respect and honor what patients have to say. Practitioners often depend on knowledge derived from experience and interaction with clients; this type of knowledge is often not formally admissible by a scientific method. These findings are consistent with work in other professions in which the central importance of clinical or practical knowledge has been supported (3,4,25–27).

> **FROM PSYCHOLOGY:** *Recognition of practice as a legitimate source of knowledge, in the tradition of Dewey . . . and Lewin [,] . . . requires a well-articulated epistemology of practical knowledge that illuminates the relationship among conceptual understanding, instrumental knowledge and professional expertise (27).*

> **FROM MEDICAL EDUCATION:** *An essential genre of knowledge used in practice is practical knowledge—"knowing how"—which is embedded in practical reasoning . . . [the study of reflective practice]. This suggests the importance of systematically eliciting the general principles and strategies embedded in the knowing-in-action of expert practitioners and articulating this knowledge-of-practice in codifications for guiding other practitioners, both novices and experts (25).*

BOX 8–1	*Key Elements of Knowledge and Clinical Reasoning Observed in Expert Physical Therapists*

Knowledge

Multidimensional

Patients provide important sources of knowledge, gathered by careful listening

Clinical specialty knowledge is a key component of evaluation

Knowledge continues to evolve through reflective processes

Clinical Reasoning

Demonstrate self-monitoring skills through selective data gathering, risk taking, and willingness to admit when they do not know

Clinical problem solving is a collaborative activity with patients

Focus on patient function and expectations, not the diagnosis

FROM NURSING: *Knowing signs and symptoms from the pathophysiology books does not guarantee that the clinician will be able to recognize the practical manifestations of the textbook accounts of an illness. The leap between the flat, singular descriptions of the textbooks must be made by more experienced clinicians who can directly point to the various manifestations in practice. Like the connoisseur, the practitioner must learn to discern the variations of signs and symptoms in practice (3).*

The experts carefully listen to patients and work hard to identify not only movement problems but also steps necessary for patients to succeed in overcoming these problems. They are proficient in knowing when to selectively gather data, ask questions, and take clinical risks. The therapists welcomed challenges of tough patients and were comfortable with uncertainty and ambiguity—that is, not knowing the answer. When asked how they know what to do, they indicated that many of their responses are based on experiences with patients with similar conditions and that they have confidence in trying alternate strategies. Being able to control and understand thinking processes and monitor problem-solving strategies is termed *metacognition* (2,11,22). Experts use metacognition to detect inconsistencies or links between gathered data and what they know from experience. This reasoning process is summarized by Sternberg and Horvath (2):

> *Research on expertise has shown that experts and novices differ in metacognitive or executive control of cognition. Experts typically spend a greater proportion of their solution time trying to understand the problem to be solved. Novices, in contrast, typically invest less time in trying to solve the problem and more in actually trying out different solutions. Experts are more likely to monitor their ongoing solutions attempts, checking for accuracy.*

In our study, a process of collaboration also seemed to occur between therapists and patients during clinical reasoning processes. Determining the correct diagnosis was not emphasized as central to patient management. What was critical was understanding patient function and the context of a patient's problem—that is, the social and psychological conditions that interfere with function. In work on clinical reasoning in physical therapy, Jones et al. (28) proposed a collaborative clinical reasoning process between physiotherapists and patients. The clinical reasoning process is thought to occur at two levels. The therapist works to frame and interpret problems with a hypothesis-oriented approach while listening to the patient and understanding the patient's needs and expectations (Figure 8-2).

As in nursing (3,14) and occupational therapy (15), the clinical reasoning process for physical therapy is not as analytical, deductive, or rational as portrayed in many clinical reasoning models. Knowing a patient, understanding his or her story, fitting the patient's story with clinical knowledge, and collaborating with the patient to problem solve are integral components of clinical reasoning, as noted in the following excerpt (3):

> *Experienced nurses reach an understanding of a person's experience with an illness, and, hence, their response to it, not through abstract labeling such as nursing diagnoses, but rather through knowing the particular patient, his typical pattern of responses, his story.*

8

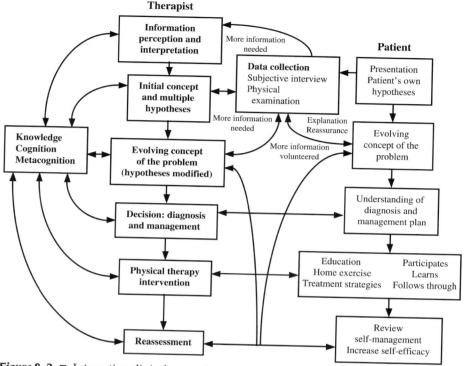

Figure 8–2 ■ Interactive clinical reasoning model. (Reprinted with permission from Jones M, Jensen GM, Edwards I. Clinical reasoning in physiotherapy. In J Higgs, M Jones (eds). *Clinical reasoning in the health professions,* ed2. Boston: Butterworth–Heinemann; 2000.)

Mattingly and Flemming (15) suggest the following about interactive reasoning in occupational therapy:

> *Creating a collaborative relationship goes beyond just being "nice" to the patient. It involves a subtle interpretation of what a person wants from therapy. Therapists interpret motives and meanings from the cues based on what patients say and do. Skilled therapists often become adept at helping patients clarify the meaning of their disability and their aspirations for the future.*

Several models of clinical reasoning have been described in efforts to represent the decision-making processes of professionals. Although these models differ somewhat among health professions, several core elements are common (3,13,15) (Table 8-2).

MOVEMENT: CENTRAL TO PRACTICE

The primary role that movement played in the clinical practice of these therapists was not surprising. Therapists exhibited manual and observational skills designed to assess functional movement. The assessment of movement dysfunction through palpation, observation, or guiding the patient's body movement was an important aspect of examination processes throughout specialties.

Table 8–2. Comparison of Clinical Reasoning Approaches in Health Professions

Health Profession	Knowledge Assumptions	Reasoning/Thinking Skills	Practitioner–Patient Interactions
Medicine			
Novices: tend to use hypothetico-deductive model (backward reasoning)	Building knowledge structures	Hypothesis generation and testing deductive thinking	History provides cues for hypothesis generation and testing
Experts: tend to use forward reasoning or a combination of backward and forward reasoning when having difficulty	Highly structured knowledge base informed by experience Specific to clinical specialty area	Pattern recognition Use of illness scripts Intuitive thinking	Listening to patient cues Illness scripts Activities
Nursing			
Cognitive and rational models limit understanding of clinical reasoning	Knowledge socially constructed	Intuitive	Listening and interpreting patients' stories
Practical reasoning part of everyday practice	Knowing the patient and family essential in clinical practice	Engaged (not disengaged) reasoning; emphasis on learning and being with others Deliberative; patient advocacy	
Occupational Therapy			
Clinical reasoning focused on human meaning involving multiple modes of reasoning	"We know more than we can tell" Tacit knowledge essential	Procedural reasoning used for and thinking about the disease and initial treatment (similar to hypothetico-deductive model) Interactive reasoning used to understand the patient; active collaboration Conditional reasoning used to understand experiences of patients (integrative form of reasoning)	Central role of narrative thinking involved in telling patient stories and story making (ways in which the therapist connects therapy to the patients' lives)

Source: Data from Benner P, Tanner CA, Chesla CA. Expertise in nursing practice. New York: Springer; 1996; Patel VL, Kaufmann D, Magder S. The acquisition of medical expertise in complex environments. In KA Ericsson (ed). *The road to excellence.* Mahwah, NJ: Lawerence Erlbaum; 1996, 127–165; and Mattingly C, Flemming MH. *Clinical reasoning.* Philadelphia: FA Davis; 1994.

8

The manual skills of the therapists appeared to be unconscious parts of their work because they often engaged in conversation with patients or family members as they worked. When the therapists were interviewed while watching videotapes of themselves, they were able to describe exactly what they were doing with their own bodies, what they felt with their hands, and their rationale for facilitating patient movement. The therapists' eyes and hands were major tools in their practices. Facilitation of patient's movement or motor performance was a critical part of prescribed exercise and home programs. Exercise programs were directly linked to the patient's function at home or work.

Focusing on restoring functional movement is consistent with the description of the scope of physical therapy practice outlined in the *Guide to Physical Therapist Practice* (29):

> **PHYSICAL THERAPISTS:** *Provide services to patients/clients who have impairments, functional limitations, disabilities, or changes in physical function and health status resulting from injury, disease, or other causes.... [I]mpairment is defined as loss or abnormality of physiological, psychological, or anatomical structure or function; functional limitation, as restriction of the ability to perform—at the level of the whole person—a physical action, activity, or task in an efficient, typically expected, or competent manner; and disability, as the inability to engage in age-specific, gender-specific, or sex-specific roles in a particular social context and physical environment.*

Many professionals have long debated the role of movement dysfunction as the unique aspect of the discipline of physical therapy (30–33). In 1988 Sahrman (33) argued that diagnoses should be made by physical therapists:

> *[J]ust as expansion of information about the nervous system led to the establishment of neuroscience . . . and the formation of doctoral programs . . . similar events are occurring with movement as the focus and with prevention and treatment of movement dysfunction as the applied science of the field. As the expertise of physical therapists grows in this area, they are increasing their ability to identify the key factors that underlie movement and movement dysfunctions that most often are separate from the medical problem that may have initiated a movement impairment.*

In 1998, in the 29th McMillan lecture, Sahrman (34) again made the case for physical therapy:

> *We have made significant strides in the transition from a technical field characterized by individuals skilled in the application of physical modalities to a profession characterized by knowledge of the movement function of the body.... [T]he profession must continue to develop the concept of movement as a physiologic system and work to get physical therapists recognized as the experts in that system.*

The expert physical therapists in our study demonstrated persistent and skillful manual and observational abilities. They were intent on designing interventions and exercise programs that were focused on functional movement specific to individual patient needs.

PROFESSIONAL VIRTUES

The experts studied had a strong inner drive to succeed and continue to learn. In addition, they were intellectually challenged by patients' problems, had their patients' best interests in mind, and focused on solving problems rather than judging or blaming a patient if a problem was not easily solved. The attributes observed in these therapists are evidence of professional virtues.

Studies in nursing (3,35) suggest that ethical expertise stems from caring practice in which recognition and respect for the other (patient or practitioner), mutual realization, and protection of vulnerability are key elements. Gastmans et al. (35) distinguish between nursing as technology and nursing as practice. In terms of techniques, the value of activities is measured by the degree of efficiency. In professional practice, activities involve competent performance of techniques and human interaction, such as establishing relationships and teaching patients and families. Professional practice cannot be measured only through efficiency; it must also consider what good is sought for the patient. Thus, nursing practice is characterized by a unique capacity to make choices in particular situations (clinical reasoning) to bring about good for a patient and his or her family. This is similar to our experts, who we described as patient advocates. Advocacy was a serious responsibility for our experts, and they believed that they had the obligation to insist on the best possible care for their patients.

Benner (3) describes well the moral dimension of clinical judgment:

Clinical judgment cannot be sound without knowing the patient's/family's situation and moral concerns. The moral perception cannot be astute without knowing and caring about the patient/family.

In physical therapy, Purtilo (36,37) has argued the importance of ethics in examining professional responsibility. Character traits or virtues, such as respect for individual differences in patients, compassion, integrity, and honesty, along with duties and rights, help guide therapists. "While duties and rights guide what one ought to do, character traits or virtues help specify ideals regarding the type of person one ought to be" (37). Therefore, the combination of the two defines professional responsibility.

PHILOSOPHY OF PRACTICE

At the heart of our theoretical model of expert practice is philosophy of practice. Philosophy of practice is not a single entity; it has elements of the four dimensions of expertise (i.e., knowledge, reasoning, movement, and virtues). Key elements in the philosophy of practice include the role of practical knowledge learned through reflective practice; core beliefs about patient-centered evaluation and treatment; collaborating and teaching patients and families to maximize function; skillful movement assessment through observation and manual skills; and shared commitment to act in the best interests of patients.

The distinction between knowing that (facts and information) and knowing how (how to do things) is derived from traditional Western philosophy. Philosophical discussion and debate continues about different approaches to generating knowledge (25,26). Some argue that the scientific method is the only way to generate knowledge and that knowing how is just more personal, non-propositional knowledge. A key point of discussion is whether knowledge can only be discovered through scientific methods or if knowledge can also be developed as part of human interaction and behavior (26,38,39). Our study incorporated an interpretive approach, using qualitative methods to understand how therapists make sense of their practice. Many authors now advocate multiple ways of generating knowledge (38–40).

Higgs and Titchen (40) have discussed multiple ways of developing knowledge in health care professions. They assert that a third dimension or category of knowledge is important for health professionals: personal knowledge. *Personal knowledge* is defined as understanding and knowledge central to an individual's sense of self. This knowledge is the result of personal experiences and reflections on these experiences. They suggest that clinicians need to develop "a personal knowledge base, including a depth of self-understanding which enable[s] them to understand complex human desires for dignity, independence and support, to appreciate the needs and frames of reference of their patients or clients, to learn to cope with pain, frailty and human endeavor and to learn to deal with ethical dilemmas within the clinical situation."

Higgs and Titchen envision three dimensions of knowledge (personal, propositional [knowing that], and procedural [knowing how]) that overlap and intersect. At the center of the intersection is what they call *influences*, which include frames of reference (e.g., philosophy, values, beliefs) (Figure 8-3). A therapist's

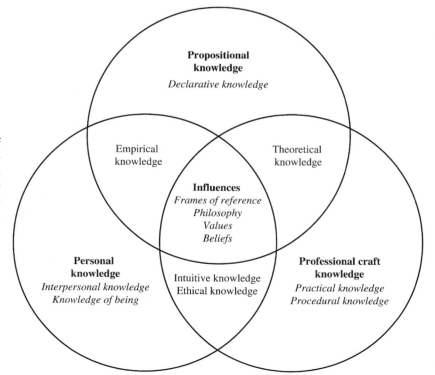

Figure **8–3** ■ Three types of knowledge used in clinical practice. (Reprinted with permission from Higgs J, Titchen A. The nature, generation and verification of knowledge. *Physiother.* 1995;81:526.)

philosophy is an extremely important and vital concept that integrates elements of knowledge, reflective clinical reasoning, professional virtues, and movement.

REFLECTIONS ON OUR MODEL OF EXPERTISE

Our findings suggest that expertise among physical therapists is some combination of multidimensional knowledge, clinical reasoning skills, skilled movement, and virtue. We propose that all four of these dimensions contribute to the therapist's philosophy or conception of practice. One of the benefits of theory development is that the theory allows one to continue to discuss, refine, and expand the model. Our grounded theory of expertise fits well into what Robert Merton first called "middle range theories" (41). Middle range theories are important tools in applied fields such as teaching, nursing, medicine, or physical therapy. These kinds of theories allow us to explore knowing more about ourselves and our work as our "knowing or knowledge base" matures through experience and understanding (42). We continue to engage in a rich discussion with our colleagues about expertise in physical therapy. Many of you have contributed to our thinking about how the model applies not only to expert practice but also to the journey that novices engage in from professional education to entry into practice. We have taken our model, as a middle range theory or working model, and proposed that novices start with working in these core dimensions of expertise as part of their professional education. Although these four elements may exist, it is likely that they are not well integrated at the novice level (Figure 8-4). As the novice continues to develop, although each of the dimensions may become stronger, they may not be well integrated for proficient practice. We propose that competent physical therapy has begun to integrate these dimensions of expertise. Our expert model then is a therapist who has fully integrated these dimensions of expertise that, in turn, leads to an explicit philosophy of practice.

This model of expertise is merely a starting point for continued dialogue and inquiry for the profession. As we continue to reflect on not only the model of expertise but what we do not know about professional learning, novice development, and expertise, we have far more questions than answers. For example: How can education be designed to address the multiple dimensions of professional competence? What kinds of knowledge should be used to teach in the classroom and laboratory? Students may be told that the solution to a patient's problem is not in the textbook, but what is necessary to facilitate the building of a knowledge base for a student that is multidimensional? What kinds of teaching strategies enhance students' abilities to listen to patients and value patients as important sources of knowledge? What evidence do we see in practice that is consistent with the core values of the profession? What is the relationship between the profession and the society we serve? As we have continued to share our work with colleagues through professional presentations, workshops, and collegial discussions, our suggestions and questions for education, practice, and research have grown. In this revised edition, we have expanded the last part of our book from one chapter of implications to three chapters of implications across research, practice, and education.

In 1989 Rose (43) called for "developing theories of practice" by going to the "trenches of practice and observing real-life situations." His claim was that

8

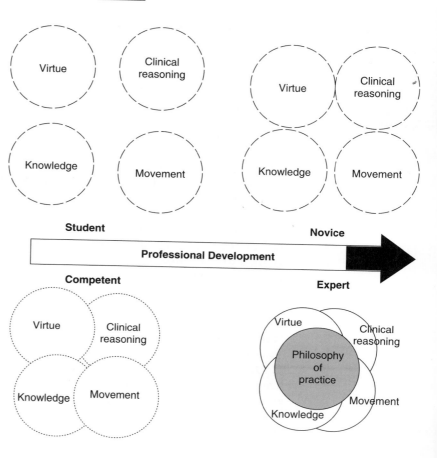

Figure 8–4 ■ As a student moves from novice status, the dimensions of the model start to come closer together but are still not sufficiently integrated for competent practice. The model for the competent therapist shows the beginning of integration of the dimensions of expertise. As these dimensions begin to overlap, the model moves toward full integration and a well-developed philosophy of practice.

doing so increases the probability that the theory has validity and will make a contribution to daily practice. His assertions hold true today. We hope that our theory of physical therapy practice helps others discuss, debate, and continue to evolve theories of physical therapy.

REFERENCES

1. Ericsson KA, Smith J (eds). *Toward a general theory of expertise.* New York: Cambridge University Press; 1991.
2. Sternberg RJ, Horvath JA. A prototype view of expert teaching. *Educ Res.* 1995:24:9–17.
3. Benner P, Tanner CA, Chesla CA. *Expertise in nursing practice.* New York: Springer; 1996.
4. Schön D. *The reflective practitioner: how professionals think in action.* New York: Basic Books; 1983.
5. Shulman L. The wisdom of practice in teaching: managing complexity in medicine and teaching. In D Berliner, B Rosenshine (eds). *Talks to teachers.* New York: Random House; 1987.
6. Rothstein JM. On defining subjective and objective measurements. *Phys Ther.* 1989;69:577–579.
7. Guralnik DB (ed). *Webster's new world dictionary of the American language,* Second College Edition. New York: Simon & Schuster; 1980.
8. Gouinlock J (ed). *The moral writings of John Dewey.* Amherst, NY: Prometheus Books; 1994.
9. Morse J (ed). Emerging from the data: the cognitive processes of analysis in qualitative inquiry. In J Morse (ed). *Critical issues in qualitative research methods.* Thousand Oaks, CA: Sage; 1994.
10. Ericsson KA (ed). *The road to excellence.* Mahwah, NJ: Lawrence Erlbaum; 1996.
11. Sternberg R. Abilities are forms of expertise. *Educ Res.* 1998;27:11–20.
12. Chi MT, Glaser R, Farr M (eds). *The nature of expertise.* Mahwah, NJ: Lawrence Erlbaum; 1988.

13. Patel VL, Kaufman D, Magder S. The acquisition of medical expertise in complex environments. In KA Ericsson (ed). *The road to excellence*. Mahwah, NJ: Lawrence Erlbaum; 1996.
14. Benner P. *From novice to expert: excellence and power in clinical nursing practice*. Menlo Park, CA: Addison-Wesley; 1982.
15. Mattingly C, Flemming MH. *Clinical reasoning*. Philadelphia: FA Davis; 1994.
16. Payton OD. Clinical reasoning process in physical therapy. *Phys Ther*. 1985;65:924–928.
17. Thomas-Edding D. Clinical problem solving in physical therapy and its implications for curriculum development. In *Proceedings of the 10th international congress of the world confederation for physical therapy*, May 17–22, 1987. Sydney, Australia; 1987, 100–104.
18. May BJ, Dennis JK. Expert decision making in physical therapy: a survey of practitioners. *Phys Ther*. 1991;71:190–202.
19. Embrey DG, Guthrie MR, White OR, et al. Clinical decision making by experienced and inexperienced pediatric physical therapists for children with diplegic cerebral palsy. *Phys Ther*. 1996;76:20–33.
20. Jensen GM, Shepard KF, Hack LM. The novice versus the experienced clinician: insights into the work of the physical therapist. *Phys Ther*. 1990;70:314–323.
21. Jensen GM, Shepard KF, Gwyer J, Hack LM. Attribute dimensions that distinguish master and novice physical therapy clinicians in orthopedic settings. *Phys Ther*. 1992;72:711–722.
22. Higgs J, Jones M (eds). *Clinical reasoning in the health professions*. Boston: Butterworth–Heinemann; 1995.
23. Elstein AS, Shulman LS, Sprafka SA. Medical problem solving: a ten year retrospective, *Eval Health Prof*. 1990;13:5–36.
24. Schmidt HG, Norman GR, Boshuizen HP. A cognitive perspective on medical expertise: theory and implications. *Acad Med*. 1990;65:611–621.
25. Harris I. New expectations for professional competence. In L Curry, J Wergin (eds). *Educating professionals: responding to new expectations for competence and accountability*. San Francisco: Jossey-Bass; 1993.
26. Hoshmand LT, Polkinghorne DE. Redefining the science-practice relationship and professional training. *Am Psychol*. 1992;47:55–66.
27. Eraut M. *Developing professional knowledge and competence*. Washington, DC: Falmer Press; 1994.
28. Jones M, Jensen GM, Edwards I. Clinical reasoning in physiotherapy. In J Higgs, M Jones (eds). *Clinical reasoning in the health professions*, ed 2. Boston: Butterworth–Heinemann; 2000.
29. American Physical Therapy Association. *Guide to physical therapist practice*. Alexandria, VA: American Physical Therapy Association; 1997.
30. Hislop HJ. Tenth Mary McMillan lecture: the not-so-impossible dream. *Phys Ther*. 1975;55:1069–1080.
31. Rothstein JM. Pathokinesiology: a name for our times? *Phys Ther*. 1986;66:364–365.
32. Winstein CJ, Knecht HG. Movement science and its relevance to physical therapy. *Phys Ther*. 1990;70:759–762.
33. Sahrman S. Diagnosis by the physical therapist—a prerequisite for treatment. *Phys Ther*. 1988;68:1703–1706.
34. Sahrman S. Paving the path to the future: 29th McMillan Lecture. *Phys Ther*. 1998;78:1208–1219.
35. Gastmans C, Dierckx de Casterle B, Schotsmans P. Nursing considered as moral practice: a philosophical-ethical interpretation of nursing, *Kennedy Inst Ethics J*. 1998;8:43–69.
36. Purtilo RB. *Ethical dimensions in the health professions*, ed 3. Philadelphia: WB Saunders; 1998.
37. Purtilo RB. Professional responsibility in physiotherapy. *Physiother*. 1986;72:579–583.
38. Bruner J. Narrative and paradigmatic modes of thought. In ED Eisner. *84th year book of the National Society for the Study of Education*. Chicago: University of Chicago Press; 1985.
39. Candib L. Way of knowing in family medicine: contributions from a feminist perspective, *Family Med*. 1998;30:672–676.
40. Higgs J, Titchen A. The nature, generation and verification of knowledge. *Physiother*. 1995;81:521–530.
41. Merton RK. *On theoretical sociology*. New York: Free Press; 1967.
42. Shulman L. *Teaching as community property: essays on higher education*. San Francisco: Jossey-Bass; 2004.
43. Rose S. Physical therapy diagnosis: role and function. *Phys Ther*. 1989;69:535–537.

8

POSTSCRIPT
The Voices of Our Experts—
10 Years Later

We have often wondered: Where and what are our "experts" doing now? How do they see their professional work now? What would we hear if we asked them to discuss their current roles in the profession? One of the concepts we have highlighted strongly in this revised edition is focus on expertise as a continuous process—not a state of achievement obtained through accumulation of years of experience or recognition through certifications or awards. We decided to ask our experts the following question and gather responses from those who were still in practice.

In the last 10 years what is/are the most significant thing(s) you have done that has/have been meaningful and/or shaped your practice?

We found the following core themes in their responses.

LIFELONG LEARNING

By far, the strongest theme from our experts was evidence of their continued commitments to learning. This pursuit of learning took different forms—from pursuing a doctor of philosophy degree (PhD) or a doctor of physical therapy degree (DPT), to obtaining additional clinical certifications and engagements in clinical research.

Recently I became certified in the administration of NNNS [NICU Network Neurobehavioral Scale]. This is the third generation assessment of neurobehavioral organization derived from the work of T. Berry Brazelton and others that can be used to evaluate high risk and drug-exposed infants.

The most significant thing(s) I have done involved making more time to read the literature, performing online searches, and sharing information with my staff that is relevant for improving patient care....Also I am starting my transitional DPT degree...

Returned to school to get my DPT....I am just finishing up my last two papers—a case study and an EBM project.

170

First of all, I'm on my own with nobody down the hall to consult with. This made me pull out every scrap of knowledge I have and also made me more aware of knowing where my limits are.

In the past 10 years, the most significant thing that has shaped my career was returning to school. I am just about to complete a PhD program focusing my coursework on epidemiology in . . . the Department of Physical Therapy and Rehabilitation Science.

REFLECTION IN AND ON PATIENT-CENTERED PRACTICE

A second theme in their responses was the centrality of reflection in and on their practices. These therapists continue to engage in an inquiry process that is focused on clinical questions arising from their practices. They certainly still do not have all the answers; they continue search for answers that are needed in patient care. Here we see their reflections on their work that bring out their passions for patient-centered care.

As a clinician, I have also become more patient in interviewing patients and really working on improving my listening skills. . . . most of my patients are complex (emotionally and from a pathological viewpoint). . . . From a basic clinical experience (treating thousands of patients) my "handling skills" have improved markedly. However, working on my communication skills (taking them to a very high level) has most likely been the greatest change in my clinical practice.

I helped write the published practice guidelines for physical therapists in the neonatal intensive care unit. . . . I am the site coordinator for a multicenter NIH-funded study to norm a new infant postural assessment.

I have done more work on developing and validating a method of treatment for the worst arm and neck pain. I consider my classroom and teachers my treatment room and more than 1,500 patients who have failed traditional PT. I have used my clinical reasoning skills, my experience, and my patients' experiences to develop a new treatment method. With the evidence-based search of the literature . . . I have clearer insight . . .

When you are seeing children in their homes, the mothers tell lots of things that they don't tell you in the clinic. For a long time I have tried my best to focus on the needs for children to have fun and to make therapy fun. What I have realized is that we need to pay attention to the parents in this respect. . . . helping them focus on how much progress their child has made.

In the past 6 years I have been slowly working toward turning my vision of building a physical therapy and fitness center specifically designed for the physically challenged into a reality. . . . My physical therapy practice has been enhanced with the influx of soldiers returning from Iraq and Afghanistan.

After years of clinical practice, I came to believe that the most significant barriers that impede the participation of people with disabilities from fully

8

participating in all aspects of life and pursuing their personal goals are environmental barriers, including physical, social, and psychological aspects of the environment...I decided to return to school to learn how to take a population view of disability and to better understand the problems experienced by people with disabilities.

GRAPPLING AND SURVIVING WITHIN THE HEALTH CARE SYSTEM

The health care system continues to change. Ethical distress is a daily occurrence because health care often is seen as a commodity driven by economic forces instead of a system for meeting the needs of those who need physical therapy care. The challenges in negotiating this system—helping patients and families receive necessary physical therapy—certainly are being felt by the experts in practice.

From a business point of view...the legislature and insurance industry has done the most to influence my practice....We have case managers and adjusters with no experience in the utilization of "Evidence Based Medicine" dictating how many visits the patient will receive....the name of the game is deny care with the hope that the patient will get better without any care or the patient or clinicians will get worn out in trying to acquire authorization for more treatment.

What a mess our health care delivery system is in this country. Dealing with private insurance companies and Medicaid takes up a lot of my time when trying to get what a child needs.

Although there is honest recognition of the seriousness of the issues they face in the health care system, this is coupled with the experts' commitments to continue to work for doing what is best for their patients and for the profession. They are not complicit, depressed, or apathetic. They have not changed career paths. They are survivors who are committed to the work they do and to the future of the profession.

I have also become in a sense a cog in a big Early Intervention Machine! I really have to coordinate what I do with state systems, child service coordinators, other interventionists.

I am quite proud of our profession in a way I wasn't before. Being in the community has shown me how well we work and how respected we are.

The most significant thing I have done involved making more time to read the literature, perform online searches, and sharing information with my staff that is relevant for improving patient care....Improving our clinical education system will help improve patient care, facilitate clinical research, improve the evidence, and improve the quality of clinicians.

Serving the soldiers with multiple joint problems and working with the Army regulations and its system of health care delivery for outpatients has been stimulating as well as challenging for my staff. We are happy to serve those who serve our country.

What can we take from these responses from our experts? Their voices lend support to key elements in the continued discussion in the health professions literature about professional preparation, professional competence, and the need for a renewed sense of professionalism. Leach describes the fully formed professional as follows:

> *"The fully-formed professional is habitually faithful to professional values in highly complex situations; it is fidelity coupled with effectiveness. Both fidelity and effectiveness are dependent on experience and reflection on experiences..."* *(2004, p. 12) (1).*

These voices of our experts verify that their core values are central to their practices and that reflection in and on practice is a critical element in their work.

Returning to Epstein and Hundert's (2) definition of professional competence—"professional competence is the habitual and judicious use of communication, knowledge, technical skills, clinical reasoning, emotions, values and reflection in daily practice for the benefit of the individual and community being served." We see our experts integrating their knowledge and skills with their *habits of mind* as they continue their work as moral agents for what is in the best interest of the patients and communities they serve.

REFERENCES

1. Leach D. Professionalism: the formation of physicians. *Am J Bioethics* 2004;4(2):11–12.
2. Epstein R, Hundert E. Defining and assessing professional competence. *JAMA.* 2002;287:226–235.

8

Part III

Lessons Learned and Applied

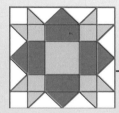

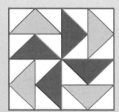

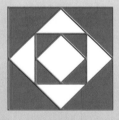

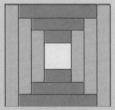

At the time of publication of our first edition of *Expertise in Physical Therapy Practice*, we could identify only a small number of colleagues who were similarly engaged in the study of expertise in physical therapy, and we invited two of them to provide work for that text in a chapter that we called "Other Views of Expertise in Physical Therapy." Today we can acknowledge a growing cadre of researchers with interest in this area, and we have invited four of them to provide the reader with a sampling of work by colleagues who have applied the model of expertise in various investigative and practice initiatives. These individuals are both deepening our understanding of expertise and provoking the next questions in this field of discovery and application. By including their work in this text, we hope to provide a unique archive of the growth of expertise research, grounded theory and applied, in physical therapy.

In Chapter 9 Linda Resnik provides an overview of a series of quantitative and qualitative investigations that combine the foundational work in two emerging theoretical fields in physical therapy, expertise and outcomes of clinical care. In Chapter 10, Ian Edwards and Mark Jones also use a qualitative grounded theory methodology to examine the nature and scope of clinical reasoning of expert physical therapists in Australia. In Chapter 11 Elizabeth Mostrom revisits her ethnographic portrait of a neurologic expert physical therapist in light of the developing grounded theory of expertise. The final chapter in this section, Chapter 12 by Ann Jampel and Mike Sullivan, presents a unique documentation of the application of the model of expertise to a professional development model for physical therapists and other hospital staff at Massachusetts General Hospital.

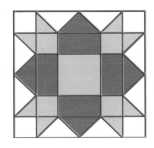

9 Expert Practice and Clinical Outcomes

Linda Resnik

Jensen, Gwyer, Hack, and Shepard's research on physical therapy expertise has been incredibly influential in my career development. The patient-centered practice model of expertise that they articulated has resonated with my own clinical experience and stimulated my interest in research on health services delivery. Their rigorous approach to qualitative research has provided a solid roadmap that guided the design and analysis of my dissertation research. Ultimately, that work stimulated me to pursue further post-graduate research training, launching me into a research career studying health service delivery in rehabilitation.—Linda Resnik, PhD, PT, OCS

CHAPTER OVERVIEW

This chapter begins with a critique of subject-selection methods in expertise research and introduces outcomes research, which has been used as an alternative way to identify expert subjects. Next, an overview of findings and implications from studies that used outcomes research to explore expertise and the relationship between therapist characteristics, service-delivery patterns, and patient outcomes in orthopedics is presented (1–4). Three studies that will be discussed examined physical therapy outcomes in the context of care of patients with low back pain. The fourth study examined physical therapy services delivery in outpatient orthopedic practice for patients with all types of impairments. The chapter ends with a discussion of limitations and opportunities of using outcomes research in studies of expertise and service delivery and provides suggestions for future research directions.

HOW DO WE IDENTIFY PHYSICAL THERAPY EXPERTS?

Researchers who study expertise must begin by identifying experts for their sample. What are the best ways to identify a sample to study, and how can researchers be sure that those they select for the sample really are experts? Historically, researchers have tackled this challenge by sampling clinicians based on their reputations and the number of years that they have practiced. This approach has face validity because professional colleagues are likely to recognize practitioners of excellence among their ranks. Thus, the theoretical models of physical therapy expertise developed prior to 2002 were based on research on therapists sampled on the basis of years of experience or reputation (5–10).

These methods of subject selection ensured a pool of subjects who were actively involved with the American Physical Therapy Association (APTA), known to APTA section leadership, and active in educational activities. For example, the 12 subjects in the Jensen et al. study had practiced in a minimum of 3 different practice settings and had 10–31 years of experience (8). Most had master's degrees, 11 out of 12 were APTA members, and all were teaching in some capacity.

Although this type of reputation is an important facet of being recognized as an expert, it was not clear if and how these attributes were related to patient outcomes. It was generally presumed that there was a relationship between a practitioner's level of expertise and patient outcomes, (6,10–12), and it was assumed that expert therapists were indeed those who achieved the best clinical outcomes. However, no prior research had actually tested this hypothesis (5–8). No prior researchers had identified and studied therapists chosen because their patients had the best outcomes, arguably one of the most important defining features of an expert.

In qualitative research, the term *transferability* is used to judge the extent to which the findings can be applied to other situations or contexts. Because the transferability of earlier theoretical models of physical therapy expertise was limited to the practice of peer-nominated experts, it was unclear if the tenets of the existing theoretical model of expertise would be transferable to expert therapists selected only because their patients achieve the best outcomes. Subject selection based on reputation and experience would, by definition, exclude therapists who might actually have the best outcomes but were not known within the APTA or were newer to the profession. Thus, there was a need to identify expert therapists based on their patients' outcomes and to compare the qualities of these experts with those of peer-nominated experts reported in the literature.

USING CLINICAL OUTCOMES TO IDENTIFY EXPERT THERAPISTS

Given the advances in the field of outcomes measurement and the availability of ample physical therapy outcomes data, assessment of patient outcomes offered a data-based alternative to identifying expert therapists based on reputation or years of experience. The methodology for evaluating outcomes of care using clinical databases is a relatively new approach in physical therapy, first introduced to the profession in the mid-1990s (13). At that time, Alan Jette advocated a shift in the dominant research paradigm in physical therapy to incorporate outcomes research, which could address disability outcomes in addition to traditional impairment outcomes (13).

Until that time, an impediment to studies on clinical outcomes of physical therapy had been lack of credible and widely accepted operational definitions of improvement following intervention (14) and the lack of a "gold standard" for patient self-reports of health status (15) to assess the outcome of intervention. By the mid-1990s substantial advances in the measurement of treatment outcomes using health-related quality of life (HRQL) instruments had occurred. HRQL measurement instruments quantify physical, psychological, and social dimensions reflecting HRQL.

HRQL data have been recommended as outcomes measures for physical therapists (PTs) (16) and have been used to assess treatment outcomes in patients with a wide variety of health conditions (17). There has been a proliferation of outcomes research in physical therapy using HRQL data (14,15, 18–29). There has also been an increased use of outcomes measurement and measurement systems in clinical settings as a component of evidence-based practice (EBP). Systematic tracking and evaluation of measures of treatment outcome are consistent with the final step of an evidence-based approach to practice: evaluation of clinical performance (30–33). Using patient HRQL to identify expert therapists does not limit participation to experienced clinicians or to those with widespread collegial recognition and has the potential to include subjects with diverse professional profiles chosen because of their level of patient outcomes.

9

THE STUDIES

USING CLINICAL OUTCOMES TO IDENTIFY EXPERTS AND EXPLORE THE THEORY OF EXPERTISE

A two-phase mixed methodology study was conducted to identify and then compare characteristics of therapists whose patients reported high levels of improvement in HRQL with those of therapists whose patients reported average HRQL improvement and thus to build on the prior theoretical framework of physical therapy expertise (1,2). This two-part study incorporated both quantitative and qualitative data, which were both considered in the development of the resulting theory of expertise. The quantitative phase of study used a retrospective analysis of the data from a large clinical database (1). The second phase involved a qualitative study of a smaller number of therapists who were identified in the quantitative phase (2). Brief summaries of these two studies are presented in the following.

In phase one, expert therapists were profiled by use of patient self-report of HRQL, and statistical methods were used to compare characteristics of therapists whose patients reported high levels of improvement in HRQL (experts) with characteristics of therapists whose patients reported average HRQL improvement (average therapists). An existing commercial database, the Focus On Therapeutic Outcomes, Inc. (FOTO) database,* containing information on patient HRQL data, along with therapist years of experience, educational degree, specialty certification, gender, and practice setting, provided an opportunity to investigate the association of these factors (34).

Because there was a need to identify therapists whose patients had the best clinical outcomes, it was essential to adjust for differences in therapists' caseload that could influence patient outcome. Otherwise, patient differences could potentially confuse or confound the results of the analysis. A statistical risk-adjustment process involving development of Generalized Linear Models (GLM) was used to control the effects of confounding variables (35–37). Residual scores were aggregated by the therapist, and the aggregated scores were used to classify therapists by their patients' outcomes because they represented the mean differences between patients' expected outcome and the actual outcomes obtained. Differences between therapist years of experience, type of professional (entry-level) degree, record of advanced orthopedic certification, region of the country, and type of practice setting were assessed.

The qualitative phase of study was guided by the grounded theory approach and used a multiple case study design (38), modeled after earlier work by Jensen et al. (8). The initial sampling decisions were made based on the analysis of the data from the FOTO database performed in phase one, in which 10% of therapists whose patients had the highest mean residual scores were identified as expert therapists and 10% of therapists whose patients had average mean residual scores were identified as average therapists. Participants were asked to provide a copy of their curriculum vitae, submit a written statement of philosophy explaining their approach to the clinical management of patients with low back pain, and schedule an appointment for a telephone interview. Participant interviews and subsequent case analyses proceeded until no new or contradictory findings were discovered and resulted in 12 participants—6 from each of the 2 groups (expert and average).

Participants from the expert group were sorted into experienced and novice subcategories based on their years of clinical experience. Because the range of experience among participants in the average group was more uniformly distributed, no subgrouping by experience was needed in the group classified as average. Data analysis started by open coding of the initial interviews, philosophy statements, and résumés. The overall research design involved three phases of data analysis: within-case, cross-case, and cross-group analysis (39–41). Credibility of the analysis was enhanced by using the following verification strategies: source triangulation, examination of researcher bias, member checks, use of

---

*Focus On Therapeutic Outcomes Inc, PO Box 11444, Knoxville, TN 37939-1444.

thick description, peer reviewing and debriefing, and an audit trail of methodologic and analytic decisions (42).

The most surprising finding from the first phase of study was that therapists classified as expert and average had similar numbers of years of clinical experience (8 and ± 8 years). Furthermore, there were no differences between groups in therapist gender, practice setting, region of the country, or professional physical therapy degree.

The primary attributes and relationships identified in the theory derived from these studies are explained in this chapter, with a synopsis of the theoretical model shown in Figure 9-1. Therapists classified as expert were distinguished by a patient-centered approach to care. In this approach, patients are viewed as active participants in therapy, and a primary goal of care is empowering patients—achieved through collaboration between therapist and patient, clinical reasoning, patient education, and establishment of a good patient–therapist relationship. The patient-centered approach results from the interplay of clinical reasoning, values,

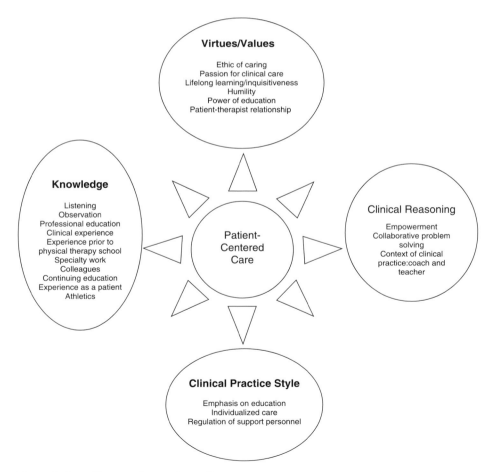

Figure **9–1** ■ Theory of expert practice.

virtues, and therapist knowledge. This approach permeates and guides the clinician's style of practice.

Excellence in patient-centered care involves clinical reasoning that is centered on the individual patient and enhanced by a strong knowledge base, skills in differential diagnosis, and self-reflection. The primary goals of empowering patients, increasing self-efficacy beliefs, and involving patients in the care process are facilitated by patient–therapist collaborative problem solving. This approach alters the therapeutic relationship and emphasizes the professional's primary role in supporting and enhancing patients' abilities to make autonomous choices (43).

In this theory, the foundation for the expert clinician's approach to care is an ethic of caring and a respect for individuality. Clinicians who value and appreciate patient individuality garner more information from and about patients. This knowledge is gained through attentive listening, trust- building, and observation. These findings suggest that therapists' passion for clinical care, their desire to continually learn and improve their skills coupled with the qualities of humility and inquisitiveness, drive their use of reflection, or thinking about practice. This combination of factors helps accelerate the acquisition and integration of knowledge.

The patient-centered approach is exemplified by the therapist's emphasis on patient education and by strong beliefs about the power of education. In this study, therapists classified as expert emphasized the patient–practitioner relationship and carefully regulated their delegation of care to support personnel. These efforts promote patient empowerment and self-efficacy, better continuity of services, more skillful care, and more individualized plans of care.

The therapists classified as expert possessed a broad, multidimensional knowledge base: a mixture of knowledge gained from entry-level education, clinical experience, specialty work, colleagues, patients, continuing education, personal experience with movement and rehabilitation, and teaching experience. Specific types of knowledge, such as years of clinical experience, were not as critical as the sum total of the knowledge base. Knowledge acquisition appears to be facilitated by work experience prior to attending physical therapy school.

The Impact of Advanced Clinical Certification

Given the growing emphasis on specialization and certification in physical therapy and the increasing number of therapists who have completed or are pursuing specialist certification and residency and manual therapy certification programs, further exploration of the association between advanced certification and patient outcomes was warranted. Only one other research team had analyzed clinical outcomes of therapists with orthopedic clinical specialist (OCS) certification (26). Little research on clinical outcomes of residency graduates or therapists with manual therapy certification or training has been published, but reports of perceptions of OCS-certified therapists (44) and program graduates from the Kaiser Permanente residency program suggest benefits (45).

The purpose of my next study, "Influence of Advanced Orthopedic Certification on Clinical Outcomes of Patients with Low Back Pain," was to assess outcomes of care, as measured by changes in patient self-report of health status, for patients with lumbar impairments treated by clinicians with and without specialization (3). This retrospective study used a sample of patients treated by physical therapists for low back pain (the same sample described in phase one). Three types of physical therapists' advanced certification were evaluated: OCS certification, graduation from residency programs approved by the American Academy of Orthopedic Manual Physical Therapists (AAOMPT), and miscellaneous manual therapy certification (MTC).

Three measures of physical function—the FOTO overall health status measure, the SF-12 (short-form 12) Physical Component Summary (PCS) (46), and SF-36 physical functioning scale (PF-10) (35)—were used as the outcomes (dependent variables) in the analyses. Statistical models were developed, which controlled for patient characteristics associated with outcomes. Linear mixed models were used to adjust for clustering of patients among therapists. Thus, a therapist identification number was added as a random variable in all models. The effect of therapist certification (OCS only, AAOMPT only, MTC only, and AAOMPT/OCS) on patient outcomes was tested by adding certification variables into the linear mixed models as fixed independent variables, using each of the three discharge outcome measurements (OHS, PCS, and PF-10) as dependent variables in three separate models.

We found no association between therapist AAOMPT residency or OCS certification on patient outcomes. In other words, patients treated by therapists with these certifications did not do better than patients treated by therapists without these certifications. However, the analysis did demonstrate that improvement of patient self-report of HRQL (i.e., clinical outcomes) was associated with therapist certification in manual therapy (MTC). Although the raw data suggested that there might be some impact of dual AAOMPT/OCS certification, there were insufficient data to estimate the effect of dual certification with statistical modeling. A larger sample of therapists with dual certification would have been required to complete the statistical analysis.

Delegation to Support Personnel

The qualitative study of expert therapists raised new questions about the impact of staffing skill mix and supervision on patient outcomes (2). What is the relationship between patient outcomes and care delegation to support personnel in physical therapy? Does the way that the therapist supervises support personnel affect patient outcomes? No prior research had examined the impact of using support personnel in physical therapy. However, numerous studies exploring the relationship between nurse staffing and patient outcomes suggest that better nurse skill mix and time spent with nurses instead was associated with decreased incidence of adverse events and shorter lengths of hospital stays (36,37,47–49).

Because expert therapists appeared to carefully control the way in which they delegated care to support personnel, it follows that the presence of external regulations governing PT and physical therapist assistant (PTA) behaviors might affect patient outcomes as well. It seemed reasonable to expect that state regulation of PT and PTA behaviors could influence the way in which a physical therapist delegates duties by mandating the maximum number of PTAs a therapist is allowed to supervise and defining the type of supervision the therapist must provide as well as the required frequency of patient reassessment after delegating portions of care to a support personnel. Thus, a further study was conducted to address these questions and test this element of the expertise theory (4). The purpose of the next study, "Delegation of Care to Support Personnel in Outpatient Physical Therapy: Implications for Quality and Efficiency," was to examine the relationship between care delegation, use of physical therapy services, and patient outcomes (4). The study sample was drawn from the FOTO database in years 2000 and 2001. The sample size, 63,900 patients treated by 2,466 therapists, was much larger than that of prior studies and included patients treated for all types of conditions. These patients were treated at 395 outpatient rehabilitation clinics in 38 states.

Two independent variables representing delegation of care to physical therapy support personnel were used. The first was "high PTA utilization," defined as the patient spending the majority of time during his or her treatment episode with a PTA; the second was the percentage of time that the patient spent with an aide (classified as 0%, 1–25%, or more than 25%). Four types of state regulations of PTs and PTAs were considered in this analysis: licensure of PTAs, regulation regarding PT/PTA ratio, requirement for re-evaluation by PTs, and type of supervisory requirement.

The association between the two independent variables representing delegation of care and the presence of state regulations governing PTAs and two dependent variables, efficiency of care and patient outcome, were examined. Efficiency of care was measured by the number of visits per treatment episode. Patient outcome was measured by the FOTO measure of functional health status. Two multilevel linear regression models were developed. In the multilevel models patients were nested within therapists, therapists nested within facility, and facilities nested within states. These models controlled for confounders at the patient level, at the facility level, and at the state level (regulation governing PT). The first model predicted number of visits in the treatment episode. The second model predicted the HRQL score. We found that delegation of care to support personnel was associated with worse treatment outcomes. Patients who spent more than 50% of their time with the PTA and those who spent any time with an aide had functional health measures that were significantly lower than those who spent less time with a PTA and no time with an aide. In addition, patients treated in states that did not have specified regulation of PTA supervision levels had functional health discharge measures that were worse than patients treated in states that specified the type of supervision a PT must provide to a PTA. These findings suggest that enhanced PT involvement leads to better quality of care. It appears that delegating physical therapy care to a support person is associated with worse outcomes and that this effect can be magnified by inadequate supervision or ameliorated with good supervision.

We also found that delegation of care to support personnel was associated with more visits per treatment episode. Specifically, any time spent in treatment with an aide and high utilization of the PTA was associated with more visits (approximately two per treatment episode). State regulations requiring that the therapist be onsite while the PTA is treating a patient (full-time onsite supervision) were associated with three more visits during the treatment episode. In contrast, state regulation of PT/PTA ratio was associated with one less visit during the treatment episode. At this point, it is unclear how the need for full-time onsite supervision alters the pattern of care delivery, leading to decreased efficiency. However, a possible mechanism for greater efficiency resulting from regulations restricting PT/PTA ratio is that therapists who supervise fewer assistants may be able to have more involvement in daily decision making.

Implications of Research

Taken together this body of research using clinical outcomes has a number of important implications for the profession and for future researchers.

Subject Selection in Studies of Expert Therapists. We found that therapists classified as expert on the basis of their patient's clinical outcomes were different from therapists studied by prior researchers of expert therapists (5,6,8–10,50–54). In reviewing the professional profiles of the participants in the group we classified as expert based on clinical outcomes, it is doubtful that all of them would be recognized as "experts" by their colleagues and communities.

Some participants had not practiced in multiple settings but had worked in the same practice environment since graduation. Their experience varied from 1.5 to 40 years; half were APTA members, and the minority had formal teaching experience. Several therapists within this group may have been considered experts by their peers. Participants from the novice subcategory, however, were the unlikely "experts" because they were not at an advanced point in their career development. In all likelihood, they had not yet been labeled as experts by their peers, and their caseloads may not have reflected the level of challenge or difficulty often reported by the experts in the prior studies (7).

These findings challenge a basic assumption that extensive experience as a physical therapist is essential for the development of physical therapy expertise (6,55). The findings also suggest that a prerequisite number of years of experience is not needed or desirable in future studies that sample physical therapy experts based on reputation. Such a requirement excludes excellent therapists with lesser amounts of experience from participation.

IMPLICATIONS FOR PHYSICAL THERAPY EDUCATION AND EMPLOYMENT

The research findings presented have implications for physical therapy program admissions, program prerequisites, and staff hiring. Together, findings from these studies suggest that the best prospective students and employees may be those with diverse work experience or with pre-physical therapy clinical experience combined with values and virtues of respect for people, inquisitiveness, and humility. Furthermore, these findings point to the influence of the professional work environment in fostering professional development, suggesting that leadership efforts to cultivate time for lifelong learning, consultation, and dialogue between therapists will pay off in improved patient care. These are areas that could be explored in future research.

Participants in the group classified as expert were distinguished from participants in the average group by one of two patterns of pre-professional preparation: diverse academic backgrounds or, for the novice therapists classified as expert, an undergraduate degree in exercise science coupled with work experience. The least experienced participant in our group classified as expert had the most pre-physical therapy clinical experience (8 years). This finding may help guide admissions decisions, for example, giving priority to those with pre-professional clinical exposure and exercise science backgrounds.

Although the professional profiles of expert participants in our research were much more diverse than those found among participants in previous studies, the theoretical model that emerged was very similar to other models of expertise (5–8). The theory supports and expands the understanding of a multidimensional knowledge base previously identified as a dimension of expertise in physical therapy (7). The model of multidimensional knowledge includes professional education, continuing education, personal knowledge, clinical experience, and pooled collegial knowledge. However, it did not appear that years of experience or clinical specialization certification were mandatory components of that knowledge base.

Instead, it appears that among experienced therapists, experts were more likely to have eclectic academic and career backgrounds, including backgrounds in veterinary science, professional dance, occupational therapy, and clinical experience in international settings. One therapist, for example, had graduated with a combined physical therapy/occupational therapy degree and had worked in both fields. Earlier in her career, she specialized in pediatrics, earned a master's degree in developmental disabilities, and was certified in both neurodevelopmental treatment and sensory integration.

Furthermore, expert therapists' values and virtues of inquisitiveness and humility were instrumental in using and gaining knowledge. All therapists in the group classified as expert valued their continued professional growth and learning. Excitement about learning was obvious as they spoke about colleagues, their "responsibility to keep up-to-date with the literature," and opportunities for growth. Coupled with this drive to learn was a sense of humility that was not evidenced in the therapists from the group classified as average. The therapists classified as expert were quick to recognize their own limitations.

Expert therapists used the rich knowledge base of colleagues who, they explained, were "all very willing to answer questions" and described how they used their peers for consultation and examination of patients. Therapists sought out knowledgeable mentors to assist them in challenging cases. Most described a work environment that offered numerous opportunities for professional growth. Regardless of the actual amount of money reimbursed for continuing education, working in a supportive atmosphere with "knowledgeable staff" apparently provided opportunities for growth. Presence of similar values and virtues was noted in prior grounded theory on expert practitioners, where expert practitioners were found to have an inner drive for lifelong learning, understand their own limitations, appreciate what they did know as well as what they needed to learn, and demonstrate a well-developed ability for self-reflection and reassessment of their own practice (6,8).

Findings from the study on the impact of specialty certification are largely consistent with the theory of expert therapists we developed (2), suggesting that specialty certification is only one component of multidimensional knowledge and by itself is not associated with improved patient outcomes or expert practice. This may be because the OCS certification process does not identify those with practical, craft knowledge in physical therapy because Board certification in physical therapy requires evidence of clinical experience and successful passage of a written examination, but it does not include testing of practical, hands-on skills. In contrast, manual therapy certification programs vary in their structure, content, intensity, and approach to practice. Some programs involve coursework only, with oral and written examinations, but they do not include a supervised clinical component. Others involve hands-on practical examination, testing practical craft knowledge as well as clinical reasoning. Further research is needed to confirm these hypotheses.

IMPLICATIONS FOR SERVICE DELIVERY

Expert therapists' emphasis on the patient–practitioner relationship appears to shape the way that they regulate delegation of care to support personnel. Delegation of care to multiple support personnel has implications for the therapeutic relationship and can interfere with patient–practitioner communication. It is likely that expert therapist's careful regulation of delegation improves outcomes of care by promoting care continuity, ensuring skillful care delivery, and providing more individualized interventions. We found that overall, the group classified as expert provided more of their own direct intervention, limited the nature of delegated tasks more stringently, and supervised their support staff more closely than members of the group classified as average. In addition, they tended to work in teams, with only a single support person. This enabled the participants classified as expert to control the episode of care and may have provided greater continuity of care to the patient.

Our analysis of the impact of care delegation in outpatient physical therapy revealed that high use of PTAs and use of aides were each independently associated with more visits per treatment episode and lower functional health outcomes. The implications of these findings for practice and for the educational preparation of PTs and PTAs are clear: There is a need for greater emphasis on PT supervisory skills and teaching of methods for PTs and PTAs to function most effectively as a team.

FUTURE DIRECTIONS IN RESEARCH

PHYSICAL THERAPY IN OTHER SETTINGS

There are many untapped opportunities for using outcomes research to enhance our understanding of the dimensions of expert practice, and it is my expectation that the body of work presented in this chapter is only the beginning. Because all of my prior research studied patients and therapists in outpatient settings, there is a need to conduct additional research exploring the characteristics of experts who achieve the best clinical outcomes in other settings, such as inpatient hospitals, nursing homes, and pediatric settings.

PRACTICE ENVIRONMENT

Additional research could explore other tenets of the theoretical model of expertise. For example, a study examining elements of the practice environment, including the use of pooled collegial knowledge, might shed light on the relationship between organizational culture and patient outcomes. This work can also be extended through the development and testing of quality-improvement initiatives. One suggestion is to evaluate the impact of quality-improvement initiatives aimed at improving continuity of patient care and enhancing the supervision of support personnel.

USE OF OUTCOMES MEASURES IN ADDITION TO OR INSTEAD OF HEALTH-RELATED QUALITY OF LIFE TO IDENTIFY EXPERT THERAPISTS

The outcomes research described in these four studies was based on the measurement of patient HRQL. The measurements that were used for calculation of the dependent variables were patients' HRQL scores at discharge from treatment. This may be the most appropriate outcome measure for patients undergoing physical therapy in a typical outpatient orthopedic practice. However, use of HRQL outcomes to measure provider effectiveness does have several limitations.

First, it is possible that aspects of physical therapy intervention, such as patient education, have lifelong health effects, which cannot be measured by examining the patient's status at discharge (7). Although these measurements may not reflect the actual long-term effect of physical therapy intervention, their use is defensible. Other research suggests that discharge scores of the SF-36, a generic HRQL, are good indicators of long-term outcomes for patients with low back pain (56).

However, there may be additional aspects of successful rehabilitation and hallmarks of an expert practitioner that are not fully captured by discharge HRQL measure. Most recognize that one of the primary goals of physical therapy is to enhance patient self-efficacy (i.e., ability and confidence in managing their own health). This is clearly an important goal of therapy in low back pain, where recurrence is likely and the patient needs problem-solving skills to handle minor setbacks. Self-efficacy and disease management skills are also of primary importance in treatment of patients with chronic diseases. Thus, change in patient self-efficacy might be another valid outcome measure to use in identifying expert therapists.

Another concern is that measurement of improvement in physical function may not be the optimal gauge of successful rehabilitation for our patients with diseases not amenable to improvement in physical function or where deterioration in function is expected. Nevertheless, we know that physical therapy can be valuable in improving quality of life in these types of patients largely by facilitating greater participation in life activities. We wouldn't expect a patient with chronic progressive multiple sclerosis or spinal cord injury, for example, to make substantial gains in physical function, yet a skillful therapist might be very helpful to such a patient by prescribing appropriate assistive technology and collaborative problem solving around issues related to access, mobility, and life activities.

This points to the potential for using measures of participation outcomes as a method of gauging therapy success and identifying expert practitioners.

CONCLUSIONS

This chapter reported on a series of four studies that explored therapist factors related to good clinical outcomes in outpatient physical therapy. The initial work consisted of a two-phase mixed methodology study that identified expert therapists based on their patient outcomes and used this sample of therapists to explore and expand on the theory of expertise in physical therapy. Several new and interesting findings from the mixed methodology study were explored in two further studies. First, an examination of patient outcomes by therapist specialty status suggested that therapist certification in manual therapy was associated with better outcomes of care for patients with low back pain but that specialty certification in orthopedics and residency training were not. Next, a follow-up study of care delegation found that use of care extenders in place of physical therapists was associated with more costly and lower quality care delivery in outpatient rehabilitation. Results of these studies suggest that years of experience or training are not sufficient to produce expertise. Therapists don't necessarily become more capable and effective with additional experience or better credentials. Instead, it is the approach to patient care and the practice patterns preferred by expert therapists that contribute to their success. The profiling of providers based on their patient outcomes and the study of therapist and service delivery factors and their association with patient outcomes have the potential to teach us a lot about how highly effective practitioners practice. There is great value in the lessons learned from these studies because this type of research can disentangle the elements of care delivery that make expert practitioners good at what they do. It is hoped that some of these elements can be taught, and this will lead to better quality of care.

9

REFERENCES

1. Resnik L, Hart DL. Using clinical outcomes to identify expert physical therapists. *Phys Ther*. 2003;83(11):990–1002.
2. Resnik L, Jensen GM. Using clinical outcomes to explore the theory of expert practice in physical therapy. *Phys Ther*. 2003;83(12):1090–1106.
3. Resnik L, Hart DL. Influence of advanced orthopedic certification on clinical outcomes of patients with low back pain. *J Manual Manip Ther*. 2004;12(1):32–41.
4. Resnik L, Feng Z, Hart DL. *Delegation of care to support personnel in outpatient physical therapy: implications for quality and efficiency*. Boston: Academy Health Annual Research Meeting; 2005.
5. Jensen GM, Shepard KF, Hack LM. The novice versus the experienced clinician: insights into the work of the physical therapist. *Phys Ther*. 1990;70(5):314–323.
6. Jensen GM, Shepard KF, Gwyer J, Hack LM. Attribute dimensions that distinguish master and novice physical therapy clinicians in orthopedic settings. *Phys Ther*. 1992;72(10):711–722.
7. Jensen GM, Gwyer J, Hack LM, Shepard KF. *expertise in physical therapy practice*. Boston: Butterworth–Heinemann; 1999.
8. Jensen GM, Gwyer J, Shepard KF, Hack LM. Expert practice in physical therapy. *Phys Ther*. 2000;80(1):28–52.
9. Embrey DG, Yates L. Clinical applications of self-monitoring by experienced and novice pediatric physical therapists. *Pediat Phys Ther*. 1996;8(4):156–164.

10. Shepard KF, Hack LM, Gwyer J, Jensen GM. Describing expert practice in physical therapy. *Qual Health Res.* 1999;9(6):746–758.
11. Rivett D, Higgs J. Experience and expertise in clinical reasoning. *NZ J Physiother.* 1995;23(1):16–21.
12. Schmidt HG, Norman GR, Boshuizen HP. A cognitive perspective on medical expertise: theory and implication. *Acad Med.* 1990;65(10):611–621.
13. Jette AM. Outcomes research: shifting the dominant research paradigm in physical therapy. *Phys Ther.* 1995;75(11):965–970.
14. Di Fabio RP. Physical therapy for patients with TMD: a descriptive study of treatment, disability, and health status. *J Orofacial Pain.* 1998;12(2):124–135.
15. Jette DU, Downing J. Health status of individuals entering a cardiac rehabilitation program as measured by the medical outcomes study 36-item short-form survey (SF-36). *Phys Ther.* 1994;74(6):521–527.
16. Jette AM. Using health-related quality of life measures in physical therapy outcomes research. *Phys Ther.* 1993;73(8):528–537.
17. Ware J, Jr., Snow KK, Kosinksi M, et al. *SF-36 health survey: manual and interpretation guide.* Boston: The Health Institute, New England Medical Center; 1993.
18. Jette AM, Delitto A. Physical therapy treatment choices for musculoskeletal impairments. *Phys Ther.* 1997;77(2):145–154.
19. Di Fabio RP, Boissonnault W. Physical therapy and health-related outcomes for patients with common orthopedic diagnoses. *J Orthop Sports Phys Ther.* 1998;27(3):219–230.
20. Patrick DL, Deyo RA, Atlas SJ, et al. Assessing health-related quality of life in patients with sciatica. *Spine.* 1995;20(17):1899–1908.
21. Everhart GS, Prince CM, Jensen GM. Physical therapy clinical residency programs: graduates' perceptions of impact and future role (Abstract). *J Orthopedic Sports Phys Ther.* 2000;30(1):A-5.
22. Amato AL, Dobrzykowski EA, Nance T. The effect of timely onset of rehabilitation on outcomes in outpatient orthopedic practice: a preliminary report. *J Rehab Outcomes Meas.* 1997;1(3):32–38.
23. Jette DU, Jette AM. Physical therapy and health outcomes in patients with spinal impairments. *Phys Ther.* 1996;76(9):930–945.
24. Gill C, Sanford J, Binkley J, et al. Low back pain: program description and outcome in a case series. *J Orthopaedic Sports Phys Ther.* 1994;20(1):11–16.
25. McIntosh G, Frank J, Hogg-Johnson S, et al. Prognostic factors for time receiving workers' compensation benefits in a cohort of patients with low back pain. 1999 Young Investigator Research Award winner. *Spine.* 2000;25(2):147–157.
26. Hart DL, Dobrzykowski EA. Influence of orthopedic clinical specialist certification on clinical outcomes. *J Orthopedic Sports Phys Ther.* 2000;30(4):183–193.
27. Jette DU, Jette AM. Professional uncertainty and treatment choices by physical therapists, *Arch Phys Med Rehab.* 1997;78(12):1346–1351.
28. Schwanz L. *Health status, goal attainment, and number of visits of knee impaired physical therapy patients: a comparison of HMO vs. fee-for-service insurance [master's]: physical therapy.* Dallas: Southwest Texas University; 1998.
29. Bruce J, Eppers B, VanHiel L. *Investigating physical therapy treatment outcomes for patients with shoulder pathology: is reimbursement type a factor? [master's]: physical therapy.* Dahlonega, GA: North Georgia College & State University; 1999.
30. Sackett DL, Rosenberg WM, Gray JA, et al. Evidence based medicine: what it is and what it isn't. *BMJ.* 1996;312(7023):71–72.
31. Lewis PS, Latney C. Achieve best practice with an evidence-based approach. Create a collaborative environment that improves patient care through consistent outcomes measurement. *Nurs Manage.* 2002;33(12):24, 26–28, 30.
32. Deaton C. Outcomes measurement and evidence-based nursing practice. *J Cardiovasc Nurs.* 2001;15(2):83–86.
33. DeLise DC, Leasure AR. Benchmarking: measuring the outcomes of evidence-based practice. *Outcomes Manag Nurs Pract.* 2001;5(2):70–74.
34. Dobrzykowski EA, Nance T. The Focus On Therapeutic Outcomes (FOTO) Outpatient Orthopedic Rehabilitation Database: results of 1994–1996. *J Rehab Outcomes Meas.* 1997;1(1):56–60.

35. Ware JE, Jr., Sherbourne CD. The MOS 36-item short-form health survey (SF-36). I. Conceptual framework and item selection. *Med Care.* 1992;30(6):473–483.
36. Aiken LH, Clarke SP, Sloane DM, et al. Hospital nurse staffing and patient mortality, nurse burnout, and job dissatisfaction. *JAMA.* 2002;288(16):1987–1993.
37. Blegen MA, Vaughn T. A multisite study of nurse staffing and patient occurrences. *Nurs Econ.* 1998;16(4):196–203.
38. Strauss AL, Corbin J. Grounded theory methodology: an overview. In NK Denzin, YS Lincoln, (eds). *Handbook of qualitative research.* Thousand Oaks, CA: Sage; 1994.
39. Muzzin LJ, Norman GR, Feightner JW, et al. Expertise in recall of clinical protocols in two specialty areas. *Proc Annu Conf Res Med Educ.* 1983;22:122–127.
40. Merriam SB. *Qualitative research and case study applications in education,* ed 2. San Francisco: Jossey-Bass; 1998.
41. Winegardner K. The case study method of scholarly research. *The Graduate School of America.* Available at: http://www.tgsa.edu/online/cybrary/case1.html. Accessed November 27, 2001.
42. Lincoln S, Guba EG. Establishing trustworthiness. In *Naturalistic inquiry.* Beverly Hills, CA: Sage Publications; 1985.
43. Law M, Baptiste S, Mills J. Client-centered practice: what does it mean and does it make a difference? *Can J Occupational Ther.* 1995;62(5):250–257.
44. APTA. Clinical specialization. Available at: https://www.apta.org/Education/specialist/whycertify/OverviewSpecCert/SpecCertOverviewDetail. Accessed May 14, 2001.
45. Smith KL, Tichenor CJ, Schroeder M. Orthopaedic residency training: a survey of the graduates' perspective. *J Orthopaedic Sports Phys Ther.* 1999;29(11):635–651.
46. Ware JE, Jr., Kosinski M, Keller SD. A 12-item short-form health survey: construction of scales and preliminary tests of reliability and validity. *Med Care.* 1996;34(3):220–233.
47. Blegen MA, Goode CJ, Reed L. Nurse staffing and patient outcomes. *Nurs Res.* 1998;47(1):43–50.
48. Czaplinski C, Diers D. The effect of staff nursing on length of stay and mortality. *Med Care.* 1998;36(12):1626–1638.
49. Kovner C, Jones C, Zhan C, et al. Nurse staffing and postsurgical adverse events: an analysis of administrative data from a sample of U.S. hospitals, 1990–1996. *Health Serv Res.* 2002;37(3):611–629.
50. Embrey DG, Yates L, Nirider B, et al. Recommendations for pediatric physical therapists: making clinical decisions for children with cerebral palsy. *Pediatr Phys Ther.* 1996;8(4):165–170.
51. Embrey DG, Hylton N. Clinical applications of movement scripts by experienced and novice pediatric physical therapists. *Pediatr Phys Ther.* 1996;8(1):3–14.
52. Embrey DG, Guthrie MR, White OR, et al. Clinical decision making by experienced and inexperienced pediatric physical therapists for children with diplegic cerebral palsy. *Phys Ther.* 1996;76(1):20–33.
53. Embrey DG, Adams LS. Clinical applications of procedural changes by experienced and novice pediatric physical therapists. *Pediatr Phys Ther.* 1996;8(3):122–132.
54. Embrey DG. Clinical applications of decision making in pediatric physical therapy: overview. *Pediatr Phys Ther.* 1996;8(1):2.
55. Noll E, Key A, Jensen GM. Clinical reasoning of an experienced physiotherapist: insight into clinician decision-making regarding low back pain. *Physiother Res Int.* 2001;6(1):40–51.
56. Gatchel RJ, Mayer T, Dersh J, et al. The association of the SF-36 health status survey with 1-year socioeconomic outcomes in a chronically disabled spinal disorder population. *Spine.* 1999;24(20):2162–2170.

9

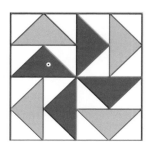

Dutchman's Puzzle — *A setting of flying geese in a puzzle that creates a new pattern.*

10 | Clinical Reasoning and Expert Practice

Ian Edwards and Mark A. Jones

CHAPTER OVERVIEW

Expertise and critical thinking theory emanating from the research and writings of Howard Barrows, Patricia Benner, Stephen Brookfield, Arthur Elstein, Jack Mezirow, and Donald Schön, to name a few, significantly influenced my subsequent interest in clinical reasoning and expert versus novice physical therapy practice. The emerging theory of expertise in physical therapy, especially the theory developed from the research of Jensen, Gwyer, Hack, and Shepard, has further assisted my awareness of the breadth of factors influencing expert physical therapists' practice and prompted my attention to highlighting these factors for students in the two Masters programs I coordinate. The impact of this evolving theory of expertise is evident in my aim to provide a curriculum that is evidence-based while fostering students' critical, reflective learning that promotes continual construction of clinically relevant knowledge along with collaborative, patient-centered clinical reasoning and ethical practice.—Mark A. Jones, MAppSc, PT

I have come to learn that it is not only what experts do but also who they are, as members and representatives of a practicing community, which leads to their peers attributing this term to them. The kind of practice that experts embody (including technical, interactive, teaching, collaborative, predictive, and ethical skills) represents what is collectively agreed to as being good for a particular practicing community. Experts, in this understanding, evoke both qualities and questions in those they mentor and teach. Expert practice also dictates a call to become a certain kind of clinician or therapist and not just to acquire a particular expertise or knowledge base (though that is certainly part of it). In all of this, such apparently "nonteachable" constructs (at least in a formal sense) as "passion," "motivation," "drive," and "love of one's work" are nurtured.—Ian Edwards, PhD, PT

Evidence-based practice has been described as "the integration of best evidence with patient values and clinical expertise" (1, p. 1). In this chapter we present a research-based model of clinical reasoning termed "clinical reasoning strategies," which we propose plays an important role in this integration process (2). The clinical reasoning strategies model describes a broad scope of reasoned clinical decisions and actions, including diagnostics through procedural interventions, teaching, and ethical conduct in clinical practice. We outline how the use of different reasoning processes enables clinicians to integrate the uniqueness of particular patient values, beliefs, and experience with more universal applicable biomedical (including evidence-based) knowledge and management strategies in areas as diverse as diagnostic decision making, teaching, and collaborative decision making.

In one sense, this chapter offers a "physiology" of clinical reasoning in that it describes the underlying processes of clinical reasoning. This chapter is structured by the explanation of the following concepts and each is, in turn, "layered" on to the reasoning model.

- *Understanding the world of the patient*: a biomedical and lived experience inquiry.
- *Clinical reasoning* in both diagnosis and management.
- *Diagnosis*: hypothetico-deductive reasoning and narrative reasoning.

■ *Management*: instrumental and communicative forms of management.
■ *Pattern recognition* and their development as a method of knowledge acquisition and storage.
■ *Critical reflection*: the examination of assumptions and the validation of decision making.
■ The *social influence* on the formation of perspectives and the implications for the practitioner on reasoning and practice.

We propose that the "dialectical" nature of the model (explained later) also helps explain the relationship between reasoning processes: how each reasoning process has its particular contribution and limits; how one influences another; and how this interplay helps generate different kinds of knowledge for use in clinical practice.

In proposing the clinical reasoning strategies model we argue that there is potential value for clinicians in several areas. First, through the notion of reasoning strategies, the model depicts the scope of reasoning "activities" in clinical practice. It therefore provides a framework for reasoning in areas of practice where the clinical reasoning literature in physical therapy has been scant and the clinical reasoning awareness of clinicians may be less. For example, how do practitioners reason rigorously through their collaboration with patients or through the nature, extent, and effectiveness of their teaching in clinical practice?

Second, by understanding the particular assumptions of the reasoning process that they may be using at a given time, we contend that clinicians can become more aware of the nature of the judgments they consciously make and also of those less conscious habitual assumptions or judgments that may not hold true under more thorough inquiry. Analogous to the combination of quantitative and qualitative assessment and analysis providing a more complete understanding than either alone, greater awareness of the sorts of reasoning required to understand patients and their problems assists clinicians' recognition of the value of different types of patient information or data to be sought or attended to.

Third, the model demonstrates how clinical reasoning can assist the integration of personal knowledge and experience with the other types of knowledge that are more traditionally valued in clinical practice, such as propositional (research derived) and professional skill-based knowledge.

CLINICAL REASONING STRATEGIES IN PHYSICAL THERAPY

This qualitative study used a grounded theory methodology, which is a field-based research approach that seeks to generate theory where little exists (3,4). The aim was to examine the nature and scope of clinical reasoning of expert physical therapists in three different practice settings: musculoskeletal or orthopedic physical therapy, neurologic physical therapy, and domiciliary care or home health physical therapy. Participants were observed during the course of their usual practice working over a period of 2 to 3 days. Data were collected in the form of audiotapes of interviews and treatment sessions and field notes. Data were analyzed by a case study analysis method (5,6) and preceded by the development of conceptual frameworks as provisional explanations of data. This initial conceptual framework included that of "attribute dimensions" from an earlier grounded theory study of expertise in physical therapy by Jensen and colleagues (5). Our methodology is described in further detail in Edwards et al. (2) and online (7).

The study's findings were that, regardless of field, each therapist reasoned in a number of focused and identifiable areas of reasoning in practice, which we term "clinical reasoning strategies" (Box 10-1). Although many of these clinical reasoning strategies had been previously identified in the clinical reasoning literature of medicine and allied health—for example, diagnostic reasoning (8) procedural reasoning (9,10), narrative reasoning (11), interactive reasoning (12), and ethical reasoning (e.g., 13,14)—this is the first they have been demonstrated to similarly exist in physical therapy practice. Throughout this literature different reasoning processes have been proposed for different aspects of clinical practice (for example, procedural—or doing something to the patient—reasoning, versus interactive—or knowing the patient—reasoning (e.g., 10,12). However, unique to this study was the finding that the various reasoning strategies were not used in isolation as a single approach to clinical decision making. Rather, physical therapists in

BOX 10–1	*Clinical Reasoning Strategies*

Diagnosis

1. *Diagnostic reasoning*: formation of a diagnosis related to physical disability/functional limitation and associated impairment(s), with consideration of associated pain mechanisms, tissue pathology, and the broad scope of potential contributing factors.
2. *Narrative reasoning*: seeks to map "the landscape" between patients' actions and their intentions or motivations. This involves understanding patients' illness experience, their "story," context, beliefs, and culture. In other words, what are patients' personal perspectives (or knowledge) regarding why they think and feel the way they do?

Management

3. *Reasoning about procedure*: decision making behind the determination and carrying out of treatment procedures.
4. *Interactive reasoning*: purposeful establishment and ongoing management of therapist–patient rapport.
5. *Collaborative reasoning*: nurturing a consensual approach toward the interpretation of examination findings, the setting of goals and priorities, and the implementation and progression of treatment.
6. *Reasoning about teaching*: planning, carrying out, and evaluating individualized and context-sensitive teaching.
7. *Predictive reasoning*: envisioning future scenarios with patients and exploring their choices and the implications of those choices.
8. *Ethical reasoning*: apprehension of ethical and pragmatic dilemmas that impinge on both the conduct of treatment and its desired goals and the resultant action toward their resolution.

10

this study were found to dialectically* move back and forth between the different reasoning processes (viz. diagnosis, procedure, interaction, collaboration, teaching, predicting, and ethics) (6).

The data from our study concerning clinical reasoning strategies and therapists' use of knowledge, in the manner of grounded theory, were constantly compared and reapplied to existing theories or literature in relevant areas such as clinical reasoning (e.g., 15,16), paradigms and typologies of knowledge (17,18), and the more formal theories of Habermas (19) and Mezirow (20) (namely, critical social theory and transformation theory, respectively). Habermas and Mezirow both theorize on the factors that either facilitate or constrain how people communicate and learn. Although the dialectical nature of the clinical reasoning strategies model represents the grounded theory produced from our study, it nevertheless also draws on the previously mentioned theories in a manner that recontextualizes them in relation to the data of this study in particular and the scope of clinical reasoning in physical therapy in general. Further explanation of Habermas's and Mezirow's theories can be found in the original thesis available online (7).

THE WORLD OF THE PATIENT: A BIOMEDICAL AND LIVED-EXPERIENCE INQUIRY

The starting point in this dialectical model of clinical reasoning is the holistic concern that the participating therapists in this study demonstrated for their patients, a concern that is corroborated by other studies of expertise in physical therapy (15,21). This world of the patient (Figure 10-1) has its biomedical and lived experience "poles." These have been well described in a variety of literature (for example, critical social theory [19], adult learning [20,22], and medical education [23]). It is not our intention or that of the authors mentioned earlier in describing these "poles" to support any false separation of body and mind. Rather, it is to emphasize the interaction of these factors.

The differentiation of knowledge into conceptions or paradigms (17,18) provides another way of expressing this polarity. Forms of knowledge that are positivist (where truth or reality is viewed as objective, observable, and measurable,

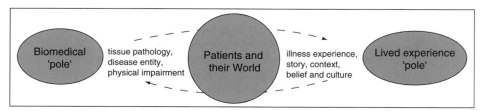

Figure 10–1 ■ The interaction of biomedical factors and lived experience in the world of the patient.

---

*A dialectic is a debate intended to reconcile a contradiction (in this case between fundamentally different processes of reasoning) without attempting to establish either view as intrinsically truer than the other.

such as tissue pathology, disease entity, and physical impairment) and nonpositivist (where truth or reality is perspective based and socially constructed and includes illness experience, belief, culture, context, and story) all have their place in this world of the patient.

Thus, tissue pathology, disease, and physical impairment as biomedical entities exist in relationship to the lived experience and particular context of the patient, shaped as it is by many cultural, social, economic, and even political factors. That is, disability is not a hard-wired outcome of illness or physical impairment where "x" amount of pathology or physical impairment equates to "x" amount of disability. As Charon and Montello (24, p. ix) put it: "Although illness is, indeed, a biological and material phenomenon, the human response to it is neither biologically determined nor arithmetical." The clinical reasoning of the therapists in the study actively addressed both "poles" of the patient's world. In doing so they drew from both the positivist and constructivist ontology of knowledge in an "appreciation" that neither the physical problem nor the person can be adequately understood without awareness of the other.

CLINICAL REASONING IN DIAGNOSIS AND MANAGEMENT

Apart from traversing the topography of the biomedical and the lived experience, clinical reasoning also stretches across inquiry (or diagnosis making) to the diverse issues of "management" (25).

Diagnosis

We define diagnosis as a broad construct that includes therapist analysis of physical disability and impairment, which is achieved through hypothetico-deductive (traditionally termed diagnostic reasoning [26,27]) and therapist–patient co-analysis of the patient's construction of meaning or coming to understand the patients' unique perspectives associated with their illness, pain, or disability experience, which is achieved through narrative reasoning (see Box 10-1).

In the hypothetico-deductive method, clinicians attend to initial cues (information) from or about the patient. From these cues, tentative hypotheses are generated. This generation of hypotheses is followed by ongoing analysis of patient information in which further data are collected and interpreted. Continued hypothesis creation and evaluation take place as examination and management are continued and the various hypotheses are confirmed or negated through empirical testing (8). Hypothetico-deductive reasoning sees diagnosis as essentially the gathering and correlation of data, which, in this context, are conceived of as measurements of a deviation from a "normal" or standard (Figure 10-2). In medicine, examples of this kind of diagnostic data are common and include the taking of blood pressure and analysis of blood counts. In physical therapy, examples of such testing (often comparing findings both with an accepted population norm and with the asymptomatic or unaffected side) would include assessing such things as gait, balance, sensation, joint complex mobility, muscle tone, strength/control and length, pulmonary function, and developmental milestones.

10

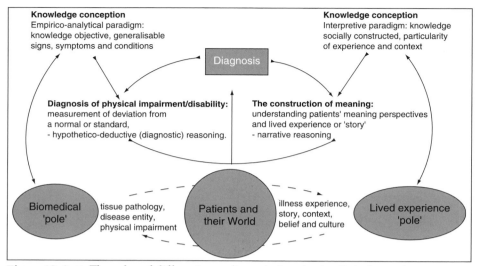

Figure 10–2 ■ The roles of different paradigms in inquiry in clinical practice.

Hypothetico-deductive reasoning is derived from an empirico-analytical (or positivist) paradigm where knowledge is not only objective but, under prescribed conditions, is also generalizable and predictive to a larger population (17). This knowledge set usually is generated out of the quantitative research paradigm where statistical probability of defined outcomes or associations is used to promote evidence-based practice guidelines for similar populations. For example, a history of sudden or forced hyperextension of the knee associated with a "snapping" sound, intraarticular effusion, and a positive Lachman's test will be common findings (i.e., a recognizable clinical pattern) in most diagnoses of ruptured anterior cruciate ligament.

The construction of meaning in diagnosis uses a *narrative reasoning* process, which seeks to understand the uniqueness of a patient's illness/disability experience (or story). In patients' (or therapists' for that matter) telling of stories or narratives there is a choice in which some elements are expressed, some elements are emphasized over others, and still other elements may not find expression (28)—that is, the particular "telling" of a story or history by patients represents their interpretation of experiences and events over time. As Thornquist (29) puts it, "histories are not taken, they are made" in the course of the interaction between physical therapist and patient. Just as the patient endeavors to emphasize what they consider important, so too, the physical therapist imputes varying significance to particular information and observations, so the clinical encounter is "structured" in particular ways. Such interpretations (albeit not necessarily consciously constructed by either patient or therapist) may not be neutral in their effects on the teller (28,30,31).

For example, using a narrative analysis, Borkan et al. (30) found that the character of injury narratives were significant prognostic indicators for a group of elderly patients following fractures of the hip—that is, those individuals who perceived their problem in a more external or mechanical way, as being caused by the environment, for example, showed greater improvement in ambulation at 3 and 6 months. This greater improvement was relative to those who showed no evidence of this thinking or perceived their problem as an internal or organic problem in terms of illness or disease. How therapists communicate either diagnostic information or management strategies to patients may have a role in the formation of patients' narratives (29). Similarly, in a qualitative phenomenologic study investigating the personal experiences and psychological processes involved in maintaining pain, distress, and disability in subjects presenting with benign chronic low back pain, Osborn and Smith (31) found participants' experiences of not being believed created for them a continual need to justify their pain and the incongruity of being mobile or appearing healthy created for them a sense that they should appear ill to conform to the expectations of others.

The nature and form of such data collection in clinical practice derives from an interpretive paradigm and a constructivist conception of knowledge (17). The interpretive paradigm describes a multiplicity of worldviews and research approaches (including symbolic interactionism, constructivism, and phenomenology, to name a few) but which generally agree that reality exists only as it is experienced and communicated (18). A patient's particular experience of illness or pain, derived as it is from a complex mixture of personal, cultural, social, economic, and even political factors, is therefore neither "normal" or "abnormal" in an absolute or empirical sense. It can be appreciated, then, that a particular interpretation of an illness or disability (for good or ill) is not readily able to be generalized to other patients even if the biomedical factors of the situation are apparently typical. In the first instance, this is because patient experiences of even typical disease syndromes and impairments may be very different and, second, physical therapists' interpretations of their patients' interpretations may vary according to such things as their own clinical experiences and personal values. A classic example is the construct "pain behavior" that is commonly assumed to be maladaptive when in reality any judgment regarding pain behaviors requires interpretation to establish their *raison d'être* (32). For this reason, the ability to understand the formation of one's personal values and assumptions is an important clinical reasoning process and is discussed later in this chapter.

Management

Management as defined in this model consists of not only the application of treatment procedures but also the broad range of clinical activities suggested by the different reasoning strategies. This includes the thinking and actions associated with interacting and collaborating effectively with patients, teaching as in educative management, predicting as both clinical prognosis and finding meaningful ways of negotiating the future in more chronic or recalcitrant conditions, and dealing with a diversity of ethical dilemmas. As with the two poles of "diagnosis" (hypothetico-deductive and narrative reasoning), the broad range of clinical activities mentioned earlier are carried out through or within different

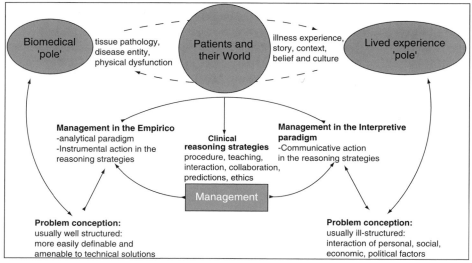

Figure 10–3 ■ The dialectical reasoning process in management.

paradigms as characterized by the two poles of *instrumental and communicative management* (Figure 10-3).

Instrumental problem solving is a term from adult learning literature (20) that describes reflection on procedure and performance in a cause and effect manner. In other words, an instrumental action in clinical practice is an action carried out using a hypothetico-deductive approach. For example, an instrumental approach to the clinical reasoning strategy of teaching might involve teaching someone to get out of a chair or teaching someone to relax facial muscles (7, p. 182). In both cases the impairments or deficit(s) preventing performance are observed, hypotheses as to the cause of the inability to perform the action are generated and tested, and actions are taken with respect to these hypotheses. For example, hypotheses related to the patient's inability to get out of the chair independently might include lack of confidence, joint stiffness, poor muscle control (either local or more global deconditioning), and problems with balance or—more simply—the patient's posture and chair ergonomics from which the action is initiated. The learning of instrumental tasks can be assessed empirically.

In contrast, underlying communicative management, according to Mezirow, is the principle that not all learning involves learning to do:

> *Of even greater significance to most adult learning is understanding the meaning [Mezirow's emphasis] of what others communicate concerning values, ideals, feelings, moral decisions, and such concepts as freedom, justice, love, labor, autonomy, commitment, and democracy (20, p. 8).*

A communicative management action in clinical practice is informed by narrative reasoning and would be exemplified (using the same examples as mentioned earlier) by first understanding and then addressing, for example, a patient's fears or decreased confidence in attempting to get out of the chair along with the unique contextual basis underpinning those feelings. In the case of increased tension in the facial muscles, communicative management might involve assisting the patient to gain insights into the behaviors or responses to stress that lead to the facial muscle tension (7, p. 184).

What is the rationale of therapists using instrumental versus communicative management? The phenomenon of therapists switching between the different forms of instrumental and communicative management (albeit often in a tacit or unconscious manner) also relates to the nature of problem conception or formulation (see Figure 10-3). The well-structured problem is more easily definable, can be cognitively framed, and is more amenable to technical solutions, lending itself, therefore, to therapists using hypothetico-deductive reasoning and instrumental action in clinical practice (20,22,33). In contrast, the ill-structured problem is a complex interaction of personal, social, economic, and even political factors and is not so easily defined, and it is not as amenable to purely technical or behaviorally orientated problem solving (viz. instrumental solutions) (22,30). This requires clinical management in an interpretive paradigm using a narratively based reasoning and communicative management to achieve a coherence of meaning between patient and therapist.

Clinical practice in physical therapy consists of both well- and ill-structured problems, with one type often embedded in another, which, itself, is suggestive of the need for clinicians to reason and take clinical actions in the dialectical manner described throughout this chapter. Hence, using the example mentioned earlier, it is necessary for the therapist to address both the inability of the patient to relax the facial muscles with instrumental management strategies and those perspective-based factors that may be contributing to the increased muscle activity through communicative management. Whereas complex problems may be physically complex or psychosocially complex, most problems in clinical practice require varying combinations, in close juxtaposition, of instrumental and communicative reasoning and action. This process occurs within each of the reasoning strategies. Take the clinical reasoning strategy of collaborative reasoning as an example. (For further discussion of how the dialectical model works in other reasoning strategies see references 6 and 34–36.)

Collaborative reasoning is the nurturing of a consensual approach toward the interpretation of examination findings, the setting of goals, and the ongoing progression of treatment. Instrumental and communicative forms of collaboration in clinical practice can be expressed as a continuum of patient autonomy. At one end of the continuum, Sim (37, p. 8) proposes that autonomy implies exercising a certain right to relinquish some autonomy and be "directed" as long as "this does not irrevocably foreclose one's future self-determination." As an example of such instrumental collaboration, consider the patient who presents for physical therapy rehabilitation following the reconstruction of an anterior cruciate ligament. The patient in this situation, having been informed previously (by the surgeon) that following surgery he will need to follow a strict protocol of exercises within particular time frames or milestones, may say something to the physical therapist like, "You're the expert. I put myself in your hands. Tell me what I've got to do and I'll do it!" The therapist is the expert (holding the power of decision making at that point) and, in the broader context of collaboration,

10

requires particular actions from the patient, although overall goals are still negotiated between therapist and patient.

This form of instrumental collaboration in which the patient's compliance to the program has an empirically "measurable" quality (e.g., the extent to which the exercises are completed) is appropriate in this context. At the other end of the autonomy continuum, consider another patient who has been off work for the last 2 years following chronic pain associated with a low back injury sustained about 3 years ago. If this patient presents and in a similar manner says something like, "Nobody has been able to help me much so far but I really believe you're the expert I have been looking for. I put myself in your hands. Do whatever you think is necessary and I'll go along with it," then such words in this different context should alert the therapist to a more communicative form of collaboration being required.

A communicative form of collaboration highlights the role of the therapist to facilitate the capacity of the patient to make constructive and achievable choices and goals in relation to a range of different areas (physical, functional, recreational, and vocational) in a gradual shift of decision-making power from therapist to patient. In other words, the therapist's efforts may be to facilitate active patient involvement in the self-management of ongoing pain and disability where the initial identification of goals are often less predetermined (than the cruciate ligament scenario), requiring greater patient–therapist co-identification and co-analysis of the patient's personal perspectives (e.g., beliefs and feelings in the context of their activity restrictions, participation limitations, and future predictions/aspirations) so that goals agreed on are not only contextualized to the patient's particular pain or disability experience but also emanate from maximal patient–therapist collaboration. The analysis of collaboration as a reasoned task that requires a considered and contextualized approach supports a central theme of Jensen et al.'s (5) model of expertise in physical therapy practice.

PATTERN RECOGNITION

A third widely accepted process in clinical reasoning is pattern recognition (16,38,39). Patel and Groen (38) describe pattern recognition as a counterpoint to the process of hypothetico-deductive reasoning in that pattern recognition involves moving from a set of specific observations to a generalization, whereas hypothetico-deductive reasoning involves moving from a generalization (i.e., hypotheses) to a specific conclusion. Patel and Groen (38) provide evidence that hypothetico-deductive reasoning, or *backward reasoning* as they termed it, is that process used by inexperienced clinicians or expert clinicians in unfamiliar or atypical cases. Barrows and Feltovich (40) propose that hypothetico-deductive reasoning is the means by which new patterns are learned, enabling clinicians, with experience, to then use forward reasoning in the future with similar clinical problems.

Consider the following examples of pattern recognition from our study. In the first two examples the therapists acknowledge the use of pattern recognition as a common feature of their practice but one that is accompanied by hypothetico-deductive testing as a method of validating the recognized pattern. It is worth stating that the physical therapists in this study had not been trained in clinical reasoning theory.

Monica (a musculoskeletal physical therapist) conducted an initial examination of a woman with chest pain following a fall who, in the course of the examination, also mentioned a shoulder problem that she had had for several months following mastectomy. Afterward, she comments:

> **MONICA:** With that lady...you could see: that's gleno-humeral capsulitis... that's stuck....But yeah I listen to what they say...often from the history, the picture that they give you, the history of the behavior, you've got a feeling of "Yeah, I think this." But then I make sure that in my examination of it, I prove it or disprove it (7, p. 114).

Neve (a neurological therapist) described recognizable patterns of tension headaches.

> **NEVE:** Say we're talking about tension headaches, I've got broad principles in my mind that seem to apply to most people in that category. With the tension headaches I've noticed over the years that they nearly all clench their teeth, that they nearly all hold their breath and breathe very shallowly, that they often also spend a lot of time frowning, and that they hunch their shoulders up. They get angry and hunch the shoulders. So I've noticed that those type of things seem to be common to them but they're not operational in all patients—you know they don't all do those things.
>
> So I suppose I've got a little framework in which I can hang my hat and say, "These things often happen and they might be happening in your case but I have to have a look and you have to see...you have to notice (i.e., test) whether they are happening and if they are happening then we can do something about it" (7, p. 122).

Danielle (a domiciliary care physical therapist) outlines an informal typology of recognizable patterns of caregiver behavior, and we see demonstrated the other property of pattern recognition: the eliciting of "rules of production." The recognition of patterns also evokes other knowledge networks held by the clinician such as treatment protocols and management options (38).

10

> **DANIELLE:** Well there's all sorts of patterns of caregivers that you can recognize...[those] that are not going to be able to manage in a very short space of time or...[those] that are not willing to, for whatever reason, accept some help. And...the whole thing can be so much more difficult because they keeping on [saying], "I can do that, I can do that, I can do that." There are the people that...can't do anything basically... you know...that's what they say from the start. Then you get the ones that seem to do amazing...amazing things...in some ways it's the ones that are doing a lot that are the ones that you need to keep more an eye on. [Because] the ones that are saying at the start they can't do things, you set things up for them (i.e., provide appropriate support and strategies). It's the other ones that you need to keep an eye on... try to maybe be there just before the crash comes (7, p. 117).

As with biomedical clinical patterns (e.g., Monica's patient with the adhesive capsulitis of the shoulder), where generated hypotheses are verified or validated hypothetico-deductively (8), therapists may also surmise (as suggested by the "patterns of caregivers") that they recognize the sound or pattern of a story (11). The intrinsic relationship between the two forms of data mentioned earlier and their contribution to the generation of clinical knowledge is conceptualized in Figure 10-4.

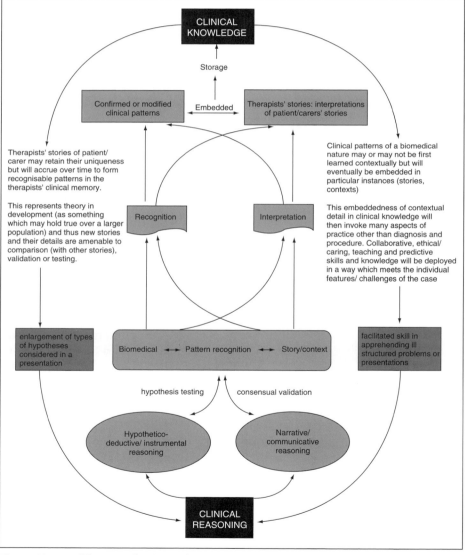

Figure 10–4 ■ The contributions of empirico-analytical and interpretive reasoning paradigms to the formation of clinical knowledge.

Figure 10-4 substantively draws on Schmidt et al.'s (16) "instantiated scripts," which describe, from a cognitive perspective and as a function of expertise, the remembering of particular patient instances (patterns) when recalling clinical information in relation to a new presentation. The extension presented here is that the contextual detail in such "instantiated scripts," for these physical therapists, contains interpretive matter related to patient/caregiver values, beliefs, and meaning perspectives. Such matter is transmitted through patient and caregiver stories. In the figure, therefore, we recognize with Charon (14) that stories must be recognized and interpreted and that interpretation must then be validated (discussed later).

The resultant clinical knowledge, then, is not only a repository of diagnostic and procedural information but also includes existential knowledge related to human experience held together in recognizable patterns accessible on their own and collectively in the form of remembered patient cases. On the one hand, biomedical clinical patterns become embedded in contextual detail and thus appear to lead to an increased repertoire of skills in apprehending ill-structured or complex problems and presentations. On the other hand, the accumulation of patients' stories in therapists' clinical experience also leads to pattern recognition and the development of a wide range of hypotheses in a presentation, which become amenable to "testing." Pattern recognition, therefore, can provide a link between generalized biomedical knowledge and the more particular knowledge found in patients' experiences and contexts.

Dianne (domiciliary care physical therapist) describes how clinical knowledge is generated by an interaction of biomedical or, as she termed it, "textbook" knowledge with the hearing of particular stories. The whole biomedical and illness/disability experience "picture" is then stored:

> **DIANNE:** When you first deal with someone with motor neuron disease you go in there with, "What did I learn in physio school? This is how you treat them and this is how they'll die..." and you've got this thing panned out. But it becomes completely different when you're actually dealing symptom by symptom and having to get over that and listen to the story before you can do anything...and you have to give some help to the caregiver who can't cope with things that are happening. So your whole picture of motor neuron disease changes dramatically and that all gets stored away (7, p. 128).

KNOWLEDGE, CRITICAL REFLECTION, AND THE VALIDATION OF ASSUMPTIONS

Although the development of clinical patterns represents an important source of knowledge for clinical practice, therapists use and are able to interpret different forms of knowledge, including:

1. Propositional, research-based biopsychosocial knowledge
2. Nonpropositional professional craft knowledge
3. Nonpropositional personal knowledge (17,41) (Figure 10-5)

Propositional biopsychosocial knowledge, as an expansion of its predecessor, biomedical knowledge, is gaining acceptance as the more appropriate

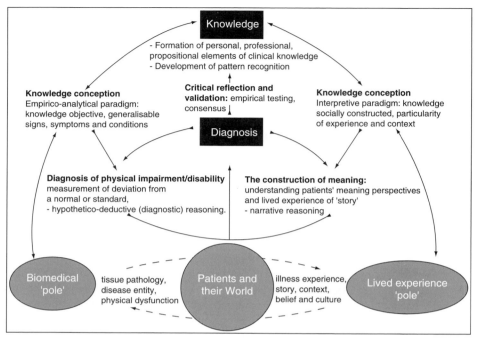

Figure 10–5 ■ Formation of knowledge through the reasoning process.

categorization of the scientific knowledge required in contemporary health care (42,43). Professional craft knowledge, comprising professional theory and procedural knowledge gained through experience as well as contextual knowledge of a particular patient and their circumstances, has been described by Cervero (44, p. 98) as a "repertoire of examples, images, practical principles, scenarios or rules of thumb (heuristics) that have been developed through prior experience." The less considered of these three forms of knowledge, personal knowledge, is that knowledge acquired through experience (life and professional) that shapes individuals' personal perspectives, values, beliefs, attitudes, likes, and dislikes and in turn influences their day-to-day cognition (e.g., attributions, expectations, personal goals), emotions (e.g., fears, anger, depression), and actions (e.g., health behaviors).

Personal knowledge, although underpinning much of what we think and do, usually is tacit knowledge rendering it less available to personal reflection, critique, and mindful change. Being shaped by our life experiences (family, societal, cultural, health, etc.), personal knowledge contributes significantly to our personality, or who we are, thereby creating a basis for the interpersonal interactions so important to patient-centered care in general and narrative reasoning/communicative action in particular.

Understanding and successfully managing patients' problems requires a rich organization of all three types of knowledge. Propositional knowledge provides us with theory and levels of substantiation enabling therapists to consider the patient's clinical presentation against research-validated theory and practice. Nonpropositional professional craft knowledge gives us the means to use that theory in the clinic while providing additional, often cutting-edge (albeit with unproven generality), clinically derived evidence. Personal knowledge is essential to gaining a deep understanding of the clinical problem within the context of the patient's particular situation, or their lived experience, thereby enabling us to practice in a holistic and caring way.

Contemporary, evidence-based physical therapy practice necessitates therapists staying abreast of the rapidly expanding body of medical and physical therapy propositional and professional craft knowledge. It is hoped that, in time, that research database will also include data pertaining to patterns of patients' personal knowledge as represented in their illness and disability experiences. However, in the meantime, therapist awareness and assessment of patients' experiences and perspectives is essential for successful application of research evidence to practice. As a result, modern physical therapy education is taking greater account of the broadening understanding of practice epistemology with curricula increasingly being designed within an adult learning framework where multiple forms of knowledge are valued and critical thinking and self-directed learning are promoted to facilitate lifelong learning (17,45,46).

Learning is at the core of both physical therapy education (formal and lifelong) and patient care. We believe that much of what physical therapy clinicians do is aimed at facilitating patient learning (e.g., improving patient understanding, promoting new perspectives and health behaviors). Both adult learning and clinical reasoning theory emphasize the importance of critical reflection of existing interpretations/perspectives, including the premises underpinning those interpretations, to foster modified interpretations and greater understanding (17,20,39). Critical reflection on the assumptions or basis of beliefs leads to what Mezirow (20) has labeled "transformative learning." Similarly, we contend that physical therapists (and patients), by being more aware of how they know what they know or believe, are better able to critically examine what are often taken-for-granted beliefs, frames of reference, and habits of mind to arrive at more reliable, constructive, and helpful views.

All forms of knowledge and practice should be open to scrutiny as is the intention of evidence-based practice. Biopsychosocial and professional craft knowledge are validated through well-designed research (in either the empirico-analytical or interpretive paradigms) and critically reflective clinical practice. In clinical practice, the biomedical component of clinical patterns may be validated (within the availability of gold standards such as, for example, Lachmann's test for anterior cruciate ligament rupture or auscultation for determining extent and quality of airflow throughout the lungs) by empirical testing.

With regard to patient narratives, such data must be consensually validated between therapist and patient rather than empirically tested (10). As Figure 10-4 suggests, it is then possible for individual cases to be compared, in one sense, by their deviations from exemplar cases. Exemplar cases may be those that have been reflected on and discussed in formal settings (e.g., articles, publications, professional conferences) or more informal ones (with colleagues in a particular practice community or interest group) (14).

In the process of consensual validation the patient needs to know that the therapist has heard the story as he or she wants it to be heard, remembering that the story may unfold over a longer period of time and involvement and not necessarily at a single sitting. Ultimately, however, as previously mentioned, the therapist does not store the patient's story itself in clinical memory; instead the therapist stores his or her interpretation of the story. Hence, there is a need for therapists to be able to evaluate the values and assumptions underlying their personal knowledge (47).

Personal knowledge (therapist's and patient's) is validated through a process of dialogue with an emphasis on finding common understanding, "trying-on" others' points of view, and assessing the justification or truth of a perspective, belief, or premise. Because one's personal knowledge (beliefs, meaning perspectives, values, frames of reference) usually is acquired unintentionally through life experiences, changing it must first involve bringing into awareness the associations, attributions, and cultural and ideological bases on which our point of view has been learned. This is often best accomplished when one's beliefs and values are exposed to new or unfamiliar beliefs and values and in situations in which one's existing perspectives don't seem to "fit" (20). For example, challenging patients' fears of pain that have become excessive and counterproductive to their recovery through education has been shown to be successful both experimentally and clinically (48,49). Similarly therapists' acceptance of alternative perspectives on practice requires critical reflection on their existing views and a willingness to hear opposing views. Critical reflection on the adequacy or reliability of our existing perspectives leads to "transformatory learning." The role of both critical reflection and validation of decision making is incorporated into the clinical reasoning model so far and is illustrated in Figure 10-5.

The therapists in our study placed great emphasis on an understanding of the development of their own values and beliefs as a factor in both relating therapeutically with their patients and their professional growth. For example:

NEVE: So I needed to have some understanding, really, of relationships....It means not just looking at the patients but looking at myself as well, looking inward as well as outward and then having some idea of what happens to me in my interaction with the patients, so that I can be aware of the dynamics of the situation and what's actually happening (7, p. 246).

MICHAEL (musculoskeletal physical therapist): I think my interaction with people and the therapeutic aspect of that has grown heaps, and that's, I think, more so coupled with my growth as a person (7, p. 246).

DENISE (domiciliary care physical therapist): I'm probably much better at dealing with all sorts of people than I ever was...difficult people and people who don't speak English and... having interpreters doesn't faze me and having people from other cultures doesn't particularly faze me anymore. You know, dealing with dying people doesn't faze me too much anymore. Although I don't know I ever want to become too dulled to that (7, p. 246).

The relevance of also identifying patients' personal knowledge (accessed by stories or narratives) is illustrated in the growing body of research demonstrating the impact personal perspectives have on a patient's disability, pain perception, health behaviors, and long-term outcome (30,31,50–52). Critical reflection of personal knowledge; exploring of the basis of personal views/beliefs; and openly considering alternative, more accurate or constructive perspectives is all part of communicative management. Although for some patients this may only require clear explanation and willingness to change, for other patients the process is more difficult because not all beliefs and feelings will be self-evident.

SOCIALLY SHAPED PERSPECTIVES, REASONING, AND PRACTICE

The dialectical model of clinical reasoning, with its interplay between empirico-analytical and interpretive knowledge paradigms, needs to be placed in a larger social context.

The reasoning that takes place in clinical practice, albeit covering a broad range of issues, needs to take account of those forces (local and global) that not only help shape the values and perspectives of therapists, patients, and families/caregivers but also the environment in which treatment takes place. This kind of knowledge is developed through societal discourses (dynamic and public "debates"), which are taken-for-granted values or frames of reference that are historically and socially produced. Figure 10-6 displays all the components of the dialectical reasoning model and is, itself, depicted as "floating" in a "sea of discourse," an expression that seeks to capture the vast and constantly evolving nature of discourses shaping society's values and attitudes. Various communities (including physical therapists) are subject to these value-shaping discourses. For example, therapists may bring to clinical practice their attitudes on issues such as a patient's sexual orientation, or generalized opinions regarding the motivation and attitude of patients with chronic pain compared with those with more acute injury (53).

We have discussed, in the context of narrative or communicative forms of clinical reasoning and management, that patients' interpretations of experience and their perspectives on their problems (helpful or unhelpful) are formed not only as a result of individual personal experiences and factors but in social and cultural ways as well (20). One important implication for physical therapy practice lies in the different capacities of patients to even engage in the process of physical therapy.

Sargeant (54) conducted a preliminary exploration of the experiences of refugee Sudanese women and their perception of exercise in relation to the increasingly common occurrence of low back pain among these women. She found that these Sudanese women have come from a very active daily life (involving a great deal of walking, for example, while fetching water, food, and fuels for cooking) to a much more sedentary lifestyle. Because their previous life was, in a sense, all exercise, the concept of exercises *per se* was, for these women, nonexistent. Even the seeking of help for problems such as low back pain is foreign to these women, particularly in the context of their previous

10

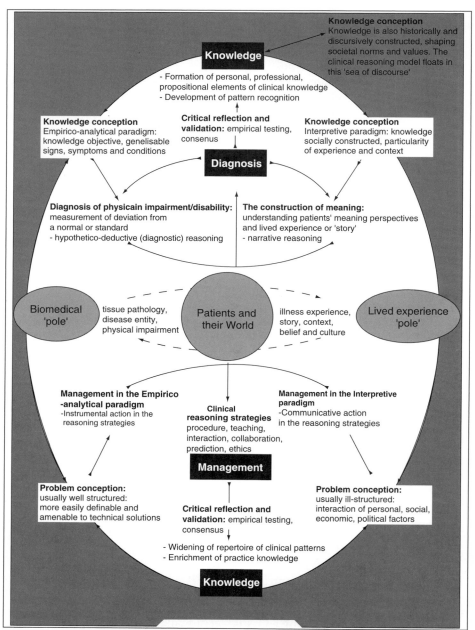

Figure 10–6 ■ The dialectical nature of clinical reasoning in physical therapy.

experience where going to the significant effort of seeking health care is normally confined to seeking help in acute illness. There are clear implications here both for what the expectations of a patient from this community/population would be in attending physical therapy (should they be aware of it as a health care option) and in how treatment should be conducted. One implication of the multi-paradigm model of clinical reasoning presented in this chapter is that clinicians need to develop ways of learning about patients and their needs in the social context of their community and its beliefs and practices and not only in the decontextualized setting of a clinic, rooms, or hospital.

CONCLUSIONS

We have outlined a model of clinical reasoning that is dialectical in nature. It holds in tension several processes of reasoning at work in the clinical reasoning of each of the observed expert physical therapists in their different fields of practice. As stated in the introduction, this model is more a physiology of clinical reasoning than a didactic, step-by-step, decision-making model. Nevertheless, we propose that an understanding of the complexity of the processes in reasoning and knowledge formation provides clinicians with a base on which to go on learning in and through the conduct of their clinical practices. This includes learning about themselves, learning from their patients, and being able to assess and assimilate as useful evidence for practice the other sources of propositional and nonpropositional knowledge that appear all around us. These conclusions concerning the nature of clinical reasoning by expert physical therapy practitioners supports the findings of the grounded theory studies by our colleagues in this book.

REFERENCES

1. Sackett D, Strauss S, Richardson W, et al. *Evidence-based medicine: how to practice and teach EBM*, ed 2. Edinburgh: Churchill Livingstone, 2000.
2. Edwards I, Jones MA, Carr J, et al. Clinical reasoning strategies in physical therapy. *Phys Ther.* 2004a;84:312–335.
3. Strauss A, Corbin J. Grounded theory methodology: an overview. In NK Denzin, YS Lincoln (eds). *Handbook of qualitative research.* London: Sage Publications, 1994.
4. Chamaz K. Grounded theory: objectivist and constructivist methods. In NK Denzin, YS Lincoln (eds). *Handbook of qualitative research.* Thousand Oaks: Sage Publications, 2000.
5. Jensen GM, Gwyer J, Hack LM, Shepard KF. *Expertise in physical therapy practice.* Boston: Butterworth–Heinemann, 1999.
6. Merriam SB. *Qualitative research and case study applications in education: a qualitative approach.* San Francisco: Jossey-Bass, 1998.
7. Edwards IC. *Clinical reasoning in three different fields of physiotherapy—a qualitative case study approach,* Vols. I and II. Unpublished thesis submitted in partial fulfillment of the Doctor of Philosophy in Health Sciences, University of South Australia, Adelaide, Australia. The Australian Digitized Theses Program, 2001. Available at: http://www.library.unisa.edu.au/adt-root/public/ adt-SUSA-20030603-090552/index.html. Accessed October 31, 2005.
8. Elstein AS, Schulman LS, Sprafka SA. *Medical problem solving: an analysis of clinical reasoning.* Cambridge, MA: Harvard University Press, 1978.
9. Fleming MH. The therapist with the three track mind. *Am J Occup Ther.* 1991;45:1007–1014.
10. Benner P, Tanner C, Chelsa C. *Expertise in nursing practice: Caring, clinical judgment and ethics.* New York: Springer Publishing, 1996.
11. Mattingly C. Clinical revision: changing the therapeutic story in midstream. In C Mattingly, MH Fleming. *Clinical reasoning: forms of inquiry in a therapeutic practice.* Philadelphia: FA Davis, 1994.
12. Fleming MH. The therapist with the three track mind. In C Mattingly, MH Fleming. *Clinical reasoning: forms of inquiry in a therapeutic practice.* Philadelphia: FA Davis, 1994.

10

13. Beauchamp T, Childress JF. *Principles of biomedical ethics*. New York: Oxford University Press, 1994.

14. Charon R. Narrative contributions to medical ethics: recognition, formulation, interpretation and validation in the practice of the ethicist. In ER DuBose, R Hamel, LJ O'Connell (eds). *A matter of principles: ferment in U.S. bioethics*. Valley Forge, PA: Trinity Press International, 1994.

15. Jensen GM, Gwyer J, Hack LM, Shepard KF. Expert practice in physical therapy. *Phys Ther*. 2000;80:28–52.

16. Schmidt HG, Boshuizen HPA, Norman GR. Reflections on the nature of expertise in medicine. In E Keravnou (ed). *Deep models for medical knowledge engineering*. Amsterdam: Elsevier, 1992.

17. Higgs J, Titchen A. Knowledge and reasoning. In J Higgs, MA Jones (eds). *Clinical reasoning in the health professions*, ed 2. New York: Butterworth–Heinemann, 2000.

18. Denzin NK, Lincoln YS: Introduction. In NK Danzin, YS Lincoln (eds). *Handbook of qualitative research*. London: Sage Publications, 1994.

19. Habermas J. *Theory of communicative action*. Boston: Beacon Press, 1984.

20. Mezirow J. *Transformative dimensions of adult learning*. San Francisco: Jossey Bass, 1991.

21. Resnik L, Jensen G. Using clinical outcomes to explore the theory of expert practice in physical therapy. *Phys Ther*. 2003;83:1090–1106.

22. Schon DA. *The reflective practitioner—how professionals think in action*. San Francisco: Jossey Bass, 1983.

23. Cassell EJ. Teaching the fundamentals of primary care: a point of view. *The Millbank Quarterly* 1995;73:373–405.

24. Charon R, Montello M. *Stories matter: the role of narrative in medical ethics*. New York: Routledge, 2002.

25. Jones MA. Clinical reasoning in manual therapy. *Phys Ther*. 1992;72:875–884.

26. Payton OD. Clinical reasoning process in physical therapy. *Phys Ther*. 1985;65:924–928.

27. Thomas-Edding D. Clinical problem solving in physical therapy and its implications for curriculum development. In *Proceedings of the Tenth International Congress of the World Confederation for Physical Therapy*, May 17–22, 1987. Sydney, Australia. London, United Kingdom: World Confederation for Physical Therapy, 1987, 100–104.

28. White M, Epston D. *Narrative means to therapeutic ends*. New York: WW Norton, 1990.

29. Thornquist E. Diagnostics in physical therapy—processes, patterns and perspectives. Part I. *Adv Phys Ther*. 2001;3:140–150.

30. Borkan JM, Quirk M, Sullivan M. Finding meaning after the fall: injury narratives from elderly hip fracture patients. *Soc Sci Med*. 1991;33:947–957.

31. Osborn M, Smith JA. The personal experience of chronic benign lower back pain: an interpretative phenomenological analysis. *Br J Health Psych*. 1988;3:65–83.

32. Turk D. Cognitive factors in chronic pain and disability. In R Gatchel, D Turk (eds). *Psychological approaches to pain management—a practitioner's handbook*. New York: The Guilford Press, 1996.

33. Greeno J. The situativity of knowing, learning and research. *Am Psych*. 1998;53:5–26.

34. Jones MA, Edwards I, Gifford L. Conceptual models for implementing biopsychosocial theory in clinical practice, *Manual Therapy* 2002;7:2–9.

35. Edwards I, Jones MA, Higgs J, et al. What is collaborative reasoning? *Adv Phys Ther*. 2004b;6:70–83.

36. Edwards I, Braunack-Mayer A, Jones MA. Ethical reasoning as a clinical reasoning strategy. *Physiother*. 2005; 91:229–236[5_AU4].

37. Sim J. Respect for autonomy: issues in neurological rehabilitation. *Clin Rehab*. 1998;12:3–10.

38. Patel VL, Groen GJ. Knowledge-based solution strategies in medical reasoning, *Cogn Sci*. 1986;10:91–116.

39. Higgs J, Jones MA. Clinical reasoning: an introduction. In J Higgs, MA Jones (eds). *Clinical reasoning in the health professions*, ed 2. New York: Butterworth–Heinemann, 2000.

40. Barrows HS, Feltovich PJ. The clinical reasoning process. *Med Educ*. 1987;21:86–91.

41. Higgs J, Jones MA, Edwards I, et al. Clinical reasoning and practice knowledge. In J Higgs, B Richardson, M Dahlgren (eds). *Developing practice knowledge for health professionals*. Edinburgh: Butterworth–Heinemann, 2004.

42. Gifford L. *Topical issues in pain 2. Biopsychosocial assessment, relationships and pain*. Falmouth, UK: CNS Press, 2000.

43. Main C, Spanswick C. Models of pain. In C Main, C Spanswick (eds). *Pain management: an interdisciplinary approach*. Edinburgh: Churchill Livingstone, 2000.

44. Cervero R. Professional practice, learning, and continuing education: an integrated perspective. *Int J Lifelong Educ*. 1992;10:91–101.
45. Higgs J, Hunt A. Rethinking the beginning practitioner: Introducing the "Interactional Professional." In J Higgs, H Edwards (eds). *Educating beginning practitioners*. Melbourne: Butterworth–Heinemann, 1999.
46. Shepard KF, Jensen GM. *Physical therapist curricula for the 1990s: Educating the reflective practitioner. Phys Ther*. 1990;70:566–577.
47. Greenhalgh T, Hurwitz B. Why study narrative? In T Greenhalgh, B Hurwitz (eds). *Narrative based medicine: dialogue and discourse in clinical practice*. London: BMJ Books, 1998.
48. Moseley L. A pain neuromatrix approach to patients with chronic pain. *Manual Therapy* 2003;8(3):130–140.
49. Waddell G. *The back pain revolution*, ed 2. Edinburgh: Churchill Livingstone, 2004.
50. Cook FM, Hassenkamp AM. Active rehabilitation for chronic low back pain: the patients' perspective. *Phys Ther*. 2000;86(2):61–68.
51. Mishler EG. Models of narrative analysis: a typology. *J Narr Life History* 1995;5:87–123.
52. Philips HC. Avoidance behavior and its role in sustaining chronic pain. *Behav Res Ther*. 1987;25(4):273–279.
53. Daykin A, Richardson B. Physiotherapists' pain beliefs and their influence on the management of patients with chronic low back pain. *Spine* 2004;29(7):783–795.
54. Sargeant N. Unpublished study as part fulfillment of Bachelor of Applied Science in Physiotherapy. University of South Australia, Adelaide, South Australia, 2004.

10

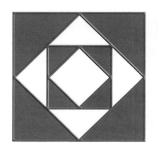

Square in a Square — A traditional Amish block that, in turning the square on point, gives a new perspective.

11

Situated Expertise: The Wisdom of Practice in a Transdisciplinary Rehabilitation Clinic

Elizabeth Mostrom

The theory of expertise in physical therapy developed and elaborated by Jensen, Gwyer, Hack, and Shepard has shaped my thinking and practice in many important ways. In my research and writing, it has provided new lenses through which I can view my inquiry into expertise. It has also provided a lexicon for description of some of the phenomena I observe as I watch experts at work—clinicians and clinical educators—while adding texture and enlarged meaning to my findings. In my work with physical therapy students, it has opened my eyes to the multiple dimensions of expertise and challenged me as a teacher to seek creative ways to sow and cultivate the seeds of emergent expertise as I engage with students in the classroom and the clinic.—Elizabeth Mostrom, PT, PhD

JOHN (on his therapy with Caitlin): She has given me a lot of confidence to go . . . I lost the words. . . . She establishes a confidence in you. She makes you . . . she made me believe in myself to a point where I thought I couldn't get past the pain, to believe that I could. And I went past the pain, and I went the distance I had to go.

BILL (on his therapy with Caitlin): I found out that I couldn't walk a straight line. . . . I was going to the right, although my perception was that I was going a straight line. . . . So I had to learn to pull back. That was interesting. . . . [Caitlin] explained what she was gonna try to do and gave me somewhat of a lesson to carry with me. And I didn't know if it was gonna work . . . but I have very little problem now. I think that the constant little things she made out for me to do helped. Now, I don't like that balance beam thing, but I can see the value in it. I can walk farther than I did before. I'm containing my balance better.

MARCIA (on her therapy with Caitlin): I've been very happy I did [have therapy with Caitlin]! Because my balance is considerably better, and . . . although I'm not one to dwell on what's wrong with me and why I feel this way, I definitely feel that I have gained a lot of knowledge [about that]. And it *did* make me feel better to know that something could be done. And Caitlin was very good about explaining the vestibular system and how there are different things that make you unbalanced and make you dizzy. So, I felt that knowing there was some reason for my dizziness—other than just a head injury—was very helpful.

This chapter tells the stories of an experienced physical therapist—Caitlin—and several of her patients—John, Marcia, and Bill—working toward mutual goals in the context of a private transdisciplinary rehabilitation clinic. The chapter also discusses some of Caitlin's work with other professionals in the clinic because her story and journey into mastery is tightly woven with her everyday interactions with members of her rehabilitation team. After the reader has come to know Caitlin, her patients, and some of her colleagues, I conclude by considering the findings of the investigation described in this chapter in light of the theory of expertise in physical therapy proposed in this volume.

This brief portrait of expertise is the result of an ethnographic and microethnographic study that spanned almost 3 years. As with all ethnographic work, a focus of the study was to seek to understand the culture of the clinic in which physical therapy and other rehabilitation services were provided. Another focus was to closely study the nature of the interaction of an experienced physical therapist (Caitlin) with patients with neurologic impairment in the cultural context of this clinic. The broader ethnographic work developed into a detailed case study of Caitlin's beliefs and day-to-day practice in physical therapy.

Data-collection methods included observation and the generation of field notes; informal and formal (audiotaped) interviews with Caitlin, other clinic associates, and patients; videotaping of patient–physical therapist sessions; and videotape review sessions with Caitlin. Videotape data were subjected to

11

detailed analysis with attention to 1) the linguistic features of discourse (message content and turn-taking [i.e., what was said and when]); 2) the paralinguistic features of discourse (how something was said [e.g., intonation, prosody, volume]); and 3) other nonverbal aspects of interaction, such as facial expressions, movement (kinesics), and the use of space (proxemics) during therapy sessions.

BACKGROUND

Caitlin was identified by several physical therapists in a variety of neurologic rehabilitation settings as someone who embodied the personal characteristics, knowledge, practical wisdom, and clinical skill associated with expertise in neurologic rehabilitation. Caitlin had been a physical therapist for 12 years when the study was initiated. She started her career in an acute-care setting, moved to an inpatient rehabilitation facility, and finally came to work in the private outpatient rehabilitation clinic described in this study in 1987. During the 6 years before the study, Caitlin had limited her practice to working with clients with neurologic impairment and had a special interest in working with adolescents and adults who had sustained head or brain injury of varying etiologies.

Caitlin is a respected and nationally recognized clinician, teacher, and speaker in her area of expertise. She received a bachelor of science degree in physical therapy and biology and later pursued a master of science degree in physical therapy, with a focus on adult education and motor learning and control. She is a frequent presenter at physical therapy conferences and continuing education courses; has published several clinical research articles; and is active in professional associations, including the neurology section of the American Physical Therapy Association (APTA). Shortly after the initiation of the study, Caitlin became a board-certified specialist in neurologic physical therapy.

Caitlin identified several motivations for moving her practice from acute care to neurologic rehabilitation. Early in her career, she was attracted to the patient relationships developed in rehabilitation and the diversity of patient problems and goals this practice area provided.

> **CAITLIN:** I liked the aspect of developing a long-term relationship with the patient. I liked the challenge of every patient being different even with the same diagnosis—having different problems, different goals.

Eventually, she became disenchanted with the institutional focus on generation of productivity units and restrictions on direct treatment time in the large rehabilitation center. She believed that frequent and direct physical therapist and patient interactions were essential to the development of therapeutic relationships and effective teaching and learning for patients and therapists. She also believed that the long-term interests of patients were not well-served by focusing on therapy goals related to what a patient could do in the hospital or rehabilitation setting as compared with the home and community. These concerns coincided with her own realization that her knowledge and understanding of what her patients were experiencing and needed was "just at a surface level. . . . I felt that there was a lot more that could be offered [to patients]."

Caitlin entered graduate school where she encountered two mentors who shaped her thinking about clinical practice in important ways. One of these individuals was her adviser, whom she described in the following manner:

> **CAITLIN:** She was a real dynamic problem solver and researcher. She really challenged me to look at the clinical process as a research process . . . to carefully look at patient problems and underlying causes and to not get into treatment and just assume old biases or standard patterns [regarding treatment regimens].

Caitlin's second mentor was her supervisor for her educational internship during her graduate studies. According to Caitlin, he "had really good insights about how to approach the adult learner, and he . . . opened my eyes to the processes of adult learning."

Having mentors and expanding her knowledge base as a result of her graduate education led to several changes in the way she approached her work:

> **CAITLIN:** I was a lot more into clinical problem solving . . . much more into looking at the inter-relationship between cognitive and movement dysfunction . . . much more into teaching . . . much more into my role as a teacher and an advocate [for patients and their families].

Caitlin's move to a private rehabilitation clinic enabled her to engage in these types of problem-solving activities and become much more involved in being a patient educator and advocate. Clients referred to the clinic are often patients with complex problems with whom other practitioners had experienced limited success. The clinic professional "associates" included physical therapists, occupational therapists, speech and language pathologists, social workers, and a neuropsychologist. In the private clinic, the therapists focused on clients' needs and concerns with respect to community reentry or returning to their home and work environments. Therapists were also able to schedule longer periods to work with patients, without having to pay attention to the number of "units" generated.

In addition to her involvement in clinical practice and research, Caitlin serves as an adjunct faculty member at a local university, where she teaches graduate-level courses in neurologic physical therapy. She spends the rest of her time juggling family responsibilities, caring for her young children, and engaging in community-oriented activities.

11

PHILOSOPHY OF PRACTICE

COMMUNAL PHILOSOPHY OF THE CLINIC AND CLINICIANS: CLIENT CENTERING

Caitlin and the other professional staff at the clinic had a shared philosophy of practice. This philosophy, which the clinicians called *client centering*, involved several key components or activities (Table 11-1). Client centering was thought to be facilitated by 1) the development of therapeutic alliances with clients; 2) a transdisciplinary team approach to care; and 3) the communal adoption of a clinic philosophy that represented the ideals, values, and beliefs of the clinicians

Table 11-1. Summary of Components and Facilitators of Client Centering

Components	Facilitators
Establishing client needs/goals; seeking meaningful, mutual goals; giving patients voice and power in decision making about care	Communal adoption of clinic philosophy; cultural beliefs, values, norms for action
Developing individualized treatment programs that address unique problems in creative ways	Establishing a therapeutic alliance with clients
Emphasis on client and family education; reciprocal teaching and learning in therapy	Transdisciplinary team approach to care
Goals of enabling and empowering clients	
Serving as an advocate for clients and families/caregivers	

and created norms for action in their sociocultural system (see Table 11-1). The following sections briefly describe, in the therapists' words, the primary components and facilitators of client centering; a subsequent section describes Caitlin's expert practice in the cultural context of this philosophy of practice.

Starting Where the Client Is

When asked what client centering meant to them, several therapists responded that first and foremost it was "important to start where the client is." One of the clinic owners explained that the clinic often receives referrals in cases in which previous attempts to work with individuals have failed. The clinic team had often discovered that other therapists "were really trying to impose their own goals on the patient or the patient's family rather than listening to the patient and the patient's family about what it is they want."

Seeking Meaning and Setting Mutual Goals: Individualizing Therapy

The search for and the development of goals meaningful to patients were described as crucial elements of client centering that went beyond carefully listening to the patient and his or her family about their problems and needs. According to one of the clinicians, it involved concerted exploration of what was most important to patients in their lives outside of rehabilitation:

> It's figuring out what are the new goals. In a lot of rehab, I think rehab is the goal . . . and here we're thinking about when you leave rehab, what are you going to do on a day-to-day basis that will be meaningful to you.

In the case of three of the clients treated by Caitlin, this information and individual patient goals formed the basis for the mutual development of therapy goals and activities that explicitly incorporated the patient's wishes regarding desired outcomes for therapy. For Bill, meaningful and functional goals included returning to work as a pharmacist and being able to bowl and golf without experiencing nausea, dizziness, and loss of balance associated with his mild head injury. For Marcia, a 73-year-old woman who had sustained a moderate head injury and multiple trauma in an automobile accident, therapy goals and activities focused on returning her to community service and church-related activities, completing daily walks, and golfing with her husband and friends.

For John, a 36-year-old man with an astrocytoma, activities and goals were directed toward allowing him to continue participating in social activities and to be engaged in some form of work that would allow him to help people, which was important to him. John also liked to cook; thus, the clinic team secured a job for him at a local soup kitchen. Participating at the kitchen became a driving force for some of John's early rehabilitation in the clinic, and the activity became a highlight of John's week. This is one example of how individualized goals and creative treatment interventions are tied to what the patient has identified as meaningful activities.

For Caitlin, the focus on the uniqueness of each patient and his or her life needs was something that made her work interesting and challenging:

> **CAITLIN:** [The clinic staff] are looking at where and how the client must function—at home, in school, at work, in their social activities—and letting *their* life needs become the guide [to the rehabilitation process].

Client centering does not require abandoning the perspectives, knowledge, and expertise of therapists in discussions about a client's rehabilitation; instead, it involves establishing partnerships with clients that provided for participation in decision making about care.

Therapy as an Educative Endeavor: The Path to Empowerment

In numerous descriptions of client centering, Caitlin and other clinic associates emphasized that teaching and learning were essential reciprocal activities in therapy sessions. The therapists learned about and from their patients and their families to allow them to develop meaningful goals for therapy. Similarly, the therapists taught patients so that the patients could function as they had before. Education and knowledge were considered tools for empowerment of clients.

Caitlin frequently discussed her roles as teacher and advocate for patients and commented on the importance of time in achieving desired educational outcomes for all involved in therapy:

> **CAITLIN:** Patient and family education takes a lot of time . . . time to let [the patient] be part of the rehab process rather than someone who is just being treated . . . or cured [by the rehabilitation team].

11

Caitlin also noted that part of the teaching and learning essential to client centering was working to alter patient and family conceptions about their roles in their rehabilitative care:

> **CAITLIN:** I think that part of the education process is letting them realize that they're the *center* of the rehab team rather than the team managing them. And I think in larger centers, that can get lost real easily.

Caitlin's emphasis on teaching and learning in therapy is consistently evident in her interactions with patients. Caitlin repeatedly spoke of and demonstrated a belief that patients participate more fully in their rehabilitation if they understand the rationale for what they are doing, the consequences of not doing specific activities, and the rehabilitation options they have available so that they can make their own choices about the care they receive. One of the clinic owners summarized this commitment to therapy as an educative endeavor and its relationship to empowerment in the following manner:

> *You can continue to see them [treat the clients] . . . or you can educate them and have them do stuff on their own. I think our whole treatment philosophy is an empowerment model—how do we empower the client? You know, the whole experience of disability is so disempowering . . . that the therapeutic philosophy has to be empowerment. You teach people how they can be back in the driver's seat again, and that takes a tremendous amount of education. And you have people coming to you with all different levels of sophistication so that you can't have a standard educational approach. . . . You can't have ready-made exercises that you just hand out and say, "Here, do 10 of these." I mean, that approach to physical therapy is anathema here.*

Importance of Advocacy

Advocacy for clients and families is also described as an essential component of client centering. Advocacy, like education, is concerned with ultimately serving client empowerment. Clinicians frequently served as advocates for clients and their families when they sought to return to activities at home or in their communities or if they needed an additional voice to assure that their needs were met in the medical or rehabilitation community.

Building Therapeutic Alliances

All clinic associates suggested that an essential facilitator, or cornerstone, of the achievement of the components of client centering was the development of therapeutic alliances with clients. One therapist described the development of an alliance in the following manner:

> *It's finding out . . . what is the language of this patient? How does this patient think? What turns this patient on? How do I then communicate in their language and in their value system and bring something to them that's valuable?*

Discovering a patient's "language" and then creating a shared language (and ultimately a shared understanding) that reflects and respects the patient's values as well as the professional's knowledge and judgment are not small tasks when working with many patients with complex brain injuries. All therapists stressed the importance of reciprocity and responsibility in therapeutic alliances. One of the associates described an alliance as "a relationship in which each participant is invested and shares responsibility for healing, learning, and change."

The collective and individual commitment to the philosophy of client centering created a framework for interpretation of activity and interaction in the clinic and raised important and interesting questions about how Caitlin (and other experienced health care professionals) worked to achieve these ideals in the complicated world of everyday clinical practice.

PHILOSOPHY IN CONSTRUCTION: CLINICAL PRACTICE THEMES

CREATING AND SUSTAINING THERAPEUTIC ALLIANCES

Caitlin believed that therapeutic alliances served as the relational foundation for the realization of client centering and successful outcomes in therapy. Thus, examining how therapists and clients develop alliances became an important focus of the study. The following sections focus on key patterns and features of interaction that seemed to foster the development of shared language and understandings. Some of these features are both facilitators for and manifestations of therapeutic alliances.

Importance of Time and Undivided Attention

Therapists emphasized that alliances could not be created in single, brief, or hurried encounters with clients. This realization was translated into a commitment by therapists to spend a relatively extended period with each client (usually 1–2 hours per visit), during which they could focus solely on a patient and his or her needs. Only one client would be seen by a therapist at any given time. In addition, after Caitlin or any other therapist initiated therapy with a particular client, only that therapist provided services within his or her discipline. In this way, continuity of care was assured for each client.

When working with her clients, Caitlin always provided her full and undivided attention. This occurred from the time she came to the waiting room to invite her patients back to the therapy gym and continued until the end of the sessions, when Caitlin would walk the patients back to the reception area to discuss scheduling future appointments.

The overall fluidity of movement and conversation during these transitions into, within, and at the end of sessions was impressive. These fluid and synchronous rhythms of therapy are part of the focused attention and respectful listening that contribute to the creation and sustenance of alliances.

Rhythms of Therapy

The smoothness of transitions into and out of treatment sessions, as well as transitions within therapy sessions (e.g., between exercise segments), was characterized by an easy interweaving of the client's and Caitlin's movements and conversations, both social and professional. In some cases, Caitlin's movements seemed to be synchronous with those of the client; in other cases they appeared to be deliberately slower and more controlled, although natural, as if to demonstrate the type of movement patterns that would be helpful for her patients.

11

Caitlin displayed an economy of movement and vocalizations that were soft and unhurried.

Although transitions into and within treatment sessions were certainly organized, they did not seem tightly structured or hurried. Sessions inevitably began with social conversations, which gradually faded into more therapist-directed and treatment-oriented discussion and activity. Some time was almost always spent gathering information from the client about how home exercises and activities were going and how they were being integrated into the client's daily functional routine. When asked about these observations, Caitlin suggested that this is something she does consciously:

> **CAITLIN:** Well, I think that's good for the patient. It's not like, "All right, let's hop on up here [and get going]." . . . I think, with patients, I'm a little different [than I usually am]. I have to very consciously slow down.

Caitlin gave an example of how, when she was working with John, she purposefully did not move around much because of his distractibility; she focuses her full attention on what information is being exchanged between them:

> **CAITLIN:** I mean, for example, if I were waiting for him to take his sweatshirt off, or this or that, you know, he's distractible. . . . I know that it takes him a long time to get his sweatshirt off, so I will use that time as an interactive time, not as a set up for this or that. . . . [I'm] trying not to interfere with the kinds of information I get from him while he is taking his sweatshirt off. As you may notice, he tends to follow me around the room, so I try to limit where I go and where I move and keep the focus on whatever information we're exchanging, whether it be how he's sleeping at night, positioning, or whatever.

Caitlin's economy, slowness, and fluidity of movement with some clients are attempts to diminish distractions in therapy and to allow her to focus on what patients are saying and doing at any point in therapy. The types of information gathered or exchanged as John removes his sweatshirt, for instance, are 1) observations of his function in this task of daily living; 2) observations of the quality of his neck, shoulder, arm, and trunk movements; and 3) reports of any pain or difficulty he is having with the task as he completes it.

Respectful Listening and Seeking Understanding

The development of an alliance and the ability to "start where the client is" are possible only in the presence of what the therapists called *respectful listening*. Such listening involved "trying to understand where the patient is coming from and where they want to go." It involved a willingness "to capture and understand the patient's sense of things . . . without passing judgment" on a patient's perceptions or views regarding his or her illness, although they might not match the therapist's perceptions.

On several occasions, Caitlin discussed the importance of accepting and respecting the client's reality and the need for nonjudgmental interaction. She found this particularly important in her work with clients who had sensory-perceptual and cognitive impairments associated with their brain or head injuries. Caitlin explained that she learned this lesson through years of experience and practice:

> **CAITLIN:** I learned never to question the patient's perceptions regarding something they're experiencing. I think that one of the things I have really learned over the years is that even if you may not believe your patient—whether it's how much pain they're having or how much time they're spending [doing home exercises]—is to realize that, to them, it seems like 2 hours or to them it seems like their pain is that intense and there's no reason to even challenge that perception.

> [I have come to realize] that not only patients but individuals in general perceive things differently. And it's not our role to question how they're perceiving things—it's valid to them. . . . You just see that perceptions don't match over and over again, but it's just their perception of the whole situation, and it's not productive to question what they are experiencing. You just need to understand where they are at and try to work from there.

Working "from there" for Caitlin, however, could mean working to alter patients' perceptions regarding certain aspects of their illness experience without disregarding, denying, or abandoning their reality or sense of things.

> **CAITLIN:** You can't deny someone else's feeling. It's what they are experiencing. But you can try to alter that experience over time. . . . You respect [their perceptions] and just gradually try to stretch the window.

Asking the Right Questions

The therapists' descriptions of respectful listening, combined with a commitment to client centering, suggests that therapists must do two things to create and sustain therapeutic alliances: they must ask clients the right questions, and they must listen to the clients' stories. Asking the right questions means asking patients about their needs, goals, and hopes for therapy. It means actively seeking what is meaningful and important to clients and using those things as a guide to therapy. Caitlin's sessions with patients were filled with questions directed at ascertaining patients' perceptions about their problems and determining their goals and expectations for therapy. The following examples are drawn from the initial evaluation session with Marcia (Table 11-2):

> **CAITLIN:** Before I start my screen, I guess what I'd like to know is what you feel, functionally, are any problems that you're having / um, that you haven't recovered fully / since the accident and the kind of rehab you've had so far?

In response to this question, Marcia discusses several areas of concern—things that bother her or things that she cannot do that she would like to do with less difficulty. These include concerns about dizziness and losses of balance (even with turning of her head when talking to friends at church), the inability to walk without a cane, her fear of walking long distances or on uneven surfaces and stairs, and her general fatigue and shortness of breath with activity. During this time, Caitlin listens intently to Marcia, occasionally records some notes, and

Table 11–2. Transcription Conventions*

Symbol	Meaning
⌈	Overlapping speech
⌐	Latching (no interturn pause)
/	Short pause (less than 1 second)
/ /	Long pause (more than 1 second)
╱	Rising intonation (often associated with interrogative)
╲	Falling intonation (often associated with "." or "!")
<u>underline</u>	Spoken with emphasis
CAPS	Very emphatic, louder
o-o-o	Dragging out of vowel sounds
/???/	Audible, but unable to make out words
. . .	Dangling sentence, feeling of more to come
∿∿	Very soft speech
∧∧∧	Harsh (often loud) speech
(smiles)	Descriptions of nonverbal behaviors accompanying talk (e.g., facial expressions, gaze direction, positional changes and movement); also used to identify chuckles or laughs and to suggest implied (but not spoken) words

*Notations illustrate features of discourse that can influence meaning and interpretation in exchanges (e.g. pauses, turn taking, and paralinguistic and nonverbal aspects of interaction).

probes intermittently for more detailed descriptions of the nature or perceived sources of the problem as described by Marcia. By asking a pointed question about what Marcia perceives to be her greatest functional losses and problems, Caitlin has obtained much information to guide both her examination and treatment program. As this 10-minute conversation concludes, Caitlin summarizes what she has heard and checks her perceptions with Marcia:

[DL] CAITLIN: So you would say that your main functional deficits that you're feeling at this point, um, since the accident, is the balance and some limitations in your walking. . .

MARCIA: ⌐Mmm hmm, and limitations in that I can't make every <u>move</u> that I used to make. You know how you just bend over to pick something up or get something off the bottom shelf down ⌈there (demonstrating).

CAITLIN: ⌊Uh hmmm

MARCIA: I'm not so sure if I can get down there by the bottom shelf and get back up again.

CAITLIN: (nodding)   ⌐So-o-o, any functional movements that really require that kind of dynamic balance // you're not so sure about / That's important to know because what I want to do is, is look at structuring the [evaluation] and, you know, rehab around the areas of function that are a problem for <u>you</u>. I mean, I might find other things/ but we really want to focus on areas that, um, are of concern for you.

In Caitlin's summary of what she has heard from Marcia (and her offer of conversational time and opportunity for additions or corrections), she also makes the idea of client centering explicit to the client. Marcia's subsequent therapy focused on the functional problems she described at the outset of therapy in addition to working toward her ability to return to playing golf—a recreational goal that emerged later in the initial session.

In addition to asking questions about patients' needs, goals, and perceptions about their problems, Caitlin also asked questions that invited their participation during treatment decisions. For instance, Caitlin believed that John would benefit from the use of an ankle–foot orthosis (AFO) and a cane to improve his gait pattern, stability, and endurance in walking. She realized that John did not think he needed these devices for safety in ambulation, but she wanted to have John involved in the final decision about using these devices. In an attempt to address John's lack of recognition or denial of the need for using an AFO or cane, Caitlin and John went for walks in the community. They walked on varying terrain, in a variety of settings, and up and down curbs and stairs. Sometimes they used an AFO and cane, and sometimes they used neither. Caitlin asked John the following types of questions:

CAITLIN: Where and when are you safe? Where and when can you clear your leg (e.g., over curbs, stairs, or obstacles)? With or without the cane? With or without the AFO?

Although this approach required several therapy sessions with John, Caitlin believed this was a way to keep the patient involved in decision making about his rehabilitation. At the same time, it permitted her to share her professional knowledge, experience, and observations with John so that he might consider her recommendations when making *his* choice about whether using a cane or AFO would make his walking easier and safer. Caitlin later discussed how she believed this approach, which involved work to align patient perceptions, expectations, and goals with actual performance and potential, differed from other prevalent models of providing treatment recommendations for clients:

CAITLIN: I think it's a different approach than going in and saying, you know, "You have to wear this. This is what I recommend. Go home and have a good day." . . . I let him be real interactive in realizing the need for the decision. And in many patients, what I often do is videotape them and let them watch themselves . . . and then ask "What do you think looks best? Where does your walking look most normal? . . . When do you feel the safest?"

Decision making in therapy becomes a collaborative process that considers the patient's perspectives and the therapist's knowledge and expertise, as they jointly make informed choices about treatment.

11

Listening to and Exchanging Stories

Asking the right questions of patients and listening to their stories are interrelated features of discourses between Caitlin and her clients that create and maintain therapeutic alliances and client centering. Many authors have written about the power of narrative and storytelling to help individuals understand the subjective experience of others (1–5); this has been postulated to be especially important in understanding the illness experience of others (6–11). Many exchanges and accounts of experience took narrative forms in therapy sessions with Caitlin.

During an initial evaluation session, Marcia shared three primary stories with Caitlin: the polio story, the driving-range story, and the tablecloth story. All of these stories had familiar narrative forms—they were situated in time and place and entailed a goal, either met, unmet, or partially met. They describe what was happening at a particular time in Marcia's life and how Marcia felt about what was happening. Thus, like most stories, they had descriptive and emotive functions. Each story lasted between 1 and 2 minutes and was not interrupted by Caitlin.

Marcia began the polio story with a statement that located the story in time:

> **MARCIA:** I was about 5 at the time. . . . Well, you know, there was an epidemic going around. . . . You know, I remember this [story] mostly by my parents retelling it.

Caitlin listened carefully to this story and then explained to Marcia how the information in the story was important because her past exposure to polio could influence her current status and level of function. The information derived from the story helped guide Caitlin's examination and evaluative judgments. Perhaps more important, Caitlin let Marcia convey this valuable information through a story, as if she recognized more can be gained from a story than information. Stories can be powerful representations of a patient's life and illness experiences, and the exchanging of stories can be powerful sources of connection and understanding between individuals. The other stories that Marcia shared with Caitlin in the initial session—the driving-range story and the golf story—provided insight into activities that were meaningful for Marcia and functional problems she had as a result of her head injury. They also provided an opportunity for shared laughter.

Stories were evident in all of Caitlin's sessions that were observed. In the case of Bill, most of the stories revolved around golf, his cottage "up north" and family activities there, or happenings at work in the pharmacy. John's stories were varied and revealing. John had a special gift for storytelling and humor. He told stories about his work at the soup kitchen, stories about family customs and celebrations on St. Patrick's Day, and stories about a friend who raised rabbits.

John told several stories that provided insight into his experiences with a life-threatening and disabling illness. John's "Las Vegas story" developed out of a description of how he responded when his neurosurgeon told him that he had a limited time to live. The neurosurgeon offered the following prescription:

"Get out and enjoy life. Do something you've always wanted to do." John's "crips" story told of a barroom brawl and the swell of emotion and activity when he and a friend, "who also happens to walk with a cane," overheard a customer tell the bartender that he "didn't want to be sittin' next to a bunch of crips." These poignant and descriptive accounts of illness experience provide insight into John's search for and creation of meaning in the context of his diagnosis with a malignant brain tumor and his subsequent disability.

Patients' stories provide an unparalleled opportunity to gain new or transformed understandings of the needs, perspectives, and experiences of patients who are ill. Caitlin's attentive listening and responding to these stories in the context of therapy sessions was an integral part of building therapeutic alliances and providing client centering.

Constructing Shared Language: The Use of Metaphor, Imagery, and Repetition

Other linguistic tools or discourse strategies, besides stories, have the potential to create connections between participants, foster conversational coherence, and facilitate the development of shared understanding. Participants in therapy sessions frequently worked to construct shared language and mental representations in therapy through metaphors, imagery, and repetition.

Several authors have discussed how figurative forms of language, such as metaphors and imagery, can serve a number of functions, including social (12); interactional (13); cognitive processing and comprehension (14–17); and, more recently, therapeutic functions (18). The latter are especially useful when metaphors are jointly created and extended by clients and therapists because metaphors can be nonthreatening ways of talking about problems, distilling thoughts and feelings, providing understanding by illustrating global insights, and facilitating the development of rapport between participants when mutual effort exists to create and interpret metaphors (18). Metaphor also has a quality that invites attention, collaborative problem solving, and interpretation by participants (18). The following is one example of the use of metaphor in therapy. In this example, Bill interrupts Caitlin toward the end of a therapy session to further describe his problems with headaches.

> **BILL:** See, right now, I'm wearing a headband / I'm wearing a hat right now.

> **CAITLIN:** Yeah (sitting more erect and looking directly at him), feels like that, huh?

> (Bill nods). And the hat just gets <u>tighter and tighter</u>.

> **BILL:** (nodding and rocking forward and back) |Tighter and tighter.

> **CAITLIN:** Right, well our goal is to try and loosen the hat / take it off altogether. (Caitlin then discusses some strategies for loosening the "hat" [i.e., diminishing Bill's headaches]).

This segment illustrates several interesting features. First, Bill interrupts Caitlin (the professional) and introduces a topic change. Caitlin does not resist the shift in topic; instead, she affirms that Bill's headaches are important enough to drop her previous topic—she accepts the invitation of Bill's metaphor. She responds non-verbally and verbally to his description of his headaches as a headband and then a hat. She then extends the metaphor by suggesting that the hat just seems to get "tighter and tighter." This suggestion arises from information Caitlin gained in earlier conversations with Bill and shows that she has been listening to Bill's concerns about his headaches. Bill responds with an *exact* repetition of her description, including the intonation and rhythm of the response. This echo (18) indicates Bill's affirmation of Caitlin's interpretation of his headaches. Finally, Caitlin invokes and extends Bill's metaphor by suggesting that a mutual goal for therapy could be to loosen or remove the "hat." One of Bill's primary goals for therapy is to diminish his headaches.

On numerous occasions, Caitlin was aware of important metaphors introduced by clients to describe something they were experiencing. She wove the metaphors into conversations within and across therapy sessions. This indicated ratification of a patient's experience and provided a shared language for the client and therapist. As Caitlin reintroduced this language in therapy sessions, Caitlin and the client co-constructed and transformed the metaphor verbally and nonverbally to gain an understanding of the patient's experiences and the tasks of therapy. In one session, Bill introduced the metaphor of a washing machine or water sloshing around in buckets to describe how he felt when doing Hallpike maneuvers for his vestibular dysfunction. This was an apt description. Caitlin appropriated and invoked these metaphors and water images as she taught Bill about the vestibular system and worked with him on various exercises. Marcia's descriptions of her balance problems became the feeling of the "earth moving under her feet"; thus, Caitlin and Marcia worked to get her back on "solid ground."

Many of the conversations that revolved around metaphors also demonstrated a great deal of what is termed *other repetition*—that is, repetition of something another conversant has said. Tannen (13) has argued that the use of repetition in discourse is an important strategy for creating conversational involvement and coherence, which serve the development of understanding among participants. Such involvement, coherence, and shared understanding are critical for the development of alliances in therapy. Repetition can also be important for the accomplishment of social and interactional goals. Repetition of others can demonstrate a willingness to listen, and ratification or appreciation of ideas can provide evidence of a speaker's evaluation of what is being discussed (i.e., repeating words or phrases indicates an important point) and can be used for humor and play in conversation. Finally, other repetition is a resource in talk that can preserve "face" (13,18,19)—that is, the need for participants to be understood, be accepted, and have their self-image appreciated and protected.

One example of other repetition in therapy was illustrated in the transcript segment regarding Bill's headaches. An important feature of repetition in that segment was echo—that is, a moment when Bill followed Caitlin's description of his hat getting "tighter and tighter" with an exact and immediate repetition of her words with the same downward intonation and rhythm. Ferrara (18) claims that echoes represent instances of insight and empathy when the client emphatically agrees with the therapist, claiming the statement as his or her own. Furthermore, Ferrara points out that it is "therapeutic to be understood so thoroughly by another that you can emphatically agree with statements they make about your life."

Another example of other repetition came from a later session with Bill. Bill discussed some of the challenges he encounters in his pharmacy when he tried to work in a busy visual environment with a computer program that has recently been changed to include additional steps for processing orders.

BILL: They inserted a new step, and it's been hard to master that.

CAITLIN: Umm hmm.

BILL: Usually I master those things really quickly like.

CAITLIN: Mmm hmm.
Does it prompt you? on the computer?

BILL: It will, but I don't wait. I can't wait for that. I got customers waiting. I've got to get those people out of there.

CAITLIN: (smiling) So you prompt the computer to hurry up!

BILL: I prompt the computer to hurry up!

CAITLIN: (laughs and smiles)

This conversation illustrates several instances of other repetition that builds to an echo when Bill repeats (with a pronoun shift) Caitlin's observation—that Bill in fact is usually so fast in his work that he prompts the computer, not the other way around.

A final example of other repetition is drawn from a session with Marcia. The following exchange takes place when Caitlin seeks further information after Marcia complains that she fatigues more quickly and easily than she did before her accident.

CAITLIN: Do you find you're taking rest breaks / during the day / not necessarily naps but . . . ?

MARCIA: Mmm, not / not a rest break / more excuses to stop and have a cup of coffee (smiling).

CAITLIN: (smiles and chuckles) That's your definition of a rest break, huh?

MARCIA: Yeah, that's my rest break! (smiling and chuckling).

Caitlin introduces the term *rest break*. An alternating repetition of the term by Marcia and Caitlin ensues, as they settle on what rest break *means* for Marcia. This is a moment of constructing joint understanding for participants and provides considerable insight into Marcia's personality and lifestyle.

Repetition, metaphor, and imagery were discourse strategies frequently used by Caitlin and her clients. Other repetition can occur without understanding,

11

however. Metaphors can emerge and be explored in conversation without the participants settling on mutually understood or compatible interpretations. Still, this does not diminish the possibilities these features of discourse offer as participants seek understanding essential to therapeutic alliances and client centering. These strategies were skillfully, although not consciously, used by Caitlin and her clients as they constructed therapy sessions together.

Therapy as an Educative Endeavor

For Caitlin, as for other professionals in the clinic, therapy is an educative endeavor. The therapists believed that knowledge and skills gained through therapy were the tools that enabled and empowered clients. Teaching and learning, however, were not considered unidirectional; instead, the educative dimension was understood to be reciprocal and interactive. Therapists are teachers *and* learners in therapy. What therapists learn about and from patients shape what and how they teach and who they are as teachers. Likewise, patients are teachers and learners. This reciprocal relationship helps lay the foundation for transformation of participants and the achievement of therapeutic outcomes.

Caitlin's Beliefs about Teaching and Learning in Clinical Practice

Caitlin believed that a therapist's role as an educator was so important, she often called her therapist–client relationships *teacher–client relationships*. Caitlin considered fostering a client's "learning about the tools to manage his recovery or to manage his disability" one of her primary tasks in therapy. Caitlin reiterated that knowledge about disorders, problems, and the tools to manage disabilities was empowering for clients and family members or other caregivers. During a videotape review session, Caitlin made the following observations about the knowledge John had gained though therapy about his problems and how to manage them:

> CAITLIN: Note how in tune he is with his own treatment, his own requirements. Whether it's instructing somebody to assist him or whether he's doing it—he <u>knows a lot</u> about . . . what works for him and what doesn't . . . and that is <u>empowering</u>, in my mind.

In addition to beliefs about the importance of teaching and learning in therapy, Caitlin had beliefs and theories about teaching, learning, and learners that influenced the way she conducted therapy sessions directed toward educational goals.

Caitlin discussed how some of her theories about teaching and learning and her practice in the clinic were the result of clinical and classroom teaching experience. After experiencing the "blank stare" of some patients, their family members, and students, she adopted a teaching strategy that she describes in the following manner:

> CAITLIN: I try to provide the big picture and then go in and do some of the pieces and then go back out to the big picture. And you always review

before you bring in new points. You tie old points to new points. You keep trying to bring it back to where they [the people learning] are. . . . You know, you just don't get so much of that blank stare like when they come in the next time and don't have any idea. You learn after that to try something different.

In the case of clients, the "big picture" includes their disorders, problems, and the functional impairments and disability these things are producing. The "pieces" are the exercises and activities that have the potential to alter the impact and extent of the problems and decrease disability. Caitlin believed that work to connect the big picture and the pieces helps establish a rationale for therapy and fosters patient understanding and cooperation.

Caitlin also believed keeping the practice on "pieces" or components of performance linked to the context of patient goals and everyday activities was critically important. At first, she did this conceptually in therapy; later, she encouraged patients to incorporate therapeutic exercises into naturally occurring and meaningful activities. Caitlin's work with clients revealed her constant efforts to contextualize the activities of therapy; she believed this was essential to establishing a rationale for therapy and for facilitating patient learning, participation, and change. For example, Marcia and Bill were avid golfers and wanted to return to that activity without dizziness, nausea, and balance loss. Thus, golf terminology, imagery, and golflike movements became very much a part of the verbal and nonverbal discourse during therapy sessions.

Caitlin frequently discussed the importance of providing a rationale for exercises. She believed her job was to help patients recognize and experience the link between what could seem to be an isolated and unrelated exercise and the functional demands of clients' lives. For example, on numerous occasions Caitlin explicitly tied Bill's visual and vestibular exercises to the requirements of his work as a pharmacist:

> **CAITLIN:** Could you imagine telling someone who wasn't as bright as Bill . . . to do all these visual exercises? And they'd go back to their spouse and say, "This lady must be crazy. I mean, why does she want me doing all these little spot checks for my eyes?" I just think it's real important to tie in rationale all the time.

Caitlin's belief that she must work to embed exercises done in therapy in the context of their usefulness (and meaningfulness) for clients is grounded in a larger theory that learning and collaboration in therapy is facilitated when activities are situated and authentic.

As illustrated earlier, Caitlin also believed it was essential to "tie old points to new points"—to work from the existing experience and understandings of learners as she works to transform or enlarge those understandings or alter experience. Constant assessment and reassessment permitted her to scaffold and build instruction according to each individual's needs and capacity at any given point. In the following quotation, Caitlin draws on her work with Bill to describe how she individualized and scaffolded instruction in therapy:

CAITLIN: In terms of going through the exercises, it just depends on each particular individual. But I try to start out with the easy ones that they can handle at first and work into the ones . . . that are more challenging. So, like, for vestibular exercises, Bill's visual exercises were pretty easy for him to comprehend and follow through with initially, not overwhelming.

I mean, if you start asking somebody to do some of the positional exercises right away and get them real dizzy [you lose them]. You've got to kind of move into those . . . move into the more challenging exercises gradually. That's probably my organizational flow. . . . As I introduce a new [exercise or category of exercises], I always review—before I introduce the new one. I say, "Okay, last week we did the visual exercises. Are they going okay? Do you have any questions?" And we try a few. And [then I say], "Now we're going to move into this." So I kind of try to tie one to the other.

To be able to individualize and scaffold instruction in therapy, Caitlin discussed how important reciprocal feedback, or what she called *interactive feedback*, between therapist and client was to the accomplishment of this task:

CAITLIN: I think the interactive feedback is really critical. I try to make sure I do that through [each exercise] and at the end as well. I think self-evaluation of the client [about his or her performance and experience] is as important as my feedback. So I always try to make sure I get that.

Caitlin's beliefs and theories about teaching and learning in clinical practice were evident in observations and detailed analyses of therapy sessions. The key organizational and interactional features that appeared in therapy sessions included constant work to situate the activities of therapy in contexts of use and meaning to the client conceptually and practically; this served to explicitly and frequently establish a rationale for therapy and the smaller exercises and activities that constituted therapy. Ongoing dynamic assessments of each client's prior, current, and emergent knowledge and skill were done through attentive observation and reciprocal feedback during sessions. She also used scaffolding of instruction in therapy—the building of supports for learning and change that permitted clients to gradually move from assisted and guided performance to independent, self-monitored, and integrated performance of skills and functional tasks.

In this regard, Caitlin seemed to be very attuned to her client's emerging potential or "zone of proximal development" (20). This zone, originally described by Russian psychologist Lev Vygotsky, based on studies of the learning and development of children (20), is defined as follows: "the distance between the actual developmental level as determined by independent problem solving and the level of potential development as determined through problem solving under adult guidance or in collaboration with more capable peers" (p. 86). A key corollary of this concept is that dynamic assessment of performance, combined with joint problem solving and learning with and through others, provides for the development and maturation of new knowledge, skill, and performance.

PERSONAL ATTRIBUTES AND PROFESSIONAL DEVELOPMENT

Caitlin is a dedicated clinician deeply committed to the philosophy of client centering. She is hard working and strives to do the best that she can in all she undertakes. She has high standards for herself and a passion for knowledge and excellence. This is balanced by her compassion, attentiveness, patience, and quiet sense of humor demonstrated when she works with clients in the clinic. She enjoys the challenges of problem solving, teaching, and learning encountered with complex patients with neurologic dysfunction (and their family members or caregivers) as they seek to return to meaningful and functional activity at home and in their communities.

Caitlin enjoyed working with the highly experienced team of clinicians who make up the transdisciplinary team at the clinic in which she worked. The 10 rehabilitation professionals that practice in the clinic had more than 150 combined years of clinical experience at the time this study was undertaken. These clinic associates had been working together for many years and were committed to a transdisciplinary approach to care in which members of the team "just do everybody else's work to some extent." The vision of a transdisciplinary team articulated by staff members involved a sharing of responsibility, knowledge, experience, and professional expertise among team members working with clients and their caregivers so that all members of the team were working to solve problems and achieve both discipline-specific and transdisciplinary goals. Roles and disciplinary boundaries between professionals were considered semi-permeable and flexible, as team members engaged in joint problem solving and work together toward therapeutic goals established with clients. For Caitlin, becoming and being a member of this highly experienced and knowledgeable team has been a driving force in her professional development. Caitlin believed that the frequent formal and informal opportunities for interaction with team members in this clinic has deepened and broadened her perspectives concerning the needs of patients and the rehabilitation process:

> **CAITLIN:** One of the things that has helped me tremendously is working with the transdisciplinary team and [working] much closer with the social worker and the speech pathologist and the neuropsychologist. They have brought me to a whole different perspective on my patients than what a PT [physical therapist] normally comes from. . . . If you're transdisciplinary— *truly transdisciplinary*—you start getting a much broader perspective. We're always trying to consult with each other about what's happening in each other's therapies and to help each other. Looking at patient problems from a multisystem perspective or multidisciplinary viewpoint is *very* different than just reporting out your findings [at a team meeting]. It's a different way of looking at the patient.

In addition to Caitlin's ongoing involvement in clinical research, university teaching, and other professional activities, her day-to-day interaction with fellow professionals and with her patients provided fertile ground for her own continued learning, reflection, and professional development. All of these activities and experiences have contributed to Caitlin's professional wisdom and growth into mastery—a mastery grounded in a commitment to the multifaceted philosophy of client centering.

11

CAITLIN—10 YEARS LATER

Like other contributors to this book (Chapters 4–7), I was curious about Caitlin's professional journey 10 years after the original investigation was completed. In a follow-up interview, I asked her to describe her journey over the past 10 years and to discuss some of the things she had done or experienced that were meaningful to her and shaped her beliefs and practice.

Caitlin continued working at the transdisciplinary clinic for about 5 years, spending approximately half of her time in clinical practice and half of her time teaching at a local university, even as her family grew. Eventually, the clinic experienced difficulty maintaining its referral base and competing as an independent practice (providing a full menu of therapy services for clients with neurologic impairment) against much larger agencies that were expanding services in this area. A decision was made, with input from all clinic associates, to shift the focus of the clinic to providing social work and counseling services to their clients. According to Caitlin, this change provided "an opportunity to look at where I wanted to go in terms of my employment at that time."

She made a decision to move into a full-time non-tenure track faculty position at the university. As it happens, the university was in the process of initiating a transition to offering the entry-level doctorate in physical therapy (DPT) degree at that time. Caitlin immediately got more involved in new course and curricular development, clinical research, and mentoring faculty-directed student research. She was the primary person involved in redesign of the neurologic components of the curriculum and saw this as a chance to spend time "looking toward what entry-level practice should look like in the new age." This responsibility was both an opportunity and challenge, and a stimulus for reflection. "So when we went to the DPT—that was real important reflective time—What are we doing well? What are we not preparing our students for?" As part of this transition, Caitlin also directed an effort across the curriculum to enhance content and student experience in the area of case management—"and it's been very successful!"

Even as Caitlin moved into the realm of academics, she held to her belief that maintaining clinical practice was absolutely essential to her ongoing development as teacher, researcher, and clinician. As she put it, "The challenge for me all along has been that I wanted to be a clinician–educator. I wanted to be both.... I felt that my strength as an educator and my strength for this program was that I was still an active practitioner." Today Caitlin is working at least 1 day per week for a hospital-affiliated agency that provides home- and community-based services for clients with neurologic impairment, with approximately 60% of those clients having sustained head injuries. She is also actively engaged in consultation and staff development for a variety of agencies in the area. She has used these connections with clinicians, patients, and clinical and community-based agencies to establish and expand her clinical research agenda, to support her teaching and the learning of her students, and to forge community–university partnerships that serve many constituents. In summary, she said she would describe her journey as "trying to maintain my clinical practice and expertise through the projects [research and outreach] I've been involved in.... I strongly believe there is a important role for the clinical specialist in the academic setting."

An example of this belief is the degree of involvement Caitlin has maintained in the Neurology Section of the APTA. "The other things I have been increasingly involved in are professional service–based activities." Over the past 10 years Caitlin has served in a variety of leadership roles for the Section and the American Board of Physical Therapy Specialists, including serving on the specialty academy of content experts and as a specialty council member. She feels that "staying very active in the Section" and maintaining the networks that evolve out of such engagement:

> ... challenges me to stay current and to make sure the curriculum in neurology stays current. It really challenges you to stay linked into what's happening and how practice is changing. For me that's vital...keeping us all dialoguing [sic] about where the profession is going in our particular content and practice areas and for our students.

When I asked Caitlin to describe some of the difficulties or distress points during the past 10 years, she identified both personal and professional challenges. From a personal standpoint, the "struggle is really where to put my energies" as she tries to devote time to multiple commitments to her family, clinical practice, teaching, research, professional involvement, and community service. From a professional standpoint, she identified a conflict between her strong commitment to clinical research and the advancement of evidence-based practice in physical therapy and her personal and deep understanding of the importance of practical (practice-based, relational, and contextual) knowledge and reasoning that is integral to clinical expertise and judgment:

> One of the struggles that I see with our move towards the emphasis on having everyone [faculty members] involved in scholarship and the push to have that be productivity in [publishing] research versus making an impact on the profession or our patients in other ways...I think there are other ways of making an impact.

She went on to express a related concern about current conceptions of evidence-based practice that relegate the role of expert opinion and judgment to some of the lowest levels of "evidence":

> With evidence-based practice we're losing some of the clinical expertise when all everybody wants to know is, you know, what level of evidence is this? And you want to say, "Wait a second"—especially in neurologic physical therapy—"It isn't all based on the number of randomized clinical trials here. There is a role for clinical judgment and expertise"...."cause my students are now asking, "What's the evidence behind this?" And that's great they're asking that, but they sort of want to throw it out if there's not a randomized trial on it.

At the conclusion of the interview, Caitlin reinforced the observation of other authors in this volume that a commitment to lifelong learning is a core theme that emerges in studies of clinical experts and expertise:

> I think I'm still pretty much in the same growing, learning mode that I was back 10 years ago, but I've shifted more to the faculty realm than the straight clinical realm.... There's always a lot to learn in our field, that's for sure!

11

Finally, Caitlin shared a story that captured her enjoyment of working with students and making a "difference" at a level that moves beyond her "own" patients to the patients that will be served by the practitioners of the future. She recounted the story of a student, recently certified as a neurologic clinical specialist, who came up to her at an APTA meeting and thanked her for modeling the kind of professional commitment and ongoing development that this former student sought to emulate. Caitlin described the encounter this way:

> It's so nice to hear, "You know what? You really made a difference. That's why I went that direction. I saw that it was really important to get beyond entry-level with my skills as a clinician." And so it's like, okay—one little person at a time—I made a difference!

So, like many of the other experts described in this volume, Caitlin exemplifies the view of expertise as a dynamic and continuous process—not an endpoint. She is truly a professional constantly in formation.

REVISITING THE CASE OF CAITLIN: CONNECTIONS TO THEORIES OF EXPERTISE IN PHYSICAL THERAPY PRACTICE

The study described in this chapter was being conducted at approximately the same time as the investigations of Jensen et al. (21), yet it was a separate endeavor. Naturally, my inquiry was informed by some of these authors' earlier work (22,23) and a growing number of investigations of emerging expertise, clinical reasoning, and professional practice in a variety of disciplines (24–34). Even so, my ethnographic and microethnographic study of practice in a transdisciplinary rehabilitation clinic had different aims than the grounded theory investigation of Jensen and colleagues (21). At the outset, I sought to explore and describe the culture of the clinic (and the beliefs and social norms associated with that culture) and provide a detailed and contextualized account of the nature of clinical expertise embedded in that culture. At the microethnographic level, this exploration led to careful analysis of interaction (verbal and nonverbal) between Caitlin and several of her patients.

What is interesting, then, about the findings in these parallel but distinct studies is how the grounded theory of expert practice in physical therapy proposed by Jensen et al. (21) (and further developed and elaborated in this volume) resonates with and informs the findings of my investigation. This connection clearly speaks to the power of their theory. At the same time, I believe that the observation and description of some of the linguistic, paralinguistic, and nonverbal features of discourse between Caitlin and her clients shed light on some of the subtle and nuanced ways that experts actually enact, moment-to-moment, the dimensions of expertise identified by Jensen and colleagues in their theory (21). In this way, the findings of these investigations complement and support each other and are an example of the process of recontextualization that Morse (35) has claimed is so critical in qualitative research. This process requires an iterative and dialectic exchange between new findings and old, between established theory and emerging theory, and between the work of other investigators and one's own work.

The linkages between the findings summarized in this chapter and the theory of expertise in physical therapy outlined in this volume are strong and clear. First and foremost, the importance of a philosophy of practice as a framework and driving force for the day-to-day work of Caitlin and the other rehabilitation professionals in my study is immediately apparent. As with the experts described by Jensen et al. (21), this philosophy permeates all the dimensions of expert practice I observed in Caitlin. In fact, I would suggest that that the communally held philosophy of client centering at the clinic created norms for action and interaction that virtually impelled practitioners toward the multifaceted form of expertise described by Jensen and her colleagues.

In the realm of knowledge, the knowledge used to inform practice in Caitlin's case was multidimensional and *always* focused on the patient. The sources of learning and knowledge were many. Certainly there were written resources such as books, journals, and the reports from colleagues in patient charts. But far more important for Caitlin were her social engagements with others that created a broad and deep network of personal, practical knowledge on which she could draw in clinical practice. Thus, professional colleagues; fellow researchers; mentors; and, very importantly, patients and their caregivers were all teachers for Caitlin and highly valued sources of knowledge. Finally, ongoing *reflection* on lessons learned from these teachers and the lessons of daily practice was another critical source of knowledge.

The descriptions of some of Caitlin's interactions with Bill, Marcia, and John, provided in this chapter, should make it clear that the clinical reasoning and decision-making process used by Caitlin is highly collaborative and engages the patient as an essential participant in this process. In fact, the descriptions of some of the features of discourse between Caitlin and her patients as she sought to create and sustain therapeutic alliances—undivided attention; careful listening and asking the "right questions"; the presence of stories in conversation; and the use of repetition, metaphor, and imagery—represent, I believe, some of the particulars of what investigators have termed collaborative reasoning (21,36), narrative reasoning (28,36–39), and interactive reasoning (29,36,40).

Key components of the philosophy of client centering adopted by Caitlin and the other practitioners in the clinic included serving as an advocate for their patients (and caregivers), a focus on client education, and goals of enabling and empowering clients to achieve their own goals and meet their needs. They, like the experts described by Jensen et al. (21), demonstrated through their actions and words that being nonjudgmental and "doing the right thing" for the good of the patient was a central moral concern in their day-to-day work with clients. Several character traits or virtues including compassion, respect for individuals and their unique perspectives and needs, and integrity are common threads that ran through many of the interactions I observed between Caitlin and her clients.

A final dimension of the theory of expert practice in physical therapy elaborated by Jensen and colleagues (21) involves a central focus on movement oriented toward meaningful function. Once again, the exceptional observation and handling skills of Caitlin in this domain were readily apparent. These skills could be seen in the way she adapted her own movements to the needs of the patients and the goals of therapy with the end result that there was a rhythmic synchronicity and fluidity that characterized the great majority of therapy

11

sessions observed. Also, as illustrated in several of the depictions of therapy in this chapter, the activities of therapy were always directed toward the aim of achieving functions that the patients desired and found meaningful in their lives.

In summary, I believe that the theory of expertise in physical therapy practice and the extensions, elaborations, and applications of this theory found in this volume offer great promise for a deeper understanding of the work of exceptional physical therapists. They also have far-reaching implications for both continued research in this fascinating area and educational practice at the professional and postprofessional level.

REFERENCES

1. Bruner J. *Actual minds, possible worlds.* Cambridge, MA: Harvard University Press, 1986.
2. Bruner J. *Acts of meaning.* Cambridge, MA: Harvard University Press, 1990.
3. Polkinghorne DE. *Narrative knowing and the human sciences.* Albany, NY: State University of New York Press, 1988.
4. Ricoeur P. The narrative function. In P Ricoeur (ed). *Hermeneutics and the human sciences.* Cambridge: Cambridge University Press, 1981.
5. Sarbin TR. The narrative as a root metaphor for psychology. In TR Sarbin (ed). *Narrative psychology: the storied nature of human conduct.* New York: Praeger, 1986.
6. Brody H. *Stories of sickness.* New Haven, CT: Yale University Press, 1987.
7. Coles R. *The call of stories.* Boston: Houghton Mifflin, 1989.
8. Frank AW. *At the will of the body: reflections on illness.* Boston: Houghton Mifflin, 1991.
9. Frank AW. *The wounded storyteller: body, illness, and ethics.* Chicago: University of Chicago Press, 1995.
10. Kleinman A. *The illness narratives: suffering, healing, and the human condition.* New York: Basic Books, 1988.
11. Reiser SJ. Foreword. In EJ Cassell. *Talking with patients: the theory of doctor-patient communication.* Cambridge, MA: MIT Press, 1985.
12. Sapir JD, Crocker JC. *The social uses of metaphor.* Philadelphia: University of Pennsylvania Press, 1977.
13. Tannen D. *Talking voices: repetition, dialogue, and imagery in conversational discourse.* Cambridge, UK: Cambridge University Press, 1989.
14. Gibbs RW. Categorization and metaphor understanding. *Psychol Rev.* 1992;99:572–577.
15. Glucksberg S, Keysar B. Understanding metaphorical comparisons: beyond similarity. *Psychol Rev.* 1990;97:3–18.
16. Lakoff G, Johnson M. *Metaphors we live by.* Chicago: University of Chicago Press, 1980.
17. Weiner B. Metaphors in motivation and attribution. *Am Psychol.* 1991;46:921–930.
18. Ferrara KW. *Therapeutic ways with words.* New York: Oxford University Press, 1994.
19. Brown P, Levinson S. *Politeness: some universals in language usage.* Cambridge, UK: Cambridge University Press, 1987.
20. Vygotsky LS. *Mind in society: the development of higher psychological processes.* Cambridge, MA: Harvard University Press, 1978.
21. Jensen GM, Gwyer J, Hack LM, Shepard KF. *Expertise in physical therapy practice.* Boston, MA: Butterworth–Heinemann, 1999.
22. Jensen GM, Shepard KF, Hack LM. The novice versus experienced clinician: insights into the work of the physical therapist. *Phys Ther.* 1990;70:314–323.
23. Jensen GM, Shepard KF, Gwyer J, Hack LM. Attribute dimensions that distinguish master and novice physical therapy clinicians in orthopedic settings. *Phys Ther.* 1992;72:711–722.
24. Benner P. *From novice to expert: excellence and power in clinical nursing practice.* Menlo Park, CA: Addison-Wesley, 1982.
25. Elstein AS, Shulman LS, Sprafka SA. Medical problem solving: a ten year retrospective. *Eval Health Professions* 1990;13:5–36.
26. Elstein AS, Shulman LS, Sprafka SA. Medical problem solving: an analysis of clinical reasoning. Cambridge, MA: Harvard University Press, 1978.

27. Dreyfus HL, Dreyfus SE, Athanasiou T. *Mind over machine: the power of human intuition and expertise in the era of the computer*. New York: Free Press, 1986.
28. Mattingly C. The narrative nature of clinical reasoning. *Am J Occ Ther*. 1991;45:998–1005.
29. Fleming M. The therapist with the three track mind. *Am J Occ Ther*. 1991;45:1007–1014.
30. Mattingly C, Fleming MH. *Clinical reasoning: forms of inquiry in a therapeutic practice*. Philadelphia: FA Davis, 1994.
31. Eraut M. *Developing professional knowledge and competence*. Washington, DC: Falmer Press, 1994.
32. Schon DA. *The reflective practitioner: how professionals think in action*. New York: Basic Books, 1983.
33. Payton OD. Clinical reasoning process in physical therapy. *Phys Ther*. 1985;65:924–928.
34. May BJ, Dennis JK. Expert decision making in physical therapy: a survey of practitioners. *Phys Ther*. 1991;71:190–202.
35. Morse J. Emerging from the data: the cognitive processes of analysis in qualitative inquiry. In J Morse (ed). *Critical issues in qualitative research methods*. Thousand Oaks, CA: Sage Publications, 1994.
36. Edwards I, Jones M, Higgs J, et al. What is collaborative reasoning? *Adv Physiother*. 2004;6:70–83.
37. Mattingly C. The narrative nature of clinical reasoning. In C Mattingly, MH Fleming. *Clinical reasoning: forms of inquiry in a therapeutic practice*. Philadelphia: FA Davis, 1994.
38. Mattingly C. Clinical revision: changing the therapeutic story midstream. In C Mattingly, MH. Fleming *Clinical reasoning: Forms of inquiry in a therapeutic practice*. Philadelphia: FA Davis, 1994.
39. Mattingly C. *Healing dramas and clinical plots: the narrative structure of experience*. Cambridge, UK: Cambridge University Press, 1998.
40. Mattingly C, Fleming MH. Interactive reasoning: collaborating with the person. In C Mattingly, MH Fleming. *Clinical reasoning: forms of inquiry in a therapeutic practice*. Philadelphia: FA Davis, 1994.

11

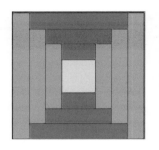

12

Implications for Practice: Applying the Dimensions of Expertise for Staff Professional Development

Michael G. Sullivan and Ann Jampel

The theories of skill acquisition and expertise in physical therapy practice provide a useful and practical model for providing guidance to staff in the development of clinical skills and professional behaviors. These models facilitate our guidance and mentoring of staff professional development as well as providing staff a continuum of behaviors and skills for self-reflection. In a very practical manner we have used the content of the 1st edition and the expert counsel of the authors to develop and implement a clinical recognition program that is very much aligned with these theories.—Michael G. Sullivan, PT, DPT, MBA, and Ann Jampel, PT, MS

CHAPTER OVERVIEW

BACKGROUND AND VISION

We were invited to contribute to this book because we have implemented a practical application of Dr. Patricia Benner's work on novice to expert theory to our professional development plan for clinicians at Massachusetts General Hospital (MGH). Dr. Benner's well-known work focuses on the critical relevance of learning from practice. Benner's work, which draws significantly from the work of Hubert and Stuart Dreyfus, helps us to understand expert practice and to develop a model that can be used for improved professional development of clinicians. Although there has been widespread discussion and acceptance of Benner's model for professional development in nursing (1), there has been very little application in physical therapy. In addition, we were able to use the research on expert practice in physical therapy as part of our program design (2). In this chapter we describe the process of design, development, and implementation of a professional development system that is centered on core concepts of novice development and expert practice. This system has been implemented over the past 4 years in the Department of Physical Therapy of MGH. The chapter also includes our own reflections on the impact of this approach on clinicians and administrators in our facility.

The Department began its efforts to apply the research on expertise in 1996 when an Interdisciplinary Practice Model was adopted at our facility. Six disciplines—nursing, physical therapy (PT), occupational therapy (OT), speech-language pathology, social services, and respiratory therapy—were reorganized under a Senior Vice President for Patient Care Services (PCS). At that time, the environment within health care was contentious with aggressive downsizing and management reorganization. It was within this context that the PCS Guiding Principles and Vision were created (Box 12-1). These principles articulated the need for clinicians to have an active voice around the care of patients as well as recognition of their contribution to patient outcomes.

CONCEPTUAL DEVELOPMENT AND PROGRAM DESIGN

In response to a staff survey that identified the need to recognize and reward staff, the Professional Development Committee was created as one portion of collaborative governance. This group was charged to develop an interdisciplinary clinical recognition program (CRP) within MGH PCS. The following assumptions were used to guide the development:

1. The essential contribution of clinicians to practice is direct patient care. Practice is enhanced through participation in activities beyond direct patient care.
2. Clinical skills evolve over time with application of knowledge and theory to individual patients and collaboration with other disciplines.
3. Self-assessment and reflection are key to the development of expertise.
4. The uniqueness of disciplines should be reflected in a model that is flexible and dynamic.
5. Clinician contribution to the care of patients should be recognized and celebrated (3).

The committee subsequently reviewed a number of theoretical models of skill development and decided to base their process on the work of Hubert and Stuart Dreyfus (4), who, through a study of skill acquisition by airline pilots and

12

BOX 12–1

Massachusetts General Hospital Guiding Documents for Patient Care Services

Guiding Principles

We are ever-alert for opportunities to improve patient care; we provide care based on the latest research findings.

We recognize the importance of encouraging patients and families to participate in the decisions affecting their care.

We are most effective as a team; we continually strengthen our relationships with each other and actively promote diversity within our staff.

We enhance patient care and the systems supporting that care as we work with others; we eagerly enter new partnerships with people inside and outside of the Massachusetts General Hospital.

We never lose sight of the needs and expectations of our patients and their families as we make clinical decisions based on the most effective use of internal and external resources.

We view learning as a lifelong process essential to the growth and development of clinicians striving to deliver quality patient care.

We acknowledge that maintaining the highest standards of patient care delivery is a never-ending process that involves the patient, family, nurse, all healthcare providers, and the community-at-large.

Vision Statement

As Nurses, Health Professionals, and Patient Care Services support staff, our every action is guided by knowledge, enabled by skill, and motivated by compassion. Patients are our primary focus, and the way we deliver care reflects that focus every day.

We believe in creating a practice environment that has no barriers, is built on a spirit of inquiry, and reflects a culturally competent workforce supportive of the patient-focused values of this institution.

It is through our professional practice model that we make our vision a demonstrable truth every day by letting our thoughts, decisions, and actions be guided by our values. As clinicians, we ensure that our practice is caring, innovative, scientific, and empowering, and is based on a foundation of leadership and entrepreneurial teamwork.

grand master chess players, developed a model that described novice to expert skills on a continuum of levels. Patricia Benner expanded and applied the Dreyfus's theoretical work to the practice of nursing (5). Benner studied clinical narratives written by nurses as a methodology to gain insight into practice and defined and described five levels of skill from novice to expert (5–7). Because of the interdisciplinary nature of the program and the clear association of nursing with the Benner model, the Dreyfus Skill Acquisition Model was selected by the committee as the overarching theoretical model for grounding the clinical recognition process.

The committee began benchmarking professional development models that were in existence within health care organizations. They found a number within the discipline of nursing and a few scattered among the various other disciplines to review. The number of models that were specifically focused on the development of clinical skills as opposed to recognizing a combination of clinical skills, good citizenship, committee participation, and leadership was even smaller. The need to develop a program that focused on clinical skills across six disciplines led the group to the use of narrative as a review methodology to help articulate clinical practice at MGH. This approach was supported by Benner's work.

The work of the committee continued with interdisciplinary review of clinical narratives. More than 100 narratives were submitted from "skilled" clinicians who had been recommended by clinical leadership from all disciplines. The entire committee reviewed these and found that they exemplified three overarching themes, previously developed by Benner, which could be adapted to guide the work of the interdisciplinary group. These themes are summarized in Table 12-1.

The interdisciplinary process proved to be vital to fully understand the differences in the ways that the various disciplines formed and presented their thoughts about patient care through narratives. Camooso (8) described that nursing narratives often focused on the Clinician–Patient Relationship with the themes of Clinical Knowledge/Decision Making and Collaboration/Teamwork less evident in their writing. Narratives for physical, occupational, and speech-language pathologists most often were written in more of a case study format. Here, the focus was on clinical decision making related to the clinical data obtained through the examination, evaluation of the data, and a description of the intervention that was provided across the episode of care. Patient–client interactions were less evident. It was during the conceptual development of the program we heard for the first time concerns whether a narrative model alone could capture the essence of clinical practice for all disciplines across practice levels.

Table 12–1. MGH Practice Committee Interdisciplinary Clinical Themes

Theme	Description
Clinician–Patient Relationship	The interpersonal or relational connection between the clinician and the patient and/or family
Clinical Knowledge and Decision Making	Understanding attained through formal and experiential learning
Collaboration/Teamwork	Through the development of effective relationships with unit colleagues and other members of the health care team, the best possible outcome is achieved for the patient and family

12

DISCIPLINE-SPECIFIC CRITERIA DEVELOPMENT

Using descriptors adapted from Benner's work, each discipline was charged with developing discipline-specific behavior/criteria for the four levels of practice that are described in Table 12-2. During 1999, a small leadership group in physical and occupational therapy began to develop criteria for each of these themes of four practice levels. Review of the literature provided some insights into theoretical models of expertise and descriptions of characteristics that distinguished novice from expert (2,9–10). However, we were challenged to describe these behaviors along a continuum that reflected practice across the three themes of practice that we identified at these four distinct levels and that

Table 12–2. Application of Benner's Criteria to Definitions for Four Development Levels of Practice

Level	Descriptive Characteristics
Entry	Learning to apply newly acquired knowledge and skills to a multitude of patient care situations. Draws on learned facts and rules to organize and guide practice. With experience, begins to modify care to meet the needs of individuals. Understands the role of other disciplines and consults with peers in designing a plan of care.
Clinician	Through experience with patients has developed a sound understanding about the care of a particular patient population. Routinely draws on learned facts and experiences as well as an understanding of possible outcomes when designing a plan of care. Recognizes patterns in clinical practice and uses this information to make clinical decisions. Displays confidence in clinical decision making. Individualizes care based on an understanding of the patient and advocates for their needs. Acts as a resource to colleagues.
Advanced Clinician	Develops in-depth knowledge about the care of a particular patient population and appreciation for the multiple factors that influence care. Constantly considers both the possibilities and the probabilities of what might be the outcomes of decisions, given the clinical and organizational factors. Uses intuition to continually modify the patient's care and to assure optimal outcomes. Values the contributions of peers and interdisciplinary colleagues. Routinely consults with and serves as a resource to others.
Clinical Scholar	Demonstrates exquisite foresight in planning patient care. Recognized as experts in their areas of specialization. Adept at negotiating conflict and collaborating with others. Responds intuitively to patients' needs and comfortably engages in clinically sound risk taking. Welcomes differing perspectives and seeks out opportunities to share knowledge. Skilled at creative problem solving, which routinely leads to efforts that strengthen organizational systems that support patient care.

From Patient Care Services Clinical Recognition Program, Massachusetts General Hospital, Copyright 2002.

could be used by staff practicing in both inpatient and ambulatory areas in an acute care teaching environment.

Using language that was consistent with the *Guide to Physical Therapist Practice* (11) as a starting point, subcategories were developed for each theme to identify entry- and expert-level behaviors. Box 12-2 shows the subcategories that were developed for each theme.

Following this process, the group stepped back to describe additional behaviors and skills that would fall along a continuum between these points. Focus groups were used to examine practice at a more "grassroots" level to better

BOX 12–2	*Subcategories Developed for Each Theme*

Clinician–Patient Relationship

Rapport and Communication
Interface with Clinical Decision Making
Advocacy
Cultural Competency

Clinical Decision Making

Self-Assessment
Clinical Reasoning
   Knowledge
   Examination
   Evaluation: Diagnosis and Prognosis
   Intervention
   Exercise Prescription
Evidence-Based Practice
Accountability
Education and Consultation
   Patient and Family
   Student
   Consultation

Collaboration/Teamwork

Interdisciplinary and Service Teams
Support Personnel
System

Movement

Motor Coordination and Skill
   Palpate
   Facilitate and Inhibit Movement
Analyze Movement and Respond
   Judgment
   Planned vs. Automatic Responses

12

articulate differences in practice. We convened two different groups of therapists who were recognized by the leadership group as practicing at different levels. One group included therapists at less than 2 years of experience, and a second group combined therapists who demonstrated more advanced levels of practice, including those who had certification through the American Board of Physical Therapist Specialists.

We asked each group similar questions, which included the following:

- How has your practice changed over time?
- How has managed care changed your practice?
- What are your most important clinical skills?
- How do you gain new knowledge and skills?
- How do you use the medical diagnosis in your clinical decision making?
- How do you handle situations where there is conflict?
- How would you describe your accountability around patient care?

Responses shaped the criteria within domains at different levels.

We have selected one subcategory to illustrate the changing expectations across the four levels. It demonstrates the expanding role of accountability across the four levels of experience (Table 12-3). Less-experienced clinicians saw this as related to the immediate needs of the patient and current intervention and often attributed the patient's lack of progress as a reflection of their limitations in providing an adequate level of care. As experience evolved, accountability was shared with the team and the clinician was able to let go of the idea that he or she could make "every patient better." Staff with more advanced skills talked about a reflective process related to patients not achieving expected outcomes, asking themselves questions such as, "What have I not yet figured out here?"

Table 12–3. Example of CRP Criteria for Clinical Decision Making: Accountability and Responsibility

	Entry Level	Clinician	Advanced Clinician	Clinical Scholar
Accountability and Responsibility	Recognizes the responsibility and accountability for his or her own clinical practice in relationship to the immediate needs of the patient	Assumes responsibility for communicating with and educating other team members, as needed, to facilitate integration of patient's PT and OT needs into current plan of care (including discharge plan)	Able to let go of the need to "make every patient better," having learned to share responsibility for care with patient	Experiences a sense of accountability for patient progress toward goals if not progressing as anticipated, asks self "What have I not figured out?"

PT = physical therapist; OT = occupational therapist.

The complete document demonstrating specific behaviors for all subcategories has become known as "The Grid." The grid is used extensively by all therapists in the Department and for many purposes (see later in this chapter).

EXTERNAL REVIEW

A review of the program planning and initial documents was done by an external group, which followed the internal review process done with clinical groups. This external review included physical therapists from other clinical and academic settings, including several of the authors of this book. Overall feedback was positive; however, we were urged to consider including another dimension from the expert practice model—movement. Not unlike their experience, we missed the need to develop movement as a central theme of the physical therapist. A small subgroup worked on developing behaviors around this theme with subcategories of the following:
■ Motor coordination and skill
■ Movement analysis
■ Modification of input to achieve desired motor response
The development of criteria in this category was challenging. Truly, movement is both "psycho" and "motor" and it is not completely possible to separate the cognitive and communication aspects from the observational and hands-on skills.

IMPLEMENTATION OF FIRST TWO LEVELS: ENTRY LEVEL AND CLINICIAN

Having reached agreement on theoretical constructs and the associated behavioral criteria for the program, the next challenge was to develop an implementation strategy to transition all eligible PCS employees into one of the program's four levels—Entry, Clinician, Advanced Clinician, or Clinical Scholar—within 1 year and to develop a mechanism to place all future new employees into the program. A key decision during implementation was the determination that achievement at the first two levels, Entry and Clinician, would be mandatory, whereas recognition at the upper two levels would be voluntary. Entry status needs to be attained within 1 year of employment. It is important to distinguish that our definition of "Entry" reflects values embedded within our culture. It is, we believe, a level of clinical practice distinct from the label "entry level" associated with licensure (minimal level of public protection) or completion of profession education. The Clinician level needs to be achieved within 2 years of employment and represents behaviors consistent with institutional values and quality standards.

Staff seeking advancement to Entry or Clinician Levels completed a clinical narrative, chosen by reflecting on a clinical experience identified by the therapist as meaningful and representative of their practice. A clinical narrative is a first-person written account of a clinical situation that stands out in the clinician's mind because of its significance. The director/manager, based on the review of the narrative and subsequent discussion with the employee, made a determination of appropriate level for entry into the program. In physical and occupational therapy, during the year-long implementation process, the director read and discussed with staff more than 100 narratives.

Following the implementation phases, entry into the CRP occurs at the completion of the orientation within 3–6 months of the date of employment. Eligible

12

employees can choose to enter at either Entry or Clinician level. The completion of a narrative, with subsequent review and discussion with the director/manager, is still required. Through this process, themes of practice and clinical behaviors are explored.

Entry into the levels of advanced clinician and clinical scholar is voluntary and seen as recognition of achievement above that required for continued employment. Achievement of either designation is rewarded by public recognition and increased salaries (5% for advanced clinicians and 10% for clinical scholars). The development group determined that a narrative alone would not fully describe practice at these two levels and determined that a combination of portfolio and interview would serve as the data that an interdisciplinary Review Board would use to make decisions for advancement.

Each applicant requires the endorsement of the director/manager. The employee then prepares and submits a portfolio that contains the following:

- A letter of endorsement from the applicant's manager
- A current curriculum vitae
- A clinical narrative
- Letters of support
  - Advanced clinician: three letters of support (two within the discipline and one outside the discipline)
  - Clinical scholar level: four letters of support (two within the discipline and two outside the discipline)

Following portfolio review by the entire review board, a three-person subgroup interviews the candidate. The discussion with the employee focuses on those themes of practice where there is limited or no evidence within the portfolio. The results of the interview are shared with the entire review board, and recommendations to advance are made by consensus.

Therapists at the Entry and Clinician Levels

In December 2005 we gathered feedback from PT and OT Entry and Clinician level staff about their experience of the CRP and the process of writing and review of narratives. Overall, they found the clinical environment engendered discussion of patients all the time. They also found the grid to be a valuable tool for organizing themes across a continuum; setting out a developmental map; and providing a common language for discussion, self-reflection, and feedback. A quote from a staff therapist hired as a new graduate to MGH is revealing:

It gave me insight into what employees were expected to be like and how we are expected to treat the patients.

Experienced therapists speak about the criteria somewhat differently:

It is a map to becoming a well-rounded clinician and included elements of clinical practice not previously applied to my own, or others', view of my practice. It provides insight into the values of the department and specifies clinical behaviors that are useful in developing goals.

Although the criteria were viewed overall in a positive light, one opinion of a therapist early in her career suggests caution:

I initially found the description of advanced clinician and clinical scholar behaviors as daunting. However, over time, as I developed skills, the criteria have helped me plot my growth.

Clinical specialists are critical to the integration of the CRP criteria into the practice environment because of their role in assessing competency (see later), but there are differences in how they used these criteria as part of their ongoing supervision. Therapists from the inpatient service described a more frequent "sitting down" and review of the behaviors with their clinical specialists and developing specific goals that were related to some of the criteria. The outpatient group described that there were more informal interactions that included aspects of the grid and less frequent use of the tool on a more formal "sit-down" basis. These style differences reflect the underlying difference in the levels of staff experience within our department. Therapists working on our inpatient service are younger and benefit from more structured and directed supervision, whereas the outpatient therapists are, in general, more experienced and thereby self-directed.

The overall perspective from the therapists is that the CRP criteria provide a constructive framework for evolving clinical practice over their career. These criteria serve as long-term objectives, but they also serve as a framework for achieving realistic short-term goals related to clinical and professional growth. When asked specifically if they thought that the CRP had advanced practice in PT and OT, the group thought that self-motivated individuals within MGH would advance their practice to a certain degree regardless of the program, especially in light of the opportunities that they have to interface with the clinical specialist resources available to them. Additionally, they felt that the organized framework of developmental stages provided an important additional structure to their practice and facilitated development of specific, individualized goals. Therapists frequently referenced an increase in their reflective processes and attributed importance to the program's interdisciplinary nature and its link to the hospital's patient care, research, and teaching missions. When asked what they would change, they talked about the potential to develop alternatives to the narrative process for those who reflected in ways other than writing.

The group had predominantly positive reactions and experiences with the narrative process and meeting with the director to discuss their patients, although some expressed concern that some therapists with the ability to achieve the two higher levels might choose not to advance based on the need to write narratives. Our therapists can differentiate between the more traditional and familiar case presentation and the narrative processes. They speak of the challenge to write and talk about the thought process behind their decision making. All agreed that themes of the patient–clinician relationship and teamwork and collaboration were much less emphasized in the case format, yet are so essential to achieving patient outcomes.

12

Reviewing the narrative with the director was described as an additional opportunity to get help with the reflective process. One staff member expressed the following:

The director got to know me and my practice better through a discussion of my patient. The discussion helped me understand the "intention" of my narrative.

Yet another staff member comments:

I felt that I was explaining my thought process versus defending what I had done with the patient. Overall, discussing was reaffirming about the care I provided my patient.

All the therapists interviewed believed the director used additional sources of input beyond the single narrative experience in making any decision about advancement.

THERAPISTS AT THE ADVANCED CLINICIAN AND CLINICAL SCHOLAR LEVELS

Discussions with clinicians across the six disciplines who have been recognized as advanced clinicians and clinical scholars provide a variety of perspectives about the program. Their experience provides others with information about sources of support to go through the process, experience of the interview, outcomes of being recognized, and thoughts about the future of the program. The clinicians involved in the development of the program through collaborative governance felt it important to champion the process by going forward themselves. Another clinician commented that the program was discussed at the time of her yearly performance review and felt encouraged by her director to go through the process. One clinician reported frequently discussing cases with her director and she felt that she understood her practice, which gave her confidence to go forward. In discussing her preparation of her portfolio another clinician describes her experience this way:

I needed to go through a narrative process with my director to really understand the role of the narrative played in the process. Initially I felt like it was another thing to do in a life that was already full. I was concerned about the effort it would take to put together the portfolio and prepare for the interview, which could have resulted in not being recognized.

She described a month-long process of getting familiar with the application process and taking the "luxury of time" to reflect on her practice.

During that time something changed and the process changed from being an expectation to something that rejuvenated my practice by helping me understand where I was and where I might like to go in the future.

One of the physical therapists reported that the CRP had been discussed during her interview process and was part of the reason that she took a position at MGH. She found the consistent use of the performance grid by both herself and her clinical specialist important for her to understand where she was on the continuum of clinical skills. She decided to engage in the review process after careful consideration of her practice in relationship to the criteria. For most, the financial rewards of the program played a role in their decision to advance.

Advanced clinicians and clinical scholars describe a variety of factors that assist them through the application and interview process. The transition from description of clinical events that is done during medical record documentation and case studies to written reflection was a challenge to many. Most advanced clinicians and clinical scholars love to talk about their patients; the difficulty for some is to transfer this into writing. For some, verbal spontaneity can get lost in the task of writing; for others it is the writing that brings out the reflection. One clinician, who worked in a very busy unit with minimal time to interact with patients, described taking notes on some of her patients and then reflecting about it afterward to tease out the details of what she was thinking. She used a clinical specialist colleague to review the document, who was able to say to her, "You seem to be working too hard. Where are you going with this?"

The nurse then chose another patient to write about, and the whole process went much more easily. In general, selecting the right patient for the narrative was challenging. A consistent experience mentioned by staff was the error of picking an unusual patient and then describing a lengthy relationship over time. This makes the process longer and challenges the clinician to describe decision making in less familiar and atypical situations. It has been hard to convince staff to demonstrate their skill at an advanced level during their practice with a more "typical" patient.

For most staff it is critical to get input from someone who has been through the program. Many advanced clinicians and clinical scholars describe difficulty "tooting their own horn" and require facilitation to put themselves in the middle of the narrative versus describing their patient from a "we" perspective. They also describe a distinct language for the program and highlight that help was needed to translate words such as "clinically sound risk" into decisions that clinicians make every day. For many, finding a mentor or coach to help guide them through the process was essential to help them complete the process.

Perspectives on the interview process vary. A general consensus is that the applicants need to fully explain their thought processes and provide a good deal of detail, even related to things that aren't evident to others in daily practice. Having a member of one's discipline as the lead interviewer was seen as helpful in interpreting discipline-specific information to the other members of the interview group. One person described the interview team as follows:

> They were clearly interested in knowing more about what I did in practice rather than "catching" me. It felt like a privilege to talk about my practice for an entire hour.

Another clinician described her challenge in describing the complexities of her practice to those who did not necessarily understand the theory behind decisions. Physical and occupational therapists have found it difficult to articulate the central importance of movement to the interview team members outside their disciplines.

Advanced clinicians and clinical scholars speak of the significance of preparation for the interview. Most have carefully reviewed the sample questions that are available, and some have gone through a mock interview process with someone within or outside their discipline.

12

The experience of being recognized in the CRP was generally positive. Those recognized speak of surprise when staff congratulated them and referred to them as "brave." A few have requested that their supervisors did not announce their advancement. On some units, tension can exist when people are advanced and other applicants are not. Many have enjoyed opportunities to be part of the further discussions and evaluation of the program that are ongoing. Most have been involved in mentoring others through the program and feel that it is a privilege to talk with other staff about their narratives and practice. All agreed that they serve an important role as a "translator" of the program's criteria and processes and in helping to demystify the experience. Some of the Advanced Clinicians we spoke with look forward in the future to being recognized at the Clinical Scholar level but felt that they needed a year or two to develop the necessary skills to "live" consistently at that level and to find the time and energy to go through the process.

THE PERSPECTIVE OF THE DIRECTOR OF THE PHYSICAL AND OCCUPATIONAL THERAPY DEPARTMENT

During the first year of implementing the program, clinical behaviors, as revealed through the narrative and the subsequent discussion with the director of the department, were the sole determinant of advancement. Thus, the narrative depicted a broad array of behaviors to "prove" practice was at a certain level. As a result both the narrative and discussion created a forum that resulted in a "summative" judgment by the director. Narratives detailed ample clinical data and decision-making rationale and frequently described an entire episode of care. The therapist's level of comfort with narrative writing was variable, as was the quality. Therapists often selected atypical patients, those not representative of their normal daily clinical work. Affective components of practice and clinical dilemmas were not evident, and the use of the narrative as reflective process was lost. Because progression to the first two levels of the CPR was mandatory, the discussion often felt interrogative and judgmental.

Reflecting on the implementation experience, we realized that it was inconsistent with our preexisting values. Specifically, practice development and the acquisition of clinical skill was a developmental and formative process that needed to be supported and guided. Although the CRP was structured as a summative process, it is the formative experiences in which the therapists engage that strongly influence the behaviors articulated in the criteria for the various levels of the CRP and ultimately influences their development as clinicians. A variety of forums and activities are used to support this process, recognizing the various preferences and stages of professional development of staff. Some staff can be self-sufficient in identifying developmental needs and structuring the associated experiences and activities, whereas others require a wide range of externally mediated stimulation to "prime" their reflective process and to underscore the central importance that self-assessment and reflection play in practice development.

Periodically through the year, therapists share a narrative or reflective writing with the director or a clinical specialist as facilitation to spur reflection and insight. The purpose of this is, as Benner describes, to "unpack" the narrative so the writer reaches further insight into practice. We have found that it is critical to suspend judgments in some cases so the narrative writer is free to explore his or her actions in a risk-free manner. Through this process we instill in the therapists the ability to ask the "what if" scenarios, knowing the complexities of daily practice require clinicians to constantly and adeptly reframe and readjust their thinking to achieve positive impacts on patient care. An excerpt from a narrative and interpretation is seen in Appendix 12-1.

The importance of reflection, a formative process, as a vibrant and active process necessary to facilitate/foster practice development is reinforced through these formative opportunities. Freed from having the narrative measure a level of practice, it now can be used as part of a reflective process. The narrative's focus is not on an entire episode of care but on moments in time, specific actions, decisions, and interactions. Changes in perspectives that we've observed in therapists and the director are summarized in Table 12-4.

Table 12–4. Therapist and Director Reflections Using Clinical Narratives

Director	During Implementation	After Implementation
	Looking for proof	Understanding why this patient was an important experience
	Validating performance	Allowing for uncertainty
	High risk	Risk free
	Focus on outcome/summation	Focus on process/formative
	Judgmental	Suspends judgments
	Final	Evolving and unfolding
	Segregated from other department functions	Integrated with other department functions
	"But"	"What else"
Staff	**During Implementation**	**After Implementation**
	Defending/proving	Self-explorations
	Precise, clear	Amorphous, explorative
	Providing answers	Exploring options
	Therapist removed from the narrative	Therapist is the center of the narrative
	Documenting what was done (past)	Think about what needs to be done (present and future)

12

The change in narrative focus has facilitated an unveiling of the therapists' underlying or emerging practice philosophies including areas of knowledge, reasoning, movement, and virtues. The focus can be on exemplary outcomes or on instances where outcomes and interventions were less optimal. The role of the director in this process is to raise consciousness among the staff about practice philosophy and to emphasize the importance of reflection in practice development.

THE REVIEW BOARD PERSPECTIVE

The Review Board is an interdisciplinary group that included clinical managers and clinical specialists from all six disciplines in the Patient Care Services unit. Like any newly formed group the Board went through a growth process that was at times painful. It took time for the group to develop trust in each other's ability to make complete and accurate assessments about an applicant's clinical practice that were consistent across the six disciplines. To arrive at a shared understanding, it is important that the entire Board reviews every portfolio and participates in the discussions that follow the interviews. This shapes understanding of the criteria and allows for the development of a shared language around the program. In this way, the different cultures and norms of each discipline can be respected, while also maintaining some consistency across the entire program.

The interview process has also evolved over the 3-year period. Initially, the candidates would be asked questions that would validate their level of practice across all of the clinical themes, although there may be evidence of all themes in the applicant's portfolio. A decision was made to focus the interview only on themes of practice where there was limited or no evidence within the portfolio. This decision seemed to better balance the relative weight of the portfolio as compared with the interview in making the decision about clinician advancement; for many candidates it has streamlined the interview process.

The anticipated workload of the Review Board has been modified over time. The original expectation of 30 portfolios per month was unrealistic; processing 5–10 applications has been more manageable. The time required to process a portfolio and interview an applicant is somewhere between 90 and 120 minutes. The interview includes: 1) the board review and development of questions, 2) lead interviewer organization and transcription of these questions for the interview team, 3) brief meetings of the interview team prior to and after the interview, 4) the actual three-person interview, and 5) review of the results by the full Board. Each Board member is involved in 1–2 interviews per month, and most all read the portfolios outside of normal practice hours.

APPLICATION TO OTHER PHYSICAL AND OCCUPATIONAL THERAPY DEPARTMENTAL FUNCTIONS

PERFORMANCE ASSESSMENT

After the original implementation, our reflection on the process forced us to reconcile the mandatory, summative use of the narrative with its potential as a formative instrument for reflection and professional development. This internal process helped integrate the summative nature of the CRP relative to the value the department has historically placed on professional and clinical development. The framework in Figure 12-1 demonstrates our attempt to conceptualize the

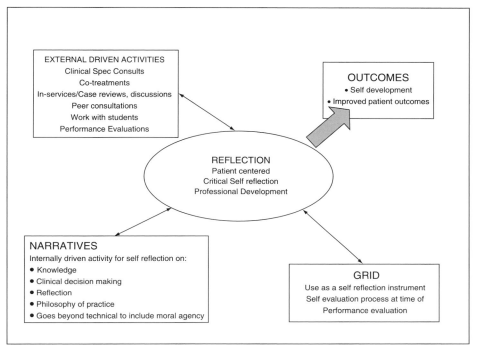

Figure 12–1 ■ Massachusetts General Hospital physical therapy and occupational therapy initial core competencies. (From MGH Department of Physical & Occupational Therapy Policy & Procedures Manual.)

integration of these historic values with the existing process used for staff developments (competency assessment, performance review, etc.) with the CRP.

We first acknowledged that therapists in supervisory roles, responsible for assessing competence and ensuring quality of care, were best suited to make the summative judgments associated with the various CRP levels. We further acknowledged that because Entry and Clinician levels were mandatory, attaining those through a singular separate process (the narrative) made little sense. We therefore began to align our preexisting employment appraisals, including competency and performance assessment, with the CRP behaviors to capture more completely the full professional role. Table 12-5 demonstrates the integration of the CRP with competency and performance assessments used in employee appraisal.

COMPETENCY ASSESSMENT

As with any health care entity providing clinical care, there must be a process that assesses the clinical provider's abilities to meet the needs of patients within a defined environment. These assessment processes occur initially during the 6-month orientation period and on an ongoing basis as practice changes,

Table 12–5. Integration of the CRP with Competency Assessment and Performance Review

	Mandatory		Voluntary	
	Competency Assessment	CRP	Performance Review	CRP
Entry	3–6 months from hire	Oral presentation of narrative 6–9 months from hire	Annually	
Clinician		Written presentation of narrative 18–24 months from hire	At 24 months from hire	
Advanced Clinician			Annually	Endorsement letter Portfolio Interview
Clinical Scholar			Annually	Endorsement letter Portfolio Interview
Conducted by:	*Clinical Specialist*	*Director*	*Clinical Director*	*Review Board*

new technologies and interventions are introduced or, as in our case, the understanding of competency evolves and expands. The clinical behaviors described by the CRP draw on collective work across disciplines (2,6,7,12) that fully articulates the scope of the professional role and reflects clinical behaviors necessary to evolve to an advanced or expert level of practice. Epstein and Hundert (12) argue for a comprehensive definition of professional competence for physicians. They define several areas of competence for physicians in the following definition: professional competence "is the habitual and judicious use of communication, knowledge, technical skills, clinical reasoning, emotions, values and reflection in daily practice to benefit individuals and communities" (Figure 12-2) (12).

This definition expands on traditional views of competence, which consider a more limited focus on cognitive, technical, and integrative (clinical reasoning) domains, and proposes that professional competence entails skills in the affective/moral relationships and "habits of mind" that include curiosity, reflection, and attentiveness. Central to their view of competence, Epstein and Hundert acknowledge that competence is dependent of context and is evaluated by the interaction of the task and the clinicians' abilities to elicit information, form therapeutic relationships, perform diagnostic/therapeutic interventions, and make client management decisions (12).

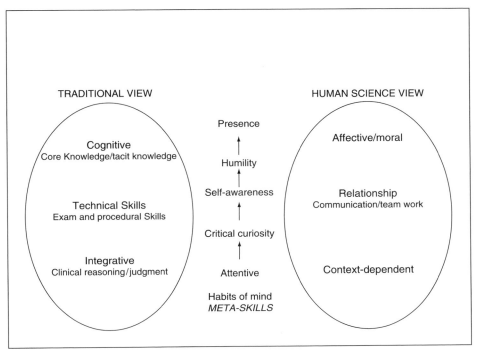

TRADITIONAL VIEW

Cognitive
Core Knowledge/tacit knowledge

Technical Skills
Exam and procedural Skills

Integrative
Clinical reasoning/judgment

Presence
↑
Humility
↑
Self-awareness
↑
Critical curiosity
↑
Attentive

Habits of mind
META-SKILLS

HUMAN SCIENCE VIEW

Affective/moral

Relationship
Communication/team work

Context-dependent

Figure **12–2** ■ Dimensions of professional competence. (From Epstein, Hundert 2002; Epstein 1999.)

Similarities are observed between the work of Epstein and Hundert and the CRP. The CRP defines a broad array of clinical behaviors that culminates in an understanding or definition of expert practice within our clinical environment. Therapists' competence and annual performance are measured against these domains and evaluated within our clinical environment. The skills to practice within our environment transcend technical abilities and require staff to possess and demonstrate skills in the affective/moral domains and demonstrate curiosity, reflection, attentiveness, and moral agency.

As therapists enter our environment we use these competencies to articulate practice and professional expectations and the values of our organization for quality of care and commitment to the patient. The competency assessment process brings to life the core values of professionalism as developed by the American Physical Therapy Association (APTA), including accountability, altruism, compassion/caring, excellence, integrity, professional duty, and social responsibility (13). The competency assessment process also helps achieve a practice aligned with the tenets of APTA's Vision 2020 (14). A sample of these competencies is depicted in Figure 12-3. The competency assessment form represents core elements of performance domains with examples of expected benchmark behaviors across each of the categories.

12

Competency	Clinical Skill/Behavior	Date Achieved
Clinician/Patient Relationship		
Rapport and communication	• Uses proper terms of respect when addressing patients/ families and appropriately drapes patient to ensure dignity. • Recognizes and values patient, family and extended family relationships and their impact on patient care. • Actively listens and attends to patient/family concerns. • Modifies communication style to meet patient's individual needs.	
Advocacy	• Recognizes and responds to patient's and families' concerns, needs, and seeks guidance appropriately. • Recognizes the need for advocacy and brings the individual patient needs to the interdisciplinary team.	
Cultural competence	• Demonstrates awareness of own value and belief and their interaction with patients/family relationships. • Recognizes that cultural issues impact that delivery of care.	

Figure 12–3 ■ Staff professional development rubric.

PERFORMANCE REVIEW

The performance review criteria were developed by the clinical leadership of the department over a period of months. Consensus was achieved among the leadership on the descriptive statements for each area of performance to achieve clarity and reliability of interpretation and to reflect a progressive trajectory for professional development, performance, and acquisition of clinical behaviors.

CLINICAL RECOGNITION PROGRAM AS A FORMATIVE STRUCTURE FOR SUPERVISION

Within our department, the therapists who are designated Clinical Specialists work closely with other therapists to develop practice skills and professional behaviors. The mandatory nature of the Entry and Clinician levels provided an opportunity to align the required annual review process with the behaviors of the CRP. A formal consultative report is done periodically throughout the year by the Clinical Specialists and is used as a forum to identify developmental needs and set appropriate goals for the individual therapist. The consultative reports provide a rich data source for the annual performance review. These reports are also reviewed among the collective clinical leadership group and provide a forum for generating ideas on methods for clinical teaching and mentoring and ensure consistency of performance expectations among leadership. See Appendix 12-2 for an excerpt from a clinical specialist.

Throughout their tenure at MGH, clinical staff members regularly refer to the CRP criteria as a tool for self-assessment. Critically assessing oneself against these criteria offers insight into areas for development and provides a vehicle to celebrate the acquisition of clinical skills/milestones. Additionally the CRP criteria and staff self-assessments serve as a forum for discussion between staff and clinical leadership. Active mentoring coupled with critical nonpunitive feedback fosters an environment that is conducive toward growth and practice development.

With clinical specialists accountable for validating the clinical behaviors of the CRP, we have achieved three benefits: 1) the CRP, at least with respect to the Entry and Clinician levels, are now seen as an integrated function; 2) those clinical experts, who best know practice, make the determinations relative to level within the CRP, providing a greater degree of credibility and meaning for the therapists; and 3) there is common language and understanding of the behaviors that surround the criteria at each level.

APPLICATION TO CLINICAL EDUCATION

Education is an integral function of the MGH mission. The physical therapy department has a long tradition of clinical education and currently works with students at all levels of observational, part-time, and full-time experiences (including internships) that range from 6 to 13 months in length. At the same time we were developing the CRP, we also set out to improve our clinical education with the following goal: identification of clear expectations for clinical performance for affiliating students at MGH at all levels of clinical experience.

This goal was driven by the continuous struggle that clinical instructors (CIs) experienced when they tried to describe appropriate levels of clinical behaviors for their students. We lacked consistency in what we expected from students at various levels, thus CIs communicated their expectations differently. We also struggled with the differences in expected outcomes that the academic programs described for students, especially as they related to reality of practice within the acute care environment. Our work with the CRP had led us to understand the benefits of describing clinical behaviors on a continuum. It has provided staff clear road signs toward the professional development journey and specific goals to work toward. It seemed that the same would be true for CIs and students. Using the CRP model, but adapting it to the educational experience, we developed the student performance grid that describes "prerequisite" skills for students' performance as they entered a particular point in clinical education.

We saw several advantages in taking this approach. From the academic program perspective, knowledge of expected levels of skill at the onset of a clinical experience allows them to match students to our environment. It also allows students to better self-assess their appropriateness for a specific clinical experience and to identify areas that they might need to focus on when they are placed at MGH. For the CIs, establishing a consistent set of behaviors that they use to assess performance during the initial phase of the experience helps focus clinical goals. It can help identify students who are struggling in one or more areas early on and provide a more comprehensive understanding of the resources required to meet their needs and assess resource availability. From a practical standpoint, using prerequisite behaviors places the emphasis on previously developed knowledge and skills and eliminates the additional complexity of the considerable variation in length of clinical experiences between academic programs. It also would provide a consistent language that would be used by CIs in their discussions around student performance.

Feedback from CIs who have used the model with students in the past year has been overwhelmingly positive. It has been helpful to have a consistent framework that crossed all domains and to view that framework as a continuum of skills. They have found it especially helpful to use during the initial assessment of student baseline skills, and it has facilitated specific focus on skill development. Having used a similar tool in the CRP, they were comfortable that students would not necessarily be compartmentalized in a single box on the grid, but they might demonstrate a range of criteria, some of which would be described above or below the current level of their clinical experience. It has been helpful in working with students who were demonstrating performance issues in one or more domains and with students who were exceeding expectations. CIs describe the benefit of being able to provide ongoing feedback against an internal departmental "standard." Those who were working with students who were exceeding expectations used the continuum described on the grid to develop ongoing goals for student performance. Goals were more easily developed that focused on the quality of the student's performance related to specific clinical processes.

CONCLUSIONS

Our early experience with the program has taught us that not all individuals attain recognition as Advanced Clinicians or Clinical Scholars. We continue to grapple with the broad and expansive behaviors that encompass the full range of being a clinician. Our experience has taught us that therapists grow across the dimensions of the CRP at different rates and that they can develop highly advanced skills within a narrow range of behaviors. The process of implementing the CRP has also helped us reach a consensus on the central importance that reflection plays in developing one's practice. We have come to appreciate that it is reflection, whether written or otherwise, that drives physical therapists to be better at taking care of patients.

Developing a CRP, based on theories of skill acquisition and expertise, has significant implications for the profession. Such models provide opportunities to implement theories and to experiment with various ways to develop clinicians. Expanded definitions of professional competence and the growing expectations of patients/consumers require us as a profession to have formal, clinically based structures and processes that guide and inform the course of professional development. Many professions, such as medicine and social work, have a dual level of licensure. These systems recognize that full independent practice is achieved after an extensive period of clinical practice that involves some element of mentorship and supervision. Current licensure in physical therapy ensures minimal protection of the public and meets a "do no harm" standard. In physical therapy, clinical specialization represents the pinnacle of clinical practice in terms of accomplishment and skill. Much development occurs between these extremes, yet we lack consensus on what that process and milestones are. The CRP offers one example of a means to support and document professional development from entry to specialization.

MGH Physical Therapy Services has long demonstrated a culture of advancing the clinical practice of individuals. A final, yet unanticipated, application of the CRP model has been the development of common language and framework among the staff and leadership to describe and understand professional development milestones and processes directed toward that development. Therapists are immersed in these processes beginning at orientation, and this continues throughout their employment. The journey toward becoming an expert clinician is just that, a journey. With practice in a state of constant evolution, our culture dissuades us from placing emphasis on reaching a destination and encourages us to prepare therapists to be in a dynamic state of analysis and reflection.

REFERENCES

1. Peden-McAlpine C. Expert thinking in nursing practice: implications for supporting expertise. *Nurs Health Sci*. 1999;1:131–137.
2. Jensen G, Gwyer J, Hack L, Shepard K. *Expertise in physical therapy practice*. Boston: Butterworth–Heinemann, 1999.
3. Massachusetts General Hospital for Children. *PCS clinical recognition program*, Boston: Massachusetts General Hospital, 2002.
4. Dreyfus HE, Dreyfus SE. *Mind over machine*. New York: The Free Press, 1996.
5. Benner P. *From novice to expert*. Menlo Park, CA: Addison-Wesley, 1982.
6. Benner P, Tanner CA, Chesla CA. *Expertise in nursing practice*. New York: Springer, 1996.
7. Benner P, Hooper-Kyriakidis P, Stannard D. *Clinical wisdom and interventions in critical care*. Philadelphia: WB Saunders, 1999.
8. Camooso C. Future trends: advancing profession practice in an interdisciplinary model. In Haig-Heitman (ed). *Clinical practice development using novice to expert theory*, Gaithersburg, MD: Aspen Publications, 1999.
9. Jensen GM, Shepard KF, Hack LM. The novice versus the experienced clinician: insights into the work of the physical therapist. *Phys Ther*. 1990;70:314–323.

12

10. Mattingly C, Flemming MHL. *Clinical reasoning*. Philadelphia: FA Davis, 1994.
11. American Physical Therapy Association. *Guide to physical therapist practice*, ed 2. Alexandria, VA: APTA, 2002.
12. Epstein RM, Hundert EM. Defining and assessing professional competence. *JAMA*. 2002;287:226–235.
13. American Physical Therapy Association. *Professionalism in physical therapy: core values*. Alexandria, VA: APTA, 2003.
14. American Physical Therapy Association. *Vision 2020*. Available at http://www.apta.org/AM/Template.cfm?Section=About_APTA & TEMPLATE=/CM/ContentDisplay.cfm& CONTENTID=19078. Accessed February 2, 2006.

APPENDIX 12–1   CLINICAL NARRATIVE

I have been a physical therapist in the inpatient PT department at MGH for about 2 ½ years, and have had the opportunity to experience working with a wide variety of patients as I have rotated through the general medical team, cardiopulmonary team, and now the surgical/trauma team.

One patient in particular stands out in my mind that represents much of what I have learned throughout my three rotations while at MGH. Mrs. R is a 69-year-old female who I was fortunate to work with during her two admissions to MGH. She initially presented to MGH with a buttock/thigh wound that was found to be necrotizing fasciitis. She is a retired nurse herself and had been very active prior to her admission, enjoying walking, traveling, hiking, and time with her family. Being a retired nurse, Mrs. R was frequently asking questions and wanted to be in control of her environment and her health. She was very knowledgeable, and it was crucial that she was aware of everything that was happening to her. Knowing this, I was cognizant of word choice, making sure I allowed her to ask all of her questions and express all of her concerns. Mrs. R had an extensive medical history, including peripheral vascular disease, CABG X4, and diabetes. During her initial admission, she underwent extensive debridement of her wound, with a VAC dressing placed.

Initially, she was seen in the SICU, during which time she was very confused due to her medications. This confusion persisted through much of her first hospitalization, limiting her participation in physical therapy. I worked with the occupational therapist, social worker, and psychiatrist to create an environment that would maximize her outcome and participation in PT. Mrs. R was discharged to an acute rehab facility and returned about 3 weeks later with ongoing wound issues. At this time, another PT completed her initial evaluation, which was limited by her need to remain in a Clinitron bed to protect her skin. Having little experience with this type of bed, I was fearful that the bed was going to be the greatest limiting factor in her progress with PT. Her mental status had cleared and had returned to baseline, and she had finally been making steady gains with her mobility with short distance ambulation with a rolling walker at rehab. She was very excited about her progress, and expressed great fear over regressing.

Mrs. R had many impairments associated with her integumentary issues and significant deconditioning due to her complicated course. Given the location of her wounds and VAC dressing, the plastic surgery team did not allow her to flex her hips due to potential for further integumentary impairment issues. I communicated with both the primary surgery team and plastic surgery team about my concerns over her bed rest. They stated that they had no plans to take her out of the Clinitron bed or to liberalize her activity, as their greatest concern was her wound healing. Understanding this, I talked with the clinical specialists in my department to problem solve the best way to mobilize Mrs. R out of the Clinitron bed while minimizing the risk of ruining the integrity of the VAC dressing, the wound and minimizing the risk of failure for the patient. I was certain that if the transfer was not successful that the patient would be very fearful about trying it again.

After exploring various options with the clinical specialist, I decided that the best approach would be to use an air pal to carefully elevate the patient over the rim of the bed and to pull her onto a tilt table. The tilt table would be crucial, as it would allow her to slowly rise from the supine position to a standing position, while carefully monitoring her hemodynamic response and pain. Given the length of time that Mrs. R had been supine, I anticipated that she would likely be orthostatic with the upright position. Knowing that she had a cardiac history, I wanted to be able to frequently monitor her blood pressure and her symptoms. In anticipation for mobilization, I instructed Mrs. R in a therapeutic exercise program, which she could complete independently in supine, which focused on increasing strength in her lower extremities. She enjoyed performing this program and religiously performed the prescribed exercises three times daily.

Prior to attempting this transfer, I had multiple discussions with the patient explaining exactly what would happen, all of the equipment, how many people would be present, and how I expected her to respond to the upright position. This helped her feel comfortable and trust me. Mrs. R was very concerned that she would experience back pain as she had an increased kyphosis and was concerned with the hard table under her back. I obtained padding from the OT department, and after showing the patient; I used this padding to line the tilt table to protect her back. The first attempt with the transfer and elevation on the tilt table was very successful. As expected, her blood pressure dropped, with only a minimal increase in her HR as she was on a beta blocker. She complained of some lightheadedness and some pain in her gastric region, secondary to the prolonged stretch in standing. Initially, she was able to tolerate about 5 minutes on the tilt table. We set daily goals to increase the elevation and time spent in the upright position.

Over the next few weeks, Mrs. R really enjoyed using the tilt table as a mode of getting out of bed, and she was very encouraged by her daily progress. I reassessed her hemodynamic response, pain, ankle range of motion, and strength regularly. I progressed her therapeutic exercise program and elevation/ time on the tilt table as appropriate. Her plan of care included incorporating functional activities in the upright position, but given her length of stay we were unable to reach this point. She expressed much thanks to me for seeking out a way to allow her to mobilize and expressed that she had lost much hope in getting better and now she felt like she could work towards independence.

Mrs. R became an advocate for her own care and had multiple discussions with the plastics team regarding rescheduling the timing of her VAC changes to allow her to participate in her PT sessions. A few days before Mrs. R was transferred to a rehab facility, she was moved into a regular air bed. Despite not working on sit-to-stand transfers and ambulation for about 1 month, she

12

was able to immediately transfer to the edge of the bed, stand up with a walker, and initiate marching in place. Her hemodynamic response was normal, and she complained of only very minimal pain. This success reinforced how important it was to work on the tilt table and find any mode for her to get out of bed, as she was able to minimize the risk of bed rest and minimize her deconditioning.

This experience reiterated to me the importance of clear communication with patients, making sure that everything is explained and agreed upon prior to performing a task. Trust is crucial, especially in situations in which success is not guaranteed, and the patient's comfort plays a big role in the outcome. It is important to consider a patient's personality, culture, and background in all aspects of evaluation and treatment.

APPENDIX 12–2

STAFF MEMBER: Barbara Darcy

FORMAT: Direct observation, documentation review, clinical discussion

DATE: November 9, 2004

- QH 72-year-old female s/p brainstem tumor resection and stroke. Devoted twin sister and husband present much of the time.
- PG 45-year-old female s/p L temporal-occipital ICH. Significant neurobehavioral issues.
- KN 48-year-old male s/p large R cerebellar bleed and ventricular extension. Presents with decreased postural control, bilateral CN III palsies, and cognitive impairments.
- SM 48-year-old Farsi-speaking woman with rapidly progressing dementia, dx. with CJD.

PATIENT–CLINICIAN RELATIONSHIP

- Demonstrates comfort in establishing rapport with patients and families. Demonstrates a genuine concern for her patients.
- Has demonstrated significant development in evaluating potential barriers to communication as well as altering her communication style as needed. Should continue to develop in this area to increase effectiveness of communication and patient performance. Examples of communication:
  - QH demonstrated decreased vision on the R. Therefore Barbara approached her from the L and positioned her bed to face visitors and the television on leaving.
  - With PG Barbara controlled the environment by closing the door; spoke quietly and calmly as she noticed signs of increased agitation.
  - With KN sometimes could be more effective with simplifying her statements and allow time for the patient to process and execute.
- Barbara consistently uses the Interpreter Service to communicate with patients as appropriate.
- Barbara demonstrated effectiveness in advocating for patient SM. The patient confided in Barbara that she felt as though some nurses were

laughing at her and she was not being addressed by her proper name. Barbara independently initiated speaking to the nurse regarding the situation and followed up with me for further discussion/advice.

■ Is working on increasing patient and family participation in their care, which I feel has improved with overall experience and clinical decision making.

CLINICAL DECISION MAKING

■ *Self-assessment:* Demonstrates accuracy in assessing limitations in knowledge and skill. Motivated to improve her practice. Barbara will seek Clinical Specialist assistance to validate her impression of her needs and assist with creating a plan. Barbara will use the plan to address her developmental needs.

■ *Patient History:* Has been working on and has demonstrated growth in performing patient interviews. As she has gained more experience with the neurologic population and her examination skills, she is gaining skill in using the patient and family as a source of information. Is also gaining skill in factoring information from the patient interview into her clinical impression, which has again supported the importance of gathering this information.

■ *Tests and Measures:* Areas that Barbara has been actively working on: examination and documentation of *motor control vision* and *balance*. Barbara consistently seeks me out for assistance with examination and/or confirmation of visual examinations. Still needs work on this area as she can describe what she observes but does not consistently effectively select or perform tests (e.g., had a patient track her pen for smooth pursuit but was switching the pen from hand to hand....hence, not smooth to pursue; e.g., could describe KN's eyes as directed downward and inward yet could not identify that this was a profound CN III palsies).

Evaluation

■ Accurately identifies primary impairments limiting the patient's functional mobility. Will seek assistance with more complex patients (e.g., sought confirmation to identify that KN had impaired motor control on the R>L and proximally>distally as the hypothesis for his decreased ability to stand and transfer).

■ Evaluations reflect the ability to integrate the pathophysiology, co-morbidities, and psychosocial issues with assistance needed for more complex patients.

■ Is gaining accuracy in predicting functional outcomes with patients but will need more experience for accuracy. Has used information from past Case Conferences to assist with variables that contribute to predicting outcomes with patients following stroke.

■ *Plan of care:* This too has been an area that Barbara has been focusing her efforts. Realizes that her plan of care is not always as specific as it could be to address the impairments identified (e.g., once she identified the primary impairments for KN she needed some assistance to come up with some reasonable but specific strategies to address the impairments that could be incorporated into a functional activity given his cognitive impairment).

TEAMWORK AND COLLABORATION

- Demonstrates comfort as a member of the neuro-peds team. Demonstrating increasing comfort in role as a team member on Ellison 12. Is demonstrating professional and effective relationships with nurses and other health care professionals.
- Identifies the need for additional consultations and institutes referrals. Works collaboratively with OT and SLP.
- Actively participates in weekly Neuro Rounds. Has needed some guidance to identify or focus her question.

MOVEMENT

- Should continue to develop skill in evaluating movement of the eyes.
- Demonstrates appropriate level of skill for analyzing movement and gait.
- Has been beginning to work more on handling skills facilitation of movement. I will usually demonstrate on her so that she can feel it. I will demonstrate on the patient and then she will try. Is beginning to see the benefits of handling skills.

OVERALL COMMENTS AND PLAN (AREAS WE'VE BEEN WORKING ON)

Overall, Barbara is doing well and steadily moving forward.

COMMUNICATION AND PROFESSIONALISM

Barbara's primary area for professional development was professional behavior including improved communication. Barbara has demonstrated significant growth in this area and consistently maintains a professional (nonjoking) demeanor while on Ellison 12. Can still have a tendency to joke around in the staff room but is not disruptive or unprofessional. I need to formally give her this feedback that she has shown much improvement in this area.

Tests and Measures

Vision: Have directed Barbara to some resources (including vision/vestibular case conference) for examining vision. Will continue to consult on patients with Barbara to confirm or assist with the examination of visual/vestibular impairments.

Balance: Continue consultation and documentation review for examination of balance.

Specificity of Plan of Care

Will continue with documentation review, direct consultation, and discussions. This is likely the focus of our discussions when I am consulted (aside from vision questions).

Part IV

Pursuing Expertise in Physical Therapy

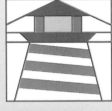

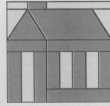

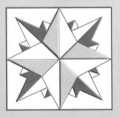

By any measure, physical therapy has grown as a profession exponentially in the latter part of the twentieth century. The work conducted on defining expertise in physical therapy over the past two decades has helped the profession broaden its view of what true professionalism means. As our profession raises its goals from technically competent to fully committed practitioners engaged in a moral contract with society to define and care for the health needs of society, the experts among us provide the models we wish to follow. Their decision making and skills are most likely to have an impact on the health needs of our patients, so we are motivated to continue to understand how these respected experts have developed as professionals.

In this section we integrate the results of our work on expertise (Part II), reflections on the work of others (Part III), and the insights developed from 15 years of teaching and discussions about expertise in physical therapy. Through valuable discussions with physical therapists across the country we have found insights into the practical application of the core concepts of the model of expertise. The purpose of these chapters is to facilitate the continued discussion and development of expertise in physical therapy.

In Chapter 13 we pose questions for future inquiry into expertise in physical therapy—both theoretical modeling and observational investigations that will further clarify this complex phenomenon. In Chapter 14 we discuss the implications of this work for doctoral-level educators and students in professional education, both Doctor of Physical Therapy (DPT) and transitional DPT educational programs. In the final chapter, Chapter 15, we share strategies for using the model of expertise to enhance the professional development of individual clinicians, teams, or managers.

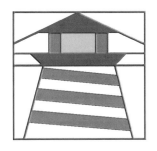

Lighthouse — A pieced block, the lighthouse beam illuminates the darkness.

13   Inquiry into Expertise: Future Directions

Since the first edition of *Expertise in Physical Therapy Practice* was published, the authors have had many opportunities for dialogue about the model of expertise. Our discussions with clinicians, students, and research colleagues have contributed to a deeper understanding of this work and have provoked many interesting questions not yet answered. In this chapter we will discuss each element of the proposed model of expertise, summarizing major research implications and suggesting new directions for inquiry.

KNOWLEDGE: A MULTI-DIMENSIONAL FOUNDATION

Through this investigation of the knowledge base of expert physical therapists we examined the process of its formation, the type of knowledge valued, and experts' sources of knowledge. Each of these aspects of the multidimensional knowledge base of experts bears further investigation.

DEVELOPMENT OF KNOWLEDGE FOR PRACTICE

The experts in this study consistently demonstrated a significant amount of self-direction in the process of building their knowledge for practice. Although not diminishing the importance of professional education, it is clear that each of these subjects exerted significant personal resources to direct the continued growth of their knowledge base. This initiative must not be overlooked, and the question remains: Can one achieve any level of expertise without this effort to grow in intellectual maturity? The documented processes we observed included pursuit of additional educational degrees, specialty certification, continuing education, teaching experience, and self-directed study. Our postscript on our original research subjects (found at the close of Part III) confirms that these individuals have continued in the pursuit of knowledge over the past decade.

Although we observed our experts frequently in pursuit of information to guide clinical decisions, what we know less about is the full range of behaviors of experts in the practice of what is now termed "evidence-based practice." Future research into the habits of experts in the area of information access and analysis is needed to determine if experts practice in a recognizable evidence-based framework. The Association of American Medical Colleges (1) and the Institute of Medicine's Health Professions Education Summit (2) have explicitly advocated the duty of all health care practitioners to use evidence-based practice and informatics. A focused research stream in this area could provide a more detailed description of whether experts use evidence-based practice more frequently than has been reported in cross-sectional research by Jette et al. (3) and if the primary barrier of lack of time for implementing evidence-based practice is reported by experts. Would our experts be considered early adopters, those individuals in a profession who are most likely to evaluate new evidence and put it into practice, serving as a model for their colleagues? Jette challenges the profession in his editorial, "Invention is Hard, but Dissemination is Even Harder" (4), to create a future that is different from the past by understanding the diffusion of innovation. Our experts seem to be well placed to influence clinical practice through diffusion of innovation (5).

An additional question raised by this element of the model concerns the frequency with which experts in physical therapy contribute to the expansion of our knowledge for practice by the dissemination of their clinical wisdom through written communications. We documented several written contributions to the evidence base of our profession among our subjects, but our subjects were much more likely to teach than to write for publication. The questions remain: To what degree is the profession benefiting from the practice knowledge held by these experts and what amount of the clinical wisdom within our profession goes untapped or undocumented? Within the last decade many additional venues for the dissemination of clinically based knowledge have emerged, including written case reports, consensus-based practice policies, and evidence for practice summaries. When expert clinicians are encouraged and enabled to communicate their clinical wisdom, we can see the creation of the scholarly practitioner who will clearly contribute to the knowledge on which the entire profession stands.

Mentors were a significant factor in the process of knowledge development used by these subjects. Investigations of the process of developing mentoring relationships may be fruitful for determining if this is a recommended part of the journey toward clinical expertise. In an unpublished qualitative investigation of 16 certified clinical specialists and their experience with mentors, all reported significant mentoring relationships that helped them improve their knowledge and clinical expertise (6). Thirteen of the sixteen clinical specialists sought out their mentor, as was found with our experts. The American Physical Therapy Association (APTA) has developed a voluntary mentoring process for its members, but to date no assessment of the effectiveness of this process has been completed. Additional studies of the outcomes of mentoring behaviors for the protégé could help us understand the role that mentors can play in the development of experts. As one's clinical career progresses, the transition from protégé to mentor was identified as a milestone for several of our subjects who were quite experienced. The skills of effective mentoring in physical therapy are yet to be defined. The pilot work by Chen and Rorher (6) with physical therapist clinical specialists found career mentoring in physical therapy to be considerably different in focus than the mentoring usually found in business fields.

The third component of this development process that intrigues us is the value of reflection to create new knowledge for the experts. Although it is doubtful that any of these subjects was familiar with the theoretical basis of reflective learning, they valued their own persistent questioning. Through constant reflection on the clinical presentations of their patients, they transformed this experience into their tacit knowledge of practice. This clinically transformed knowledge is so context rich that recall and use with new patients is rapid, whereas some other, less contextual knowledge may have to be referenced. We would like to understand more about this process of building the tacit knowledge for clinical practice and how expert clinicians make linkages that are useful for future problem solving. What part of this process is consciously driven and what signs and symptoms or knowledge of the patient facilitate retrieval of useful information? Can reflection on practice be facilitated through journaling or recordings? Is reflection on practice most effective when done alone or with colleagues?

13

TYPES AND SOURCES OF KNOWLEDGE VALUED BY EXPERTS

Our experts built a deep and quickly accessible foundation of biomedical and technical knowledge in their specialty area. They benefited from the ability to focus their practice, which provided some limits to the quantity of knowledge to be monitored. Our youngest subject had 10 years of experience, so it was not surprising to find that none of these experts mentioned a traditional type of procedural knowledge that most informed their practice. By this point in their career, other, more interactional types of knowledge were more highly valued. A longitudinal investigation of clinicians could help us understand if such a movement away from the value of procedural knowledge toward interactive knowledge is common to clinicians.

Specifically, the types of knowledge our experts valued included self-knowledge, knowledge of the patient, knowledge of the systems that affect their patient, and knowledge of normal and abnormal movement. *Self-knowledge* remains very much undefined in our data but was included because it appeared as a consistent theme. Subjects would recount that as their maturity and self-awareness grew, they believed they became better clinicians. The aspects of self-awareness that are most crucial should be identified through more focused interviewing, so that we might discover whether the process can be facilitated. There may be a link between the clinicians' self-knowledge and their ability to solicit the next important type of knowledge: knowledge of the patient.

Knowledge of the patient and the *systems that affect them* are two types of knowledge that grow the most quickly in any clinician's practice. However, the importance of building this knowledge, learned from the patient, is one of the clearest themes in our work. This finding can be enhanced by learning more about what information is crucial to obtain from each patient. Listening to patients was identified as the primary skill required to enhance this part of the knowledge base, so studies of focused, active listening may also advance our practice in this area. The experts also showed initiative in expanding the scope of their role with their patients by deepening their knowledge of all the systems that affect their patient or families.

From many different perspectives, our experts in four specialty areas identified the importance of their *knowledge of normal and abnormal movement*. This knowledge ranged from focused and detailed analyses of very small amplitude movements of the spine to gross functional assessments of the quantity and quality of movement in the sit to stand task. The growth in this knowledge base through observational analysis and kinesthetic awareness was pursued consistently, and the experts were always seeking greater proficiency through practice. As the ability of physical therapists to assess movement both with and without technological assistance increases, our patients will be better served. The experts demonstrate that this will only happen with concerted efforts to practice and improve movement analysis knowledge. What do the experts see that the average physical therapist does not? Does a more accurate description of abnormal movement lead to better patient outcomes? Is knowledge of and skilled observation of movement abnormalities a key to expert practice?

BOX 13–1	*Questions for Future Research*

> **Knowledge**
>
> 1. How do experts most efficiently develop their knowledge for practice?
> 2. Do experts use an evidence-based framework for their practice decisions differently than do novices?
> 3. What types of evidence available in the literature are of most use to experts?
> 4. Are experts considered to be early adopters of evidence for practice?
> 5. To what extent do experts in physical therapy contribute their knowledge of clinical practice to their peers?
> 6. What are the principle effective skills of a mentor to improve the expertise of a physical therapist?
> 7. How can clinicians learn to reflect on their knowledge and make it more useful to them?
> 8. What types of knowledge become most useful to clinicians as they gain expertise?
> 9. Are there questions used by experts during patient histories that elicit crucial knowledge of the patient?
> 10. How are experts different from novices in their ability to identify abnormal movement in their patients?

CLINICAL REASONING: COMPLEX, COLLABORATIVE, AND PATIENT FOCUSED

The clinical reasoning element of the model of expertise has been addressed by us and other authors in this text, yet it is clear that we are just beginning to develop theories that may help us understand how expert clinicians make decisions and evaluate the outcomes of those decisions. Since the publication of our first edition, the health care context for critical clinical decisions has only become more challenging, placing even more pressure on the need for accurate and timely decisions. Many avenues for further inquiry exist for those interested in the clinical or practical reasoning processes of physical therapists, including the scope and type of clinical reasoning required, the collaborative context and use of knowledge for clinical reasoning, and the use of narrative in describing practical reasoning in physical therapy.

THE SCOPE AND TYPE OF CLINICAL REASONING REQUIRED

The intense observations of experts reported by several authors in this text provide compelling evidence for the broad range of performance in clinical reasoning required of physical therapists. Edwards and Jones in Chapter 10 observed eight clinical reasoning strategies in two broad categories of the patient management model—diagnosis and patient management. In each of these categories, well-structured and easily identified problems are approached in one manner

13

(instrumental management), and less easily understood problems are approached in another manner (communicative management). Throughout an interaction with a patient, experts demonstrated movement among the different clinical reasoning strategies as their need to gain information or to instruct or consult changed. Additional investigations into these clinical reasoning strategies, through observations with novices, students, and experts, should continue to strengthen our understanding of the complex interplay of problem solving between patient and therapist.

We also found our expert subjects to be adept in various types of clinical reasoning: large decisions about whether or not a client needs care and minute-to-minute decisions about adjusting hand placement or choosing a teaching tool for a patient. The experts have a large capacity for clinical reasoning and do not seem to illustrate the reasoning fatigue that novices or students might. In fact, it is the challenge of the "difficult" patient that motivates many experts, calling on their advanced repertoire of reasoning tools. Experts can determine what knowledge is needed in the situation and have available to them a variety of reasoning patterns to help them obtain the information. What personal characteristics motivate these experts to persevere until an acceptable plan of care is identified?

THE COLLABORATIVE CONTEXT FOR CLINICAL REASONING IN PHYSICAL THERAPY

The study of experts in physical therapy demonstrates repeatedly the high value held by the experts for patient-focused care, perhaps nowhere more strongly than in the collaborative problem-solving process between patient and therapist. Patients hold the knowledge that the experts value highly and need to help them perform their diagnostic, care management, and educational roles. The identification of narrative reasoning, or the collection of narratives from the patient, has been identified in this text as a critical tool for expert practitioners. Questions remain, however, about how narrative reasoning can be used in today's fast-paced health care environment when time with patients continues to be limited. Knowing when to use narrative reasoning in the course of care of a patient, early or later, may also help transfer this behavior to novices.

Although varying interpretations exist of these first-generation models of clinical reasoning in physical therapy, the need to understand successful practice remains important to the entire profession. As commented by Rothstein (7), we know too little about clinical reasoning and we should know more. "The mystery should not persist, because this is a topic that lends itself to research, and, most importantly, to inquiry using a variety of methods from myriad points of view" (7).

PRACTICAL REASONING AND THE ROLE OF NARRATIVE

One of the struggles with our model is that it is difficult to artificially separate the dimensions of expertise (knowledge, clinical reasoning, movement, and virtue). For example, we have described knowledge in physical therapy expert practice as being multidimensional and derived from various sources. We have also talked about the critical role of reflection and metacognitive skills in the clinical reasoning process. Without a doubt, expert clinical reasoning creates new knowledge for practice. This new knowledge is then evaluated in an interactive and context-rich process with subsequent patients to assess its value to practice. In this manner, reflection on practice leads to new understandings and building of clinical knowledge. This argument is an important one for us if we believe that knowledge in physical therapy can be created in several ways, from experimentally designed clinical research studies to reflections on everyday practice.

William Sullivan, senior scholar at the Carnegie Foundation for the Advancement of Teaching, is one of the lead scholars in Carnegie's comparative study of professional education in medicine, law, engineering, and clergy. In his book, *Work and Integrity* (8), he urges us to reconsider the central importance of practical reasoning in professional expertise. At the core of practical reasoning is the ability for the practitioner to apply inquiry skills and engage in a reflective process. Sullivan defines practical reasoning as a threefold pattern that includes: 1) the analytical reasoning of a detached scientist using evidence, knowledge, and objectivity; 2) application of the inquiry skills of a professional as they apply the knowledge to the particular condition; and 3) consideration of the relationship between the patient and professional as an integral part of being a healer. Professional expertise embodies this threefold pattern of practical reasoning as practitioners not only bring knowledge and inquiry skills, but must also bring the relationship and their role as healer—all done in the context of practice. This relationship is depicted in Figure 13-1.

Our model of expert practice in physical therapy with a focus on knowledge, clinical reasoning, movement, and virtue is consistent with these elements that are part of practical reasoning. The question is, then: How do we best understand or capture the knowledge that may be embedded in this process? Benner

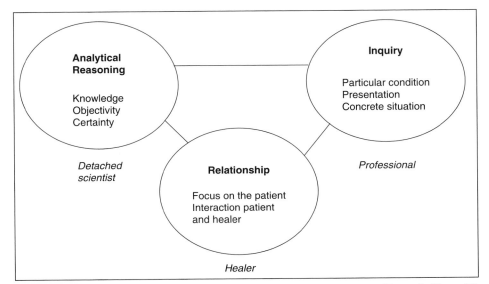

Figure 13-1 ■ Model of the threefold circuit of practical reasoning. (From Sullivan W. *Work and integrity: the crisis and promise of professionalism in America*. San Francisco: Jossey-Bass; 2005.)

and colleagues have used clinical narratives in the study of nursing (9,10). They have used clinical narratives as a core tool in their study of critical care nursing and have used clinical narratives as a teaching tool. Narrative descriptions or reflective accounts from practitioners can uncover greater understanding of the context of practice, including insights into the relationship and interaction with patients, the work, and the inquiry process of the practitioner (11). Stories from practice across levels of experience and expertise can provide a framework for reflective discussion or could illustrate exceptional or challenging practice situations. We have seen little use of narrative as a tool in physical therapy for exploring knowledge or reasoning. A useful structure for clinical narratives is Benner's guidelines for clinical exemplars (Table 13-1). In Chapter 12, Jampal and colleagues discuss how they have used narratives as part of their professional development program at Massachusetts General Hospital.

In physical therapy research, these narratives could be seen by a different name: case reports. Rothstein presented the need for case reports in our professional literature eloquently in 2002, stating:

> In physical therapy, we lack a literature that describes—in replicable detail—what we do with patients. Without such a literature, the world cannot possibly understand the patient management of which we are so proud, colleagues cannot engage in dialogue designed to improve patient care, and researchers are deprived

Table 13-1 Guidelines for Writing Clinical Narratives

Selecting the Exemplar	Writing the Exemplar	Evaluating the Exemplar
A situation that stands out in your mind because of the significance in how you think or practice. Consider these prompts about situations: 1. An example of good physical therapy practice. 2. Where the situation taught you something new, you discovered new ways of interventions, noticed something new. 3. A memorable exchange or interaction that taught you something new. 4. A situation where you made a difference. 5. A situation where there was a breakdown, an error, or a moral dilemma.	Exemplars are to be written as a narrative account. Consider the following: 1. Write in first person. 2. Tell your story. 3. You may want to record your oral description of the story first because this is less linear than writing. 4. Try to complete the story first before you start editing. 5. Avoid summary sentences. 6. Try to include dialogue to give a firsthand account of what happened. 7. Include your concerns about your judgment and your actions. 8. Change names and identifying information to protect confidentiality.	These rich stories of clinical practice contain clinical knowledge that is not well described in current practice. Suggestions for evaluating narratives: 1. Remember to build trust because narratives are examples of risk taking. 2. Consider criteria such as vividness of description, veracity, clarity and new coherence, and good use of first- or you person accounts. 3. Students or clinicians should have an opportunity to reflect on their narrative account because the presentation and discussion of the account can provide additional insights.

Sullivan W. *Work and integrity: the crisis and promise of professionalism in America.* San Francisco: Jossey-Bass; 2005.

of knowledge about the nuances of practice—which means that the research they conduct cannot be as applicable to practice as it needs to be (12, p 1062).

Documenting the narrative reasoning of our clinical experts is now a well-accepted means of contributing to the knowledge needed both for practice and for meaningful clinical research.

BOX 13–2	*Questions for Future Research*

> **Clinical Reasoning**
>
> 1. What are the most common types of clinical decisions confronting physical therapists and which clinical reasoning strategies are most effective for each?
> 2. Do students, novices, and experts all demonstrate multiple clinical reasoning strategies during an interaction with a patient? When in the process of professional development does this ability develop?
> 3. What are the best ways to help students gain skills in a variety of clinical reasoning strategies?
> 4. Can practice policies (guidelines or documentation rubrics) help novice practitioners develop broader methods of reasoning?
> 5. How is clinical knowledge developed from practical reasoning and how is it evaluated?
> 6. Can narratives be used to enhance the clinical reasoning of physical therapists?

MOVEMENT: OUR CENTRAL FOCUS

Ours is the first work on expertise to identify the element of movement as a unique aspect of the expertise of physical therapists. Movement is what we do as physical therapists and the focus of our work with our patients. Movement is what we know, what we see, what we measure, and what we value. Many aspects of this element of the model are intriguing for further study.

MOVEMENT AS A PHYSIOLOGIC SYSTEM

One of our most respected colleagues in physical therapy, Shirley Sahrmann, has published many scientific papers in which normal and abnormal movement patterns in patients with various diagnoses are studied (13,14). Often viewed as a movement expert, we were not surprised to find her using a creative movement analogy as a theme for her 1998 Mary McMillan Lecture, entitled, "Moving Precisely? Or Taking the Path of Least Resistance?" (15). In this lecture, Sahrmann exhorts physical therapists to continue to develop the concept of movement as a physiologic system and physical therapists as experts in that system. Commenting on her 40 years of experience in patient care Sahrmann states:

> *One lesson that I learned from working with patients is that it is very easy to overlook the subtle changes in the path of movement, but if the changes*

13

are addressed early and precise movement is restored, a desirable outcome is relatively easy to obtain (15, p. 1210).

Also in this lecture, Sahrmann encourages physical therapists to build a firm knowledge base in movement sciences and to use more precise language in communicating about movement dysfunction. The language of movement analysis has both a laboratory and a clinical dialect, and neither is likely well-understood by physical therapists fluent in one or the other. The clinician who wishes to enhance his or her knowledge base in movement analysis often must seek assistance in the form of graduate education to comprehend laboratory measures of movement. Researchers who use discrete measures of movement in multiple dimensions contribute valuable assessments to studies of the effectiveness of our interventions but may fail to leave the clinician with a clinically useful measure. The research agenda in both the laboratory and the clinic can help us define movement as a physiologic system. Our experts are the type of physical therapists who can contribute to these goals for the profession. They display a primary commitment to understand the movement they observe, all the systems that affect movement, and all the systems that abnormal movement subsequently affects. They can articulate their analysis of movement dysfunction as a physiologic system. Further study of the language used by novices and experts to diagnose movement dysfunction as a finite impairment of some system pathology, or as a physiologically integrated system enabling other body systems, is needed.

MOVEMENT AS PHYSICAL THERAPIST INTERVENTION AND ASSESSMENT

The experts in four practice domains were observed to use movement to treat patients and to assess the effects of their movements in a seamless dimension of touching. They discussed the confidence they had in the information they gained from their touch or movement of a patient's body. The movement element of the model of expertise could be further studied by assessing the appropriateness or accuracy of this confidence. Little research exists that assesses the accuracy of movement analysis decisions made by physical therapists. Cook and colleagues, in a study of 134 orthopedic certified specialists, found that 74% reported that they felt confident or very confident in diagnosing lumbar clinical spine instability, using a variety of movement assessments, including "hesitancy of motion during movement assessment," "observable or palpable abnormalities of motion during movement assessment," and "observed motion disparity," among other criteria used for diagnosis (16). More confirmation is needed of the accuracy of experts' movement assessments in their roles of diagnosing and evaluating the effectiveness of the plan of care.

These experts expressed a great value for the repetitive practice necessary to achieve the skilled movement they used to treat their patients. Whereas the assessment of psychomotor skills is difficult in professional education and postprofessional education, evaluative rubrics should be developed that will allow clinicians to evaluate their progress toward the goal of skilled direct interventions. If we developed such standardized assessments we would be forced to organize how we think about movement in terms of efficiency, safety, comfort, and effectiveness for both clinician and patient. We have gone too long in a profession so centered in movement to ignore the goal of developing best movement practices. To develop their motor skills our experts often sought out mentors who could give them "hands-on" feedback on the desired psychomotor skill set, and this begs the question as to whether psychomotor skills can be improved in isolated practice.

BOX 13–3

Questions for Future Research

Movement

1. How accurately and thoroughly do novice physical therapists diagnose movement dysfunction in patients as compared with experts?
2. Is self-study or mentored study better to assist novice physical therapists to improve their manual skills in patient interventions?
3. Must a physical therapist be able to move to have good outcomes with patients? What are the implications of this component of expertise for physical therapists who are disabled?
4. How important is visual observation of movement to the diagnostic accuracy of physical therapists' clinical decisions?
5. What elements should be included in an evaluative rubric for assessing the quality of physical therapists' movement during direct interventions?

VIRTUE: CARING COMMITMENT

The experts observed in our study could be characterized as observing the highest level of ethical sensitivity, as first described by Pellegrino (17) and later by Swisher and Krueger-Brophy—the practice of virtue (18). He describes an ascending order of ethical sensitivity starting from observance of the laws, followed by observance of rights and fulfillment of duties, and finally the practice of virtue. The virtues observed in our experts clearly provide the motivation for excellence in the other three elements of the model and likewise require a sacrifice on behalf of the subject. Each virtue identified in this model bears further study of the unique contribution to the development of expertise.

CARE AND COMPASSION

Each therapist demonstrated actions and behaviors that communicated a strong sense of caring and compassion for each of their patients. One of the behaviors we saw most consistently was a nonjudgmental approach with patients. One expert was very clear that when he did not have success with an intervention with patients, it was not the patient's fault but only that he did not know enough. What are the elements in a clinical setting that support therapists' withholding judgment and demonstrating respectful language for patients regardless of clinical presentation or background? What role does the community of practice play in promoting these kinds of behaviors?

Recent efforts in medical education are focused on promoting professionalism—and on not only describing these behaviors but attempting to measure them as well. McGaghie and colleagues developed a conceptual model for altruism and

13

compassion (19). They see compassion as a fundamental element of the overt behavior of altruism—putting the needs of others before your own. In their conceptual model, they hypothesize that altruistic acts are the behavioral expressions motivated by one's compassionate core. This compassionate core includes inner resources; awareness of self and others; and influences from personal, professional, and social situations. This model of altruism is a good example for work that could be done in physical therapy. Although we may begin with a description of virtuous qualities we hope to see in practice, there needs to be far more research and model development of professional attributes and behaviors.

COMMITMENT TO EXCELLENCE

Our experts were highly motivated to become the best practitioner possible. They actively sought mentors who might assist them in their pursuit of learning. For them, learning is a continual process because they never feel that they have the answers to address those tough questions and challenging cases. Whereas we have stated that our experts were highly motivated and committed to excellence, we do not know much about the kinds of motivation that may be at work. Is this all internal motivation that comes from a strong sense of self-efficacy (20)? What kinds of internal and external support and reward system contribute to this motivation? Is motivation a central aspect of a "calling to a profession?"

AUTHENTIC SELF

We found that our experts were consistently honest and forthcoming with their patients. They were willing to admit when a mistake had been made and take responsibility for the error. They had confidence in their ability to have an honest conversation with their patients. With the current concern and emphasis in health care on safety and reduction of errors, this finding is timely. Ruth Purtilo, in a recent editorial, "Beyond Disclosure: Seeking Forgiveness" (21), wrote this:

> Why is the idea of apologizing absent from the health care professions at a time when taking precautions to prevent mistakes, being reflective, and being accountable are increasing in the literature and guidelines about professionalism?.... [D]enial is so pervasive in our profession that I have long thought that every curriculum should require a course in dealing with avoidance and denial, so that breaking through them in difficult circumstances can become part of the professional physical therapist's competencies.

Our experts seemed to show evidence of this competency that Purtilo is advocating for in the profession. How did these therapists come to this understanding and confidence in being humble and willing to admit mistakes? What kinds of learning experiences and curricular innovations would support such actions?

MORAL ACTION

We found our experts willing to assume responsibility for their patients and the care they needed. This would often include advocating for patients so that they could receive the resources they needed, whether that was equipment or additional therapy. Not only did our experts work at the individual level of patient care, they also took seriously their role as a member of a profession that must self-regulate. We had experts who were willing to identify and report unethical behaviors of colleagues or other health professionals. These acts of whistle blowing are examples of moral courage.

Purtilo defines moral courage as a readiness for voluntary, purposive action in situations that engender realistic fear and anxiety to uphold something of great moral value (22). What are acts of moral courage in the physical therapy profession? We often talk about the importance of role models, but we rarely describe, explore, or publicly share the experiences, actions, and achievements of such role models (21).

We also may need to consider what precedes the moral action we have observed in these therapists to understand more about their thinking and reasoning processes that lead to virtuous action (23). Benner and colleagues' research on nursing practice reveals that engaged ethical reasoning linked with clinical reasoning is part of the craft of the expert nurse clinician. She calls this integration of reasoning and judgment in a context that is often charged with emotion

---

BOX 13–4

Questions for Future Research

Virtue

1. What are the elements in a clinical setting that support therapists' withholding of judgment and demonstrating respectful language regardless of patient presentation or background?
2. Are expert individuals free from bias and judgment, or do they simply learn to restrain these human qualities?
3. What role does the community of practice play in promoting virtuous or nonvirtuous behaviors?
4. What kind of models could be developed that represent professional attributes and behaviors in physical therapy?
5. What is the balance between internal and external motivation in promising young novices and expert practitioners?
6. What are successful internal and external support and reward systems that contribute to this motivation?
7. Is motivation a central aspect of a "calling to a profession"? What are the elements of a calling in the physical therapy profession?
8. What are the critical factors in supporting physical therapists' ability to be humble and admit mistakes? What kinds of learning experiences support such actions?
9. What are acts of moral courage in the physical therapy profession? What are the experiences, actions, and achievement of such role models?
10. How is ethical reasoning integrated into case management?
11. When and where do novices acquire skills and abilities to engage in ethical reasoning?
12. What would skilled ethical comportment look like in physical therapy?

13

and complexity "skilled ethical comportment" (24). In Chapter 10, Edwards and colleagues propose several different reasoning strategies used by physical therapists, including ethical reasoning. They also have argued that there is a need for further research exploring just how ethical reasoning is a central part of a clinical reasoning strategy in physical therapy (25). There is much to be explored in this area. For example: How is ethical reasoning integrated into case management? When and where do novices acquire skills and abilities to engage in ethical reasoning? What would skilled ethical comportment look like in physical therapy?

ADDITIONAL TOPICS FOR THE EXPERTISE RESEARCH AGENDA

As we have met with various colleagues to discuss the important next steps in this field of inquiry, many suggestions integrated several elements of the model of expertise or took a broader approach. These potential areas for research are summarized here with the hope that many future investigators will find questions of interest.

A sign of the maturation of our profession as a scholarly field is the development of research agenda in various areas of practice. The authors of this text have contributed suggestions for research questions based on this work in expertise, but more research questions may be found in or adapted from APTA's Clinical Research Agenda, the APTA's Educational Research Agenda, and the APTA's Health Services Research Agenda.

We have long been interested in the merits of longitudinal research into the career paths of promising novice clinicians. These individuals may be identified during professional education or in the early years of practice through a nomination format. Scholarship winners selected by schools or APTA may also serve as research subjects for such an endeavor. A longitudinal design would allow a more accurate tracking of significant events and influences in the practitioners' career and could carefully examine the influence of critical reflection as a component of expertise. There is a potential to include novice therapists as collaborators/investigators in such a project.

Our work and that of others support a central role for teaching that seems ready for further exploration, looking at both the motor learning aspect and social cognitive learning theory.

The integration of the elements of expertise in the model has been termed the "development of a philosophy of practice". Such a philosophy, honed over years of clinical practice, likely results in the wisdom of practice that remains an untapped source for investigation. Case studies of wise practitioners could provide insights into both the aspects of expertise and the developmental processes used in the journey.

Resnik has tackled the thorny question of the outcomes of care achieved by experts and average clinicians. This question is the question most often asked about the work on expert practice in physical therapy. As new measures of outcomes that matter to patients and to the health care system are developed, they will provide the additional tools needed to assess outcomes of care for all physical therapists. Explorations of expertise will not only benefit from the use of these measures; they will inform the development of the measures.

REFERENCES

1. Association of American Medical Colleges. Learning objectives for medical student education: guidelines for medical schools. In *Medical school objectives project.* Washington, DC: AAMC; 1998.
2. NAS. *Health professions education: a bridge to quality.* Washington, DC: Institute of Medicine; 2003.
3. Jette DU, Bacon K, Batty C, et al: Evidence-based practice: beliefs, attitudes, knowledge, and behaviors of physical therapists. *Phys Ther.* 2003;83(9):786–805.
4. Jette AM. Invention is hard, but dissemination is even harder. *Phys Ther.* 2005;85(5):394–403.
5. Rogers E. *Diffusion of innovations*, ed 4. New York: Free Press; 1995.
6. Chen M, Rohrer B. The role that mentoring plays in the development of clinical specialists in physical therapy." Unpublished Master's Thesis, Division of Physical Therapy, Duke University, Durham, NC; 2000.
7. Rothstein JM. The difference between knowing and applying. *Phys Ther.* 2004;84(4):310–311.
8. Sullivan W. *Work and integrity: the crisis and promise of professionalism in America.* San Francisco: Jossey-Bass; 2005.
9. Benner P, Tanner CA, Chesla CA. *Expertise in nursing practice.* New York: Springer; 1996.
10. Benner PE, Hooper-Kyriakidis PL, Stannard D. *Clinical wisdom and interventions in critical care.* Philadelphia: WB Saunders; 1999.
11. Hatem D, Rider EA. Sharing stories: narrative medicine in an evidence-based world. *Patient Educ Couns.* 2004;54(3):251–253.
12. Rothstein J. Case reports: still a priority. *Phys Ther.* 2002;82(11):1062–1063.
13. Norton BJ, Sahrmann SA, Van Dillen LR. Differences in measurements of lumbar curvature related to gender and low back pain. *J Orthop Sports Phys Ther.* 2004;34(9):524–534.
14. Van Dillen LR, Sahrmann SA, Wagner JM. Classification, intervention, and outcomes for a person with lumbar rotation with flexion syndrome. *Phys Ther.* 2005;85(4):336–351.
15. Sahrmann SA. The twenty-ninth Mary McMillan lecture: Moving precisely? Or taking the path of least resistance? *Phys Ther.* 1998;78(11):1208–1218.
16. Cook C, Brismee JM, Sizer PS. Factors associated with physiotherapists' confidence during assessment of clinical cervical and lumbar spine instability. *Physiother Res Int.* 2005;10(2):59–71.
17. Pellegrino E. The virtuous physician and the ethics of medicine. In EE Shelp (ed). *Virtue and medicine: explorations in the character of medicine.* Dordrecht, Holland: Reidel Publishing; 1985.
18. Swisher L, Krueger-Brophy C. *Legal and ethical issues in physical therapy.* Boston: Butterworth–Heinemann; 1998.
19. McGaghie WC, Mytko JJ, Brown WM, et al. Altruism and compassion in the health professions: a search for clarity and precision. *Med Teach.* 2002;24(4):374–378.
20. Sternberg RJ. Abilities are forms of developing expertise. *Educ Res.* 1998;27:11–20.
21. Purtilo R. Beyond disclosure: seeking forgiveness. *Phys Ther.* 2005;85(11):1124–1126.
22. Purtilo R. Moral courage: unsung resources for health professional as healer. In D Thomasma, J Kissell (eds). *The healthcare professional as friend and healer: building on the work of Edmund D. Pellegrino.* Washington, DC: Georgetown University Press; 2000.
23. Purtilo R, Jensen GM, Royeen CB (eds). *Educating for moral action: a sourcebook in health and rehabilitation ethics.* FA Davis Company, 2005.
24. Benner P. Learning through experience and expression: skillful ethical comportment in nursing practice. In D Thomasma, J Kissell (eds). *The healthcare professional as friend and healer: building on the work of Edmund D. Pellegrino.* Washington, DC: Georgetown University Press; 2000.
25. Edwards IA, Braunack-Mayer, Jones M. Ethical reasoning as a clinical reasoning strategy in physiotherapy. *Physiother.* 2005;91:229–236.

13

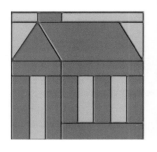

School House — A simple block school house represents learning.

14 Implications for Doctoral-Level Education in Physical Therapy

The original work on expertise has sparked many discussions about the role of formalized educational programs in facilitating the development of expertise. The stories of these expert clinicians, their career paths, and their skills and knowledge provide a rich stimulus for educators to contemplate as they plan educational curricula. When we read these stories, a sense of familiarity strikes us as we recognize shared experiences of exceptional learning and mentoring opportunities. As academic and clinical educators, we want to direct our efforts toward producing more clinicians who will achieve these exceptional levels of practice. How can the lessons learned from these physical therapists be used to improve the educational process for new doctors of physical therapy?

In this chapter, we will share the implications we have gleaned from our work and that of others in this text for doctoral-level educational programs in physical therapy, both professional preparation of physical therapists (DPT) and postprofessional transitional doctoral programs (tDPT). Individualized postprofessional development, in the formats of staff development, continuing education, residencies, fellowships, and self-study, will be covered in Chapter 15.

STRATEGIES FOR USE IN DOCTORAL EDUCATION IN PHYSICAL THERAPY

Throughout years of presentation of the model of expertise, we have collected suggestions for strategies that may be used in the classroom or clinical setting to facilitate the development of each element of the model. Five categories of such strategies are provided in Box 14-1. These strategies cross the elements of the model and may be useful in developing in the doctoral learner one or more elements of the model of expertise. The five strategies listed include some of the research methods used by us and other researchers in this text to elicit expertise data for interpretation. It was not uncommon for us to find our research subjects to be fascinated with these methods and eager to respond. More novice learners may find some of the strategies intimidating but can be encouraged to use them to document the growth of their practice skills.

Wouldn't many experienced physical therapists appreciate seeing a video recording of themselves as a new practitioner? Although some learners will come to the classroom or clinic with well-developed writing or reflecting skills, others will need the guidance of a skilled teacher/mentor to facilitate the ease with which they perform these assessments of the model elements. Our experience is

---

BOX 14–1

Strategies To Be Used in Didactic or Clinical Learning Experiences

1. **Reflect**: provocative questions for discussion.
2. **Read:** literature that explores the elements of expertise and answers clinical questions.
3. **Interview:** with novice, mid-career, and experienced practitioners and faculty.
4. **Record performance:** audio or video stimulus for reflection.
5. **Model/Practice**: aspects of expertise in the classroom or clinic.

that even reluctant students find a measure of appreciation in developing skill in the strategy and in facilitating a younger learner in a peer or mentored relationship—for example, a tDPT and a DPT student paired to perform an assessment. The reader will find a similar set of strategies suggested for use in Chapter 15 for professional development.

Also included in each of the following sections discussing the primary elements of the model of expertise are four Expertise Assessment boxes (Boxes 14-2 through 14-5). In these boxes, the reader will find more explicit examples of learning experiences that might be planned in either professional or postprofessional education programs to assess the learner's development along the path to expertise. These suggestions have been informed by colleagues across the country who have shared successful ideas for promoting the development of expertise in students or novice practitioners. We include these boxes to inspire the thinking of all those charged with developing the professional values or clinical competencies of doctoral students in physical therapy.

THE MODEL OF EXPERTISE USED BY EDUCATORS

KNOWLEDGE: FROM PROCEDURAL TO PRACTICAL THROUGH REFLECTION

Through our research we have found that expert clinicians have mixed responses to their professional education as physical therapists. Some encountered teachers who became mentors and role models. Others believed that their academic classes did not prepare them to think like clinicians or think about patients in a useful manner; they deliberately had to reformulate everything they had learned to make it useful to them as clinicians. All valued learning throughout their lives, however, and all clearly identified that they needed to continue to learn. Assuming that entry-level education is not important to these practitioners is a mistake, however. In fact, it is the base on which the rest of their knowledge is built. It serves as the foundation for learning and practice. The real question is: What can be done in the educational process to facilitate the path from an entry-level education to expertise?

As in practice abilities, experts improved in their ability to learn throughout their careers in structured formal and clinical learning experiences. They described themselves as different learners than they were in their professional education programs. They have developed the metacognitive skills so necessary to monitor their own understandings and to transform procedural knowledge into practical knowledge (1).

Our data are supportive of the different assumptions on which professional education and graduate education are based. Students in postprofessional graduate education in physical therapy usually are learners with a rich contextual background on which to build a depth of knowledge that is the hallmark of graduate studies. Students in professional education programs are learning theoretical knowledge while building the contextual framework in which to use this knowledge. The strategies suggested to foster the development of expertise in this chapter can be structured along this continuum for DPT or tDPT learners. Especially for DPT learners, there is the need for education *for* practice to be rooted *in* practice. It must be taught around patient care by people who understand patient care and the relevance of scientific advancement. It must truly be *professional* education (2). Learners in tDPT programs will be more able to structure their learning experiences toward self-identified goals, and this should be expected of them.

Professional education for physical therapists today should facilitate the development of the kinds of self-directed learning skills that are spoken of by our experts, so that the transition from student to clinician will be smoother. Such self-directed segments of professional education may be considered to sacrifice breadth for depth in overall student learning. The educational community today continues to struggle with the question of generalist preparation of new graduates, characterized by value statements such as, "We can't let the students graduate without seeing this type of patient." Perhaps students can be given foundational knowledge that, coupled with strong discovery and analytical skills, will allow them to transfer basic patient clinical decisions safely from one patient diagnostic category to another. The study of expert practice does not solve this question for entry-level professional education, but clearly postprofessional education should allow for the development of specialized knowledge.

Does this investigation provide any insight into what to teach in professional education curricula? As in every field, the knowledge base necessary for the practice of physical therapy is increasing exponentially. The brief time spent in initial professional education must be planned wisely to maximize the ability of students to safely provide the best possible care to patients treated by new graduates. The experts provided little insight into what content knowledge to remove from the curriculum. Clearly only a fraction of available scientific knowledge can be included in DPT curricula, and we cannot account for the quantity of new knowledge that is formed daily. Instead, students should be helped to learn how to find knowledge, how to judge its usefulness to their practice, and how to embed it into their daily practice so that it becomes knowledge-in-action.

Knowledge is not only transmitted to students; students are also actively involved in constructing their evolving knowledge of physical therapy. They must learn to value a spectrum of sources of knowledge-in-action and build skills to tap reservoirs of knowledge to meet their needs for particular problems. The most valued source of knowledge to these experts was their patients, so students must build the skills necessary to learn from patients, to hear the patient's voice. Epstein describes this as mindfulness or being present and hearing your patient in a very specific, nonjudgmental way (3). He proposes five levels of mindful practice that range from denial and externalization, at the extreme level of mindless practice, to generalization, incorporation, and presence at the highest level of insightful and reflective practice. In our early work we observed distinct differences between novice and experienced clinicians in their ability to focus and listen to their patients in very busy clinical settings (4).

This is not to resurrect the old aphorism that encourages a young therapist simply to see each patient as an individual. Our experts have learned that they have a crucial partner in their work, the patient. They must listen hard; question clearly; know themselves; and, most important, value the perspective of the problem given to them by the patient. The skills physical therapy students must master to do this were also identified in a study of physicians by Dunn et al. (5). As compared with third-year medical students, experienced physicians could help

14

patients stay focused on their primary issues during the history, gather important information during the history while under time constraints, keep track of important information during the history without taking notes, evaluate the patient as a historian, and enlist family members as sources of knowledge. These focused communication skills can provide the physical therapist with a complete description of a patient's problem from the patient's perspective.

The experts valued their knowledge of teaching as one of their most important physical therapy interventions. All of the subjects had a deep understanding of the significant factors involved in changing health behaviors or in adjusting to a major change in functional ability. For many of the experts, the success of the total patient encounter depended on the ability to successfully teach patients and their families. They learned how to teach by pursuing postprofessional education and through trial and error in the clinic. Because teaching performance includes knowledge and skill components, professional curricula must address both types of learning activities.

A student's knowledge of the effective components of teaching and learning must be enhanced. Students must develop an understanding of the difficult process of changing health behaviors, perhaps through experiential learning. Box 14-2 identifies key knowledge assessment strategies to consider. Repeated exposure to patient education learning experiences that are focused on evaluation of the student's teaching performance must also be provided. Two potential attitudinal

---

BOX 14–2   *Knowledge Assessments in the Model of Expertise*

1. **Reflect**
   a. What types of knowledge do you value? What types do you avoid and why?
   b. What sources of knowledge might you consider in your patient evaluation?
   c. How would you rate your access to and ability to interpret knowledge for practice?
   d. Think of one example of a time when you transformed basic or procedural knowledge into clinical knowledge by reflection.
   e. During this clinical rotation, describe a time when you pursued additional knowledge and how you applied it to your patient.
   f. How are you planning on organizing your knowledge so that you can recall it efficiently?
   g. How will you use technology to help you master the volume of knowledge you wish to access?
   h. How is your knowledge of yourself? How have you changed the most since you began this program?
   i. What life lessons have affected your knowledge as a physical therapist?

(Continued)

BOX 14–2   *Knowledge Assessments in the Model of Expertise—Continued*

2. **Read**
   a. Develop skills in accessing literature using current technology.
   b. Develop skills in assessing literature for its applicability to specific clinical questions.

3. **Interview**
   a. Interview faculty and experienced clinicians about what type of knowledge is most valuable to them (which journals, web resources do they favor?).
   b. Interview faculty and experienced clinicians about how they organize their knowledge for practice and how technology can assist with access to important resources.

4. ***Record Performance (with proper permission)***
   a. Audio record your first patient history–taking episode, review it, and find examples of active listening and examples of missed opportunities to hear the patient's story.
   b. Video record a patient history with five patients who represent culturally different backgrounds. Review these records and look for evidence of your ability to acknowledge or uncover culturally significant beliefs of your patients for use in your care of them.
   c. Show students a video recording of an exceptionally insightful patient history or an exceptional interviewer to illustrate active listening and demonstration of the patient as an important source of knowledge.

5. ***Model/Practice***
   a. Tell a story in class about how you developed some tacit knowledge. Show a video record of yourself practicing with a client and answer learner questions such as, "Why did you do that?"
   b. Place students in the role of teacher for more novice students and then reflect on "how did you know that?"
   c. Use "think out loud" as a method to explain the knowledge you used in your evaluation of a patient to a student.

barriers to overcome with many entry-level students as they approach this content are as follows: 1) they believe that treating the patient is more important than teaching the patient, and 2) they believe that even as novices they are effective patient educators. Interviews with experienced clinicians can help instill an equal value for teaching and treating. Observation of skilled patient educators can help students understand the magnitude of changes that can be facilitated in their patients.

14

CLINICAL REASONING: ENHANCING COLLABORATION, RISK TAKING, AND PATIENT FOCUS

Students must learn the initial skills of clinical decision analysis and understand how to critically analyze their own treatment decisions. They must be willing and motivated to develop metacognitive skills and to examine their thought processes, and they must be able to constantly judge their outcomes. Efforts of the profession to define practice and the underlying educational requirements for practice have described physical therapists with increasingly high responsibilities for clinical decision making and clinical judgment. Our study supports this description of physical therapist practice and provides insight into the various types of clinical decisions required of physical therapists.

The curriculum must give students an accurate forecast of three types of clinical decisions: 1) diagnostic and prognostic determinations, 2) moment-by-moment intervention decisions, and 3) broad-based patient management decisions. Various types of clinical decisions must be practiced in classrooms and clinical settings. Expert practitioners must provide examples of their decision-making processes for students. Although the experts have significant amounts of tacit knowledge and know more than they can tell, they can tell enough about their decisions to begin to describe the processes for students. They can help students practice the techniques of problem identification and problem solving and can show students how to gather patient and family contextual data and use those data in clinical reasoning.

Professional education can be enhanced by a context-rich environment in each didactic class and by clinical education experiences guided by an experienced mentor. By being exposed to reflection in action in every class, students learn to risk thinking broadly about a problem and give voices to their hunches, without the penalty of providing an incorrect answer. If this process is used repeatedly, students can be better equipped to think on their feet in clinical settings. A clinical mentor can reinforce this pattern by thinking out loud with students as they solve patient problems. The clinical decision-making processes documented by our expert clinicians were uncovered by requiring such a process of the experts as they viewed their own performance on videotape. Box 14-3 shows many of the clinical reasoning assessments that should be considered for expert clinical decision making. The use of recorded performance and other strategies could provide a rich learning opportunity for students in clinical settings.

Proficiency in clinical decision making is a necessary component of expert practice in physical therapy. The link between proficient clinical decision making and specialty practice, although not tested in our study, appeared to be supported such that expert clinical decisions might not be expected from these subjects if they practiced outside of their specialty areas. The majority of professional educational programs continue to educate physical therapists for general practice. Without the ability to focus the professional education program into an area of practice, students at graduation cannot be expected to have proficiency in clinical decision making. This supports the importance of continued professional development efforts to the improvement of practice in physical therapy.

BOX 14–3 *Clinical Reasoning Assessments in the Model of Expertise*

1. **Reflect**
   a. What types of decisions do physical therapists make?
   b. What type of a decision maker are you at this point in your life?
   c. What types of decisions in physical therapy will you be/are you comfortable with? Which ones will/make you uncomfortable?
   d. How much of a risk taker are you in your personal life? With your patient's care?
   e. Draw a model of your typical clinical reasoning pattern.
   f. Think of a mistake you have made with a patient. Analyze what contributed to this mistake and predict the impact of your error.
   g. How often do you feel you are guessing in making diagnoses?
   h. Are there problematic patterns of behavior in your clinical reasoning, such as overestimating or underestimating patient potential?

2. **Read**
   a. Identify readings on clinical reasoning theory.
   b. Read examples of the clinical reasoning in use by OT, PT, Nursing, and Medicine.
   c. Read patient case reports that describe physical therapists' clinical decision making.

3. **Interview**
   a. Conduct a clinical reasoning interview with an experienced PT and a physician, using an interview guide.
   b. Ask an experienced clinician to discuss how his or her clinical reasoning has changed over time.
   c. Select a patient for telephone follow-up, several months after care has ceased, to further evaluate the clinical decisions you have made.

4. **Record Performance (with proper permission)**
   a. Review a video of your evaluation of a standardized patient and chart your clinical reasoning. Then view a video of an expert evaluating the same standardized patient and chart the clinical reasoning of the expert with this patient. Compare your paths to a diagnosis.
   b. Videotape two evaluations you perform with patients with similar initial complaints or referring diagnoses. Review the videos to chart your clinical reasoning path and compare the two experiences for similarities and differences.
   c. Watch a video of an expert clinician performing an evaluation with a difficult case and chart his or her clinical reasoning.

5. **Model/Practice**
   a. Use "thinking-out-loud" as a way to explain a specific aspect of your practice to a peer.
   b. Write a case report that documents your clinical reasoning that leads to a clinical decision.

14

MOVEMENT: TAKING PRACTICE SERIOUSLY

No one doubts the importance of movement to the practice of a physical therapist. The understanding of normal and abnormal movement comprises a large percentage of the knowledge covered in a typical physical therapy curriculum. The experts each displayed a depth of understanding of movement analysis in their patients, evidenced by data gleaned from visual and tactile inputs. Rose (6), an anthropologist teaching in a physical therapist educational program, gives this beautiful description of the psychomotor skills of the physical therapist:

> *The body becomes the physical therapist's instrument in several metaphoric senses of the word....first of all, the means by which physical therapists perform a technique, whether for diagnostic or treatment purposes...the body is the physical therapist's instrument: it is the primary means by which they get "good information" about a patient's condition—through feeling and seeing and listening to a patient's response.*

Our experts demonstrated an understanding of the movement capabilities of their own bodies and an ease of use of their bodies in patient interventions and teaching. Students should be encouraged to set their sights high when mastering psychomotor skills in physical therapy curricula. They should repeatedly watch the skilled, fluid movement of an expert clinician and his or her patient, observing closely the palpation techniques; the touch; the handling; the stabilizing; the facilitation; the support; and the simple, caring gestures. Opportunities to deconstruct with the skilled clinician the pattern of movements that are included in one treatment session can allow students to define the gaps between their fledgling movement skills and their personal goals. Novices require practice to perfect their movement skills; patients again are excellent teachers for therapists. Intimate access to a patient's body is a gift that is offered to therapists from which they are obliged to learn and improve. Box 14-4 illustrates movement assessment items for academic and clinical educators to consider.

VIRTUE: SELF-KNOWLEDGE AND SELF-IMPROVEMENT

The experts are uniquely virtuous practitioners. Their personal characteristics added to all dimensions of their clinical practices and, most important, enabled them to act as moral agents for their patients. The values of honesty, integrity, compassion, and determination provided the experts foundations on which to build pillars of ethical practice. When faced with ethical dilemmas, they recognized the ethical components of each situation and possessed courage to act in highly ethical manners. Their nonjudgmental approach to their patients enhanced their effectiveness with a wide variety of patients. Their stories serve as excellent teaching tools because students can reflect and test their personal determination against the model of ethical action.

The personal characteristics of these experts are not unlike those qualities that professional program admissions committees use to screen applicants to physical therapy programs. If students are admitted with these virtues, is any place available in the curriculum to foster the deepening or testing of a student's personal

BOX 14–4   *Movement Assessments in the Model of Expertise*

1. **Reflect**
   a. How do you use your body in achieving patient goals?
   b. How fluid is your movement?
   c. How much do you trust what your touch tells you as compared with your eyes? Ears?
   d. What is your best movement skill as a physical therapist? Who taught you this?
   e. Are there movements or positions required of you that remain awkward for you?
   f. What movement patterns in patients are the most difficult for you to evaluate?

2. **Read**
   a. Review reading on acquisition of motor skill and motor learning.
   b. Read current literature on motion analysis techniques used in laboratories.

3. **Interview**
   a. Review development of skills with physical therapy colleagues.
   b. Discuss the role of movement in practice with an occupational therapist.

4. **Record Performance (with proper permission)**
   a. Video record the learner's performance of an intervention with a patient in each year of education. Review and write a reflective paper comparing the aspects of their movement.
   b. View a video recording of patient movement and identify abnormal movement. Increase the difficulty of the stimulus and reduce the time or repetitions available for the task.
   c. Watch a video recording of expert clinician performance and critique with learners.
   d. Use new performance recording technology (telephones, personal digital assistants, iPods) to increase opportunities for viewing practice.

5. **Model/Practice**
   a. Provide peer-to-peer opportunities to practice new skills and to provide feedback.
   b. Describe a patient movement pattern using contemporary motion analysis terminology.
   c. Share a case report of a patient in which you compare the link between the impairments in movement and functional abilities.

14

values structure? Some might argue that the professional education experience is losing sight of the importance of values education in the values-neutral climate into which higher education has drifted. Much could be gained by including learning experiences that could strengthen students' senses of themselves as moral practitioners. The stories of these experts provide examples of attaining such virtues and how these values can grow and change when actively practiced.

Is moral action and agency a professional competency that should be expected of doctorally prepared physical therapists? Several authors would agree that it is (7,8). Jensen (9) describes the use of standardized patients as a means to provide learners with questions and performance feedback as they identify central ethical issues during an interview. Davis (10) recommends documenting one's own moral history as a means to move learners from positions of self-interest to positions of the patient's best interest and reading examples of moral courage to instill a sense of moral agency in professional physical therapists. Eight additional physical and occupational therapist authors expose strategies for ethics education that are appropriate for entry-level students and tDPT students (8). A summary of strategies for virtue assessment are described in Box 14-5.

A Philosophy of Practice: Integrating the Elements of Professional Expertise

Most notable among the findings of this investigation of expert practice in physical therapy is the presence of philosophies of practice. What is this concept, philosophy of practice, and is it taught in our current curricula? Unique philosophies of practice were held by experts within each specialty area we studied, composed of the assumptions that informed their clinical judgment and their personally defined roles. How can young physical therapists be taught to develop a philosophy of practice? Two clear elements emerge from the research to date: 1) students must be challenged to develop a deep sense of self-knowledge and 2) there should be a definable role as a physical therapist.

Students in doctoral education must be challenged to use the educational experience to learn more about themselves as thinking, feeling health care practitioners. Self-knowledge was important to our experts and was an integral part of the values that could be observed in all their patient interactions. Epstein has encouraged self-awareness as a key component of professional development and excellent practice for physicians (3). Professional learning is not only a process of change for the individual but also serves as their enculturation process into the profession. If they are successful in establishing their professional identity, the entire profession will benefit. If students in doctoral education do not value self-reflection or believe themselves to be fully mature professionals, they likely will miss many opportunities to grow along the path to expertise. Physical therapist students are admitted to professional education at a similar age as are medical students, but they perhaps do not encounter as many life-critical episodes with patients as do medical students. Such episodes are more difficult to ignore as stimuli for self-reflection about one's role with patients, and so more purposeful educational experiences may be necessary to foster the type of self-reflection skills that will serve the physical therapist well throughout a career.

BOX 14–5 | *Virtue Assessments in the Model of Expertise*

1. **Reflect**
   a. What are your personal values?
   b. What are your professional values?
   c. Where are your personal and professional values in conflict?
   d. Do your behaviors reflect your values? When and where?
   e. What is the clinical situation that will most significantly test your values as a physical therapist?
   f. What will you consider a sacrifice for your profession? What sacrifices will you make and which won't you make?

2. **Read**
   a. Review readings on ethics, virtuous practice, and moral courage.
   b. Discuss readings with ethicists and other members of the health care team.

3. **Interview**
   a. Conduct an interview with a virtuous practitioner using an interview guide to extract examples of moral courage observed or performed.
   b. Interview an expert practitioner about the APTA Core Values of the profession.
   c. Interview a member of your state licensure committee or chapter ethics committee and discuss the nature of whistle blowing in physical therapy.

4. **Model/Practice**
   a. Develop and discuss a case study that illustrates virtuous practice.
   b. Distinguish virtuous practice from merely ethical practice.
   c. Reward virtuous actions among learners through the development of awards, bulletin boards, or peer acknowledgements.

Panel discussions with skilled reflective practitioners, writing assignments and the use of narratives (11), and interviews can be used to facilitate a student's growth in self-awareness. Another recommendation is purposeful reflection on one clinical incident over time, documenting the meaning learned from the incident with each new period of reflection. The facts of the incident remain consistent, whereas the meaning attached to the facts change as the practitioner changes. Classroom and clinical instructors can share their journey in discussion with students, using revealing questions, such as, Who am I becoming as a physical therapist? Who is responsible for patient outcomes? Who controls my encounters with my patients? In what ways ought physical therapy enhance the quality of life of patients?

The experts in this study have all developed an expansive sense of their roles with patients and their families, enabled by their conception of physical therapy. They are the most remarkable patient advocates—roles they never dreamed of

14

playing during their professional education. The expansive role statement is developed over time with the accumulation of knowledge and the confidence to take risks in defining who they will be with their patients. As can be seen in the Postscript on our experts, this expansion of their roles continues and experts are the ones among us who push themselves to do and be more for their patients. Experts are those who help us believe that our vision for our profession can be realized.

For doctoral students to understand this expectation of developing a role that they wish to play in health care, they must hear and discuss this concept with experienced practitioners. They must work to see differences in roles adopted by various physical therapists and use these observations to inform their current or hoped-for role. The conscientious pursuit of a professional identity will facilitate the transfer from learner to practitioner or from novice to expert practitioner. Rose comments:

> *Competence and identity—the concept of practice recognizes that the acquisition of knowledge or skill is part of the construction of an identity or a person. As expertise develops, it brings with it a socialization into the traditions and values of a community of practice, beliefs about self, an orientation toward the world, a sense of possibility (6).*

The use of case studies and practitioner biographies may help students learn about different practitioner's sense of their roles and use this in developing a philosophy of practice. The expert's knowledge of the health care system allows her to provide many services to her patients, but it is her philosophy of practice that incorporates her personal values, and virtues, and will enable her to persist when the going is difficult.

Exposing students to practitioners who profess distinctly different philosophies of practice can help to demonstrate how a philosophy of practice influences all clinical decisions. It also can encourage students to formulate philosophies and reflect on how they will be formed by external health care influences and internal values and desires for patients. A novice practitioner may feel ill equipped to face the difficult ethical, legal, and fiscal challenges to his or her clinical judgments without having developed the internal "barometer" on which experts rely.

CONCLUSION

Countless numbers of professionals bear the responsibility of educating and socializing new physical therapists. The potential for positive interactions is tremendous, but how should these encounters be structured? Although much is known about best educational practice for teaching procedural knowledge, less is known about how best to set new entrants on the path toward expertise and nurture their motivation for excellence. We hope the strategies shared in this chapter will prove a valuable resource for all our colleagues in all disciplines who contribute their energies to the teaching and mentoring of physical therapists.

REFERENCES

1. Higgs J, Jones M. Clinical reasoning in the health professions. In J Higgs, M Jones (eds). *Clinical reasoning in the health professions.* Boston: Butterworth–Heinemann; 2000.
2. Schon D. *The reflective practitioner: how professionals think in action.* New York: Basic Books; 1983.

3. Epstein R. Mindful practice. *JAMA*. 1999;282(9):833–839.

4. Jensen G, Shepard KF, Gwyer J, Hack LM. Attribute dimensions that distinguish master and novice physical therapy clinicians in orthopedic settings. *Phys Ther*. 1992;72:711–722.

5. Dunn T, Taylor C, Lipsky M. An investigation of physician knowledge-in-action. *Teaching Learning Med*. 1996;8(2):90–97.

6. Rose M. Our hands will know: the development of tactile diagnostic skill-teaching, learning and situated cognition in a physical therapy program. *Anthro Educ*. 1999;30(2):1330–1160.

7. Huddle T. Teaching professionalism: is medical morality a competency? *Acad Med*. 2005;80(10):885–891.

8. Purtilo R, Jensen G, Royeen C (eds). *Education for moral action: a sourcebook in health and rehabilitation ethics*. Philadelphia: FA Davis; 2005.

9. Jensen G. Mindfulness: Applications for teaching and learning in ethics education. In R Purtilo, G Jensen, C Royeen (eds). *Educating for moral action: a sourcebook in health and rehabilitation ethics*. Philadelphia: F.A. Davis, 2005.

10. Davis C. Educating adult health professionals for moral action: in search of moral courage. In R, Purtilo G, Jensen C Royeen (eds). *Educating for moral action: a sourcebook in health and rehabilitation ethics*. Philadelphia: F.A. Davis; 2005.

11. Hatem D, Rider E. Sharing stories: narrative medicine in an evidence-based world. *Pat Educ Counsel*. 2004;54:251–253.

14

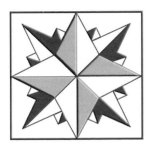

15 Implications for Practice and Professional Development

PRACTICE AND PROFESSIONAL DEVELOPMENT

Although our work has many implications for future research on expertise (Chapter 13) and for education of physical therapists (Chapter 14), it is in reflecting on practice that our work particularly resonates. We have certainly had this confirmed in our many conversations with clinicians about our work. The descriptions from our experts that show all that practice can be have provided us a rich opportunity for discovering ways to improve practice for all of us. Those interested in our work in the clinical community serve in administrative and in direct patient care roles. It appears that all physical therapists are concerned about both their own professional development and that of others—including those they supervise, manage, or teach or those who are peers and colleagues in other disciplines. This chapter holds useful ideas for individual clinicians who are guiding their own professional development, managers, and clinical specialists who teach in residency or fellowship programs of professional development.

We have identified some specific strategies that can be used in any practice setting to help encourage the development of expertise in all clinicians (Box 15-1). Throughout the chapter we offer some specific suggestions about ways to encourage the development of expertise in practice. Many of these suggestions are similar to those provided in Chapter 14 for development of students, with the important addition of peers across many disciplines as part of the development process.

From our expert clinicians, we have learned that physical therapy practice is the following:

■ Patient centered
■ Complex
■ Broadly based
■ Exciting

Most of us have experienced these positive feelings about our practice, although perhaps not as often as we might like. All clinicians, even our experts, sometimes find aspects of their work boring, uninteresting, or overly challenging. For the most part, however, our subjects love what they do. What makes them different from those of us who feel these more negative aspects more often? Or from the occasional young graduate who says, "Why did I waste all that money on school to be doing this?" Or from the reluctant clinician we have all encountered who has practiced for 15–20 years and says, "I'm tired of seeing the

BOX 15–1

Strategies to Be Used in Clinical Practice Experiences

Reflect: proactive questions for discussion
Read: literature that explores the elements of expertise and answers clinical questions
Interview: peers across disciplines during collaborative patient care
Recorded performance: audio or visual stimulus for reflection
Model/practice: mentorship and professional development programs

same problems every day. If you've seen one back, you've seen them all!" Although answers to these differences sometimes lie in the therapists themselves, we can find many opportunities to encourage positive practice by structuring the environments in which we work.

KNOWLEDGE

Expert clinicians possess a thirst for knowledge and are able to put this knowledge to work in direct patient care. These clinicians seem to have been in the "right place at the right time" because they have met educational mentors and had opportunities to work with expert clinicians and specific patient populations. This is not mere coincidence, however. These clinicians have made specific career choices. When they could not find colleagues to help them grow and develop, they moved on in search of more. As we have learned from our clinicians, knowledge is not learned solely, or even primarily, in the structured lectures of didactic education. Certainly, more formal education provides a base, but the knowledge our subjects best recalled was learned by practice—the doing of the craft of physical therapy with patients in the presence of other clinicians who helped guide their thinking and taught them to refine their clinical decision making.

Our practice environments must find mechanisms to provide what has become perhaps the scarcest resource of all—time. Therapists need time with their patients, time with their colleagues, time for reflection, and time to return to the literature if they are to develop what is called knowledge in practice that results from becoming better clinicians (1). Our subjects found this time in a variety of ways. One mechanism they used was to become busy people—to make time in their days to accomplish many things. They also worked efficiently, managing more than one task at a time.

It seems unrealistic, even unhealthy, however, to expect every therapist to carry an increased desire for more time for professional activities as a personal responsibility. Instead, ways to support effective use of time within practices must be found. Managers should value time for learning as a necessary part of practice. Just as physicians are expected to participate in rounds, review the literature, and serve as clinical mentors for physicians-in-training, physical therapists must have this expectation. Mentoring colleagues, serving as clinical instructors, and interacting in interdisciplinary discussions help therapists providing instruction and the therapists receiving the instruction increase their knowledge. Managers have many options to support such activities. Formal mentorship programs can be established to bring therapists together. Journal clubs, in-service presentations, and grand rounds, especially those built on the principles of evidence-based practice (EBP), are activities that offer opportunities to learn within the context of practice. Many of our subjects reported participating in these activities throughout their professional lives in a wide variety of settings.

Many clinicians have chosen a particular form of professional development, specialization, to help themselves improve their knowledge about patient care. We refer here to formal specialization, recognized by certification, such as those sponsored by the American Board of Physical Therapy Specialties (ABPTS). Other programs exist for manual therapists, hand therapists, and other areas of practice. The preparation for the ABPTS specialist examination requires the therapist to spend a certain amount of time in reflective clinical practice. The examination itself is based on skills identified as necessary for advanced practice clinicians in the clinical setting.

Many clinical sites have developed formal programs to assist in this acquisition of knowledge in clinical practice. These generally take the form of residencies, which usually are designed to lead to recognition as a Board-certified specialist, and fellowships, which usually are designed for more in-depth study in a specialty or subspecialty. One of the salient features of these types of programs is that they are based in the practice setting, thereby capitalizing on patients and colleagues as the major sources of knowledge.

Patients are a primary source of knowledge, so time must be made to learn from them. The time allocated for examination must be sufficient to allow accurate data collection, and the time allocated for intervention must be sufficient to allow evaluation of the success of the intervention. The treatment time must not be the only thing considered; therapists need time to review collected data, integrate their findings with the knowledge gathered from the literature and colleagues, and document their activities clearly. Again, managers must make choices that allow this to occur. There must be recognition that all of these activities constitute legitimate uses of a therapist's time. The idea of so-called billable time—that is, only the time spent in face-to-face interaction with the patient—as the only acceptable time spent must be abandoned. Physicians have found many ways to improve their efficiency while maintaining time for reflection. Many ways can be found to improve efficiency in documentation without reducing it to repetitive phrases. Dictation and the use of scribes are two means by which the quality of documentation can be preserved with reduced practitioner time. Our subjects did not offer many complaints about the burden of documentation but seemed to recognize the importance of spending time in accurately detailing care.

One of the ways not used as a mechanism to gain time was the delegation of activities to physical therapist assistants (PTAs) or other technical workers. The concept of a PTA was developed as a mechanism for improving the efficiency of physical therapists in their practices (2). Certainly, increased delegation to PTAs is frequently offered as an answer to the ever-increasing press from managed care. Why, therefore, did we not see a wise and judicious use of PTAs in the practices of our expert clinicians? Because we had no observations of this behavior and our original study focus was not on the concept of delegation, we did not discuss the issue of delegation with our subjects. In retrospect, this would have indeed been an enlightening discussion. Because delegation plays such an important role in practice, future research should be done to explore this issue. The absence of any PTAs, however, is certainly food for thought. Aides were used in the practices we visited, and we observed that our subjects interacted with these aides. These observations were made after we completed our original work, but the issue of the role of the PTA in the practice of the physical therapist has not yet reached any higher degree of consensus. It remains to be understood if and how PTAs contribute to the practice of expert physical therapists.

The plea for more time may initially seem naive and unrealistic in an ever-tightening health care market. Ignoring the need for adequate time to develop sound knowledge in practice, however, is shortsighted and defeating. Physical therapists, like other health care practitioners, have responsibilities on at least

15

three levels. First, they are responsible for individual patients. Second, they have responsibility for groups of patients. Whether by writing practice policies or actually having a financial risk in providing care for a group of patients over time, more and more therapists should apply knowledge gained from one patient to the decisions made for many. Certainly, efficiency in decision making only improves as we are able to apply knowledge from one patient to other, similar patients. Third, therapists have a responsibility to improve the health care system to assure that future patients receive the best care possible. This responsibility can take the form of critical inquiry, research, or advocacy.

These three levels of responsibility can only be met when time and opportunity exist to develop knowledge deeply rooted in practice. These abilities are not and cannot be fully formed in the initial education for practice; they are developed over time. If therapists do not assume these responsibilities, society can rightly question the necessity of physical therapy for maintaining and acquiring good health. By finding ways to ensure that time is available to address all responsibilities, we can provide the opportunity for physical therapy to continue its development as an integral part of the health care system.

We encourage managers and therapists to provide as many opportunities for reflection as possible. Box 15-2 identifies strategies that can be used across practice settings to aid in this activity. They are written as behaviors for the individual therapist; practice managers will also see immediate application to their professional development programs.

| BOX 15–2 | *Strategies for Increasing the Knowledge Dimension in Practicing Clinicians* |

1. **Reflect**
   a. What types of knowledge do you value? What types do you avoid and why?
   b. What sources of knowledge do you use in making your clinical decisions?
   c. How would you rate your access to and ability to interpret knowledge for practice?
   d. Think of one example of a time when you transformed basic or procedural knowledge into clinical knowledge by reflection.
   e. Describe a time when you pursued additional knowledge and how you applied it to your patient.
   f. How do you organize your knowledge so that you can recall it efficiently?
   g. How do you use technology to help you master the volume of knowledge you wish to access?
   h. How is your knowledge of yourself? How have you changed the most since you began practice?

(Continued)

BOX 15–2	*Strategies for Increasing the Knowledge Dimension in Practicing Clinicians—Continued*

    i. What life lessons have affected your knowledge as a health care provider?

    j. What knowledge would have helped you prevent a practice error?

2. Read

    a. Develop skills in accessing literature using current technology.

    b. Develop skills in assessing literature for its applicability to specific clinical questions.

    c. Read and discuss with peers a variety of literature that encompasses not only clinical practice, but also includes basic science, theory development, and health care delivery.

3. Interview

    a. Ask peers across disciplines how they organize their knowledge and use technology to help them master the volume of applicable knowledge.

    b. Ask information specialists how to use technology to help organize the volume of applicable knowledge in a way that supports clinical care.

4. Recording Performance (with proper permission)

    a. Audio record a patient history–taking episode, review it, and find examples of active listening and examples of missed opportunities to hear the patient's story.

    b. Video record a patient history with five patients who represent culturally different backgrounds. Review these records and look for evidence of your ability to acknowledge or uncover culturally significant beliefs of your patients for use in your care of them.

    c. Show students a video record of an exceptionally insightful patient history or an exceptional interviewer to illustrate active listening and demonstration of the patient as an important source of knowledge.

5. Model/Practice

    a. Use "thinking out loud" as a way to explain a specific aspect of your practice to a peer or a student.

    b. Exchange peer assessments with a colleague to identify ways to improve access to the literature needed to improve care.

    c. Design your own knowledge self-assessments ("quizzes") on clinical topics useful in your practice to use in mentoring peers or supervising students.

CLINICAL REASONING

Our therapists demonstrated complex clinical reasoning. They understood that patients are the center of clinical decision-making processes but highly respected the need to examine other sources of knowledge (e.g., the literature, teachers, mentors, colleagues) in making decisions. They also demonstrated an ability to make decisions quickly based on the data they had gathered from these many sources, a flexibility in revisiting their decisions when new data demonstrated a need for change, and a tenacity when acting as advocates for decisions they knew to be right.

How can a novice clinician move to this level of clinical reasoning? How can experienced but less than expert therapists move to this level of clinical reasoning? One of the lessons we have learned is deeply rooted in the expert therapists' conception of practice. For them, practice was not simply doing something to a patient in a given moment. It was contextual and continual over the entire time that a specific patient needed the therapist's attention and thought and across the patient's full range of needs. These experts recognized the links between pathology, impairments, and function and the need to think across the patient's life span, whether they were explicitly aware of articulated disablement models or not.

As discussed, these therapists also did not contemplate only one patient at a time. They were cognizant of their surroundings and aware of other patients' and colleagues' needs, yet they were not distracted by them. They were able to remain focused on the patient with whom they were working, while also balancing the needs of their environment.

At any point, the expert clinician gathers data from a specific patient, recalling pertinent information from the databank of previous cases as they applied to this patient, adding this patient's information to that databank, and recognizing the implications of the collective information for good policy. This databank is sometimes formal and documented, but most often it is an integral part of the therapist's cognition. The therapist is able to take the bits and pieces, the various data items, and store them in a way that allows a contextual understanding, most often related to the patient's function.

Identifying trends in the delivery of physical therapy services that seriously detract from the ability of a therapist to learn to practice expertly is relatively easy. For example, if the role of a physical therapist is considered entirely as a person who performs an initial examination of a patient, designs a plan of care, and turns the patient over to another provider, the therapist is denied the opportunity to learn about ongoing changes that occur in the patient as a result of the interventions provided. Doing this blocks the ability to understand fully the accuracy of prognoses. The role of the practitioner as an evaluator of the patient's progress is eliminated. As discussed in the following section, examinations and interventions are about movement. If the qualitative changes in movement that result from our interventions are not observed, building a databank and learning from patients cannot occur.

Similarly, if delivery is structured such that no continuity of care is provided, the therapist's ability to develop sound clinical reasoning is seriously truncated (3). This takes many forms in clinical environments: assigning therapists on a "first come, first served" basis, assigning outpatients certain days to be seen without specific appointment times, or arranging for weekend and evening coverage without providing adequate documentation on the patient's progress. All of these indicate the absence of continuity of care. Perhaps one of the most blatant examples of this is placing therapists on a per-hour call basis. In this form of organization, therapists are called in each day for the number of hours needed for the specific number of patient visits scheduled that day. Although this is tempting because of the obvious short-term economic implications, it completely negates the concept of a physical therapy practice. Certainly neither the patient nor the therapist has any assurance of continuity. In fact, they can be almost certainly assured that no opportunity will be provided for the reflective clinical reasoning that was displayed by the expert therapists.

If these negative methods of organizing services can be identified, however, more positive ones can also be described. Clinical environments that encourage access to varied sources of knowledge are good examples. Grand rounds journal clubs, access to on-line search engines and databases, and in-service programs are all ways to give therapists access to the literature. The program for development and recognition of clinical competence described in Chapter 12 is an example of a program that encourages clinicians to reflect on their clinical reasoning. Support of continuing education, in all of its forms, is another. The learning component most desired by clinicians and most strongly emphasized by our therapists, however, is the opportunity to interact regularly with other clinicians who are also questioning and reflecting. Time should be found in a clinical day to interact with other therapists. This discourse takes many forms: one-to-one conversations, group discussions, reviewing documentation, or using electronic media and communication. Whatever the form, the ability to have this discourse returns again to the use of time, the most valuable of commodities.

If reduced cost is a primary goal of the health care system, even of American society, why should resources be spent to achieve a system for delivery of services that allows for development of clinical reasoning? First, because the optimum intervention for every patient encountered is not known, this clinical reasoning should be developed to provide optimal interventions. Our research should be grounded in clinical reasoning that understands individual patients and their relationship to similar patients. Without this grounding, research exists in a vacuum, and without research, the efficacy of our care cannot be improved. Reducing costs by providing a certain intervention in a certain way is useless unless a particular intervention is known to be right for a specific patient. Efficiency matters little if efficacy is not provided. Short-term cost reductions may actually result in long-term cost increases as mistakes made in the name of expediency are discovered. As Edwards and Jones support in Chapter 10, experts who use sound clinical reasoning are the primary sources for the right questions that should be asked to best understand the long-term implications of physical therapy care.

A second reason that society might care about improving the opportunity for sound clinical reasoning is that optimum interventions may depend heavily on the knowledge in practice that the expert therapists displayed. Indeed, if patients are the primary sources of data, each time a new therapist approaches a patient, a new database should be built. That database can never be sufficiently complete if it includes only occasional, or even single, contact with the patient. Much of this is true for many professions in health care, but it becomes more essential in the management of chronic problems. Can a plan be developed for a lifetime of care for a child with profound disability based on one discussion with that child and his or her parents? Can a decision be made about the need for nursing home intervention because of functional loss made on the basis of data gathered at only one point in time? Can a rehabilitation admission be denied for a person with a head injury based on one examination of that patient? Can a manual therapist effectively make an intervention based on data gathered by putting hands to the patient's joint only one time? Such things can be considered because they occur in today's health care system. The expert therapists, however, remind us that these are all decisions that improve by having multiple data points. Only a reflective therapist who has developed craft knowledge can put a patient into the context needed to make good decisions.

Box 15-3 offers strategies that clinicians and managers can use across clinical settings to help expand this dimension of expertise. They are written as behaviors for the individual therapist; practice managers will also see immediate application to their professional development programs.

BOX 15–3

Strategies for Increasing the Clinical Reasoning Dimension in Practicing Clinicians

1. **Reflect**
   a. What types of decisions do physical therapists make?
   b. What type of a decision maker are you at this point in your life?
   c. What types of decisions in physical therapy are you comfortable with? Which ones make you uncomfortable?
   d. How much of a risk taker are you in your personal life? With your patient's care?
   e. Draw a model of your typical clinical reasoning pattern.
   f. Think of a mistake you have made with a patient. Analyze what contributed to this mistake and predict the impact of your error.
   g. How often do you feel you are guessing in making diagnoses?
   h. Are there problematic patterns of behavior in your clinical reasoning, such as overestimating or underestimating patient potential?

2. **Read**
   a. Identify readings on clinical reasoning theory across disciplines.
   b. Read examples of clinical reasoning across multiple disciplines.
   c. Read patient case reports that describe physical therapists' clinical decision making.

3. **Interview**
   a. Ask experienced clinicians from physical therapy and other disciplines to discuss how their clinical reasoning has changed over their experience.

(Continued)

BOX 15–3	*Strategies for Increasing the Clinical Reasoning Dimension in Practicing Clinicians—Continued*

    b. Select a patient for telephone follow-up, several months after care has ceased, to further evaluate the clinical decisions you have made.

4. *Recording Performances (with proper permission)*

    a. Review a video of an evaluation of a standardized patient, and chart your clinical reasoning. Then view the model video and chart the clinical reasoning of the expert with this patient. Compare your paths to a diagnosis.

    b. Videotape two evaluations you perform with patients with similar initial complaints or referring diagnoses. Review the videos to chart your clinical reasoning path and compare the two experiences for similarities and differences.

    c. Watch a video of an expert clinician performing an evaluation with a difficult case and chart their clinical reasoning.

5. *Model/Practice*

    a. Use "thinking out loud" as a way to explain a specific aspect of your practice to a peer or a student.

    b. Share a case report with peers that documents the clinical reasoning that led to specific clinical decisions.

MOVEMENT

Because the use of movement by physical therapists is intrinsic to their practices, it might be overlooked in thinking about them as experts. That would be a great loss, however, because the beauty seen in their use of movement also would be overlooked. Our therapists used movement naturally and seamlessly in their interactions with patients. It was also woven into their clinical reasoning because they used data gathered from observing and feeling their patients move as primary sources of their knowledge. They also used their own movement in guiding patients. The illustrations of specific cases, which were taken from videotapes of the therapists interacting with patients, provide at least a small indication of the fluidity and naturalness of the movement of these therapists.

    The ability to perform in such a beautiful manner is not the skill of a novice. It takes deliberate, focused, and intense practice (4). Practice is used here in several senses. Therapists should engage in repetition of a specific skill to gain motor control, as in "I should practice my manual muscle testing positions." Therapists also should incorporate the use of their own movement and the

15

patient's movement into their conception of the practice of physical therapy, as in "The practice of physical therapy is based on movement analysis."

We should ensure that clinical environments provide opportunities for both sorts of practice. Because we cannot become skilled clinicians without learning by doing, time should be allotted for practice to occur. Therapists also should have access to more skilled clinicians to mentor this psychomotor development. This is especially important because movement often can place patients at risk. Asking a patient to progress a little more, walk a little faster or farther, or lift more weight more often places the patient at risk. If the physiologic and anatomic status of the patient has been misjudged, these requests can result in cardiopulmonary incidents, fracture, muscle strain, skin lesions, or worse.

As to the development of physical therapy as a practice that uniquely uses movement, watching the more recent developments in the definition of physical therapy that have relied less and less on the adjunctive modalities and more and more on descriptions of the movement activities with which therapists engage patients has been heartening. Movement has been characterized as its own system, which has a physiologic and anatomic basis and crosses many organ systems of the body (5). Certainly, the experts in this study reinforce this concept of practice. Box 15-4 offers suggestions for managers and clinicians to develop this often hidden, but vital, dimension of practice.

VIRTUE

One of the most obvious things about the therapists studied is that they are good people. They demonstrate strong values, including commitment to others and a passion for excellence. As mentioned before, they would bring this goodness to any occupation. Yet, there are many ways that they display these characteristics specifically in physical therapy. They are advocates ensuring that patients receive adequate care, they demonstrate professional generosity to their colleagues and patients (always providing extra time), and they display compassion and empathy. These experts clearly displayed the virtue of moral courage—that is, they were aware of the need to act morally and they took that action, despite the presence of some risk for themselves (6,7).

These are personal values that the therapists bring with them to their practices. What can be done, then, to help move more therapists to this level of care? Perhaps the most important thing to learn from these therapists is to set high standards for other therapists. When lesser behavior is observed in colleagues, it must not be tolerated. A cultural norm that requires advocacy, generosity, and compassion can be established. People's personal values cannot be changed, but their behavior can be altered, or they can be made to feel so uncomfortable that they choose to leave.

Although this is certainly an extreme, small examples of unacceptable behavior occur each day. Use of language that demeans patients, refusal to help a colleague, and shoddy workmanship in documentation diminish the practice of physical therapy and reflect a meanness of spirit that is quite the opposite from that of the expert therapists.

Glaser has discussed the three realms of ethics, especially as applied to health care (8). He describes these as the realm of the individual, the realm of

BOX 15–4

Strategies for Increasing the Movement Assessments in the Model of Expertise

1. **Reflect**
   a. How do you use your body in achieving patient goals?
   b. How fluidly do you feel movement?
   c. How much do you trust what your touch tells you as compared with your eyes? Ears?
   d. What is your best movement skill as a physical therapist? Who taught you this?
   e. Are there movements or positions required of you that remain awkward for you?
   f. What movement patterns in patients are the most difficult for you to evaluate?

2. **Read**
   a. Review reading on acquisition of motor skill and motor learning.
   b. Review current literature on motion analysis techniques and findings.

3. **Interview**
   a. Review development of skill with physical therapy colleagues.
   b. Discuss role of movement in practice with peers from other disciplines.

4. **Record Performance (with proper permission)**
   a. Video record your performance of an intervention with a patient as you develop more skill with a new technique. Review and think reflectively about changes in your movement over time.
   b. View video records of patient movements and identify abnormal movement.
   c. Watch videos records of expert clinician performance and critique with peers.
   d. Use new performance recording technology (telephones, personal digital assistants, iPods) to increase opportunities for viewing practice.

5. **Model/Practice**
   a. Provide peer-to-peer opportunities to practice new skills and to provide feedback.
   b. Describe a patient's movement patterns using contemporary motion analysis terminology.
   c. Share a case report with peers describing the links between a patient's impairment in movement with the patient's functional abilities.

the institution, and the realm of society. He goes on to describe the interconnection between these three realms. Each exists in relationship to the other, and actions within each realm must be understood to fully comprehend an ethical situation, especially in the area of health care. An individual's actions are colored by the decisions made at the institutional level, which is in turn colored by the decisions made at the societal environment. Certainly, individual actions also affect institutional actions and institutional actions affect societal actions. This model makes clear that we need to understand the impact each realm has on the other. It may be that the institutional imperative (the ethical choices made in the institutional realm) can lead to these reflexive behaviors that are a response to external pressures and that are disconnected from espoused ethical beliefs (9).

On a more positive note, those who demonstrate virtuous characteristics can be rewarded. This responsibility for censure and reward lies most heavily on those in leadership positions. Whether this leadership arises from an organizational position (being the "boss") or from personal power and characteristics, the expert therapists have demonstrated the great benefits of positive traits. One other finding from our study must be remembered—these therapists love their work because they are routinely challenged by the problems they encounter in practice. Box 15-5 offers ideas for helping to develop this most elusive of the qualities displayed by our expert practitioners. They are written as behaviors for the individual therapist; practice managers will also see immediate application to their professional development programs.

PHILOSOPHY OF PRACTICE

We have described the work of many experts from many different perspectives in Chapters 4–7 and in Chapters 9–12. A consistent finding, across all settings and all research approaches, is that these therapists had a unifying philosophy of their practice. Their choices about practice were "of a whole." This cohesiveness means that development of each of the four dimensions of expertise strengthens the whole, just as solidifying the philosophy augments each of the dimensions.

The philosophy of practice transcends particular patient types and settings, but it is difficult to imagine how a new therapist develops a cohesive philosophy without some stability in his or her practice. If a therapist is constantly rotated to new services before basic knowledge can be gained, then no higher-level skills will be developed. One of the strengths of the profession of physical therapy is the variety of patients and settings available for practice. Most of the therapists in our study have treated a variety of patients and many continue to do so, but they have recognized the end for a deep understanding of patient care for all of these patients.

Each of the strategies offered for the four separate practice dimensions can help therapists develop a cohesive practice philosophy. In addition, we suggest that therapists routinely ask themselves these questions:

■ Who am I becoming, or how am I changing as a physical therapist?
■ What do I expect of myself in regard to my patient's outcomes?
■ Who is in control of my encounters with my patient?
■ In what ways ought physical therapy care enhance the life of my patient?

BOX 15–5

Strategies for Increasing the Virtue Assessments in the Model of Expertise

1. **Reflect**
   a. What are your personal values?
   b. What are your professional values?
   c. Where are your personal and professional values in conflict?
   d. Do your behaviors reflect your values? When and where?
   e. What clinical situations most significantly test your values as a physical therapist?
   f. What sacrifices have you made for your profession? What sacrifices will you make and which won't you make?

2. **Reading**
   a. Review reading on ethics, virtuous practice, and moral courage.
   b. Discuss readings with ethicists and other clinicians across disciplines.

3. **Interview**
   a. Conduct an interview with a virtuous practitioner to discuss examples of moral courage observed or performed.
   b. Interview an expert practitioner about the American Physical Therapy Association's stated Core Values.
   c. Interview a member of your state licensure board or Chapter Ethics Committee to discuss the nature of whistle blowing in physical therapy.

4. **Model/Practice**
   a. Identify with colleagues strategies to work collaboratively to take action that supports ethical patient care.
   b. Discuss a case study that illustrates virtuous practice.
   c. Distinguish moral courage from merely ethical practice.
   d. Reward virtuous actions among peers.

CONCLUSIONS

The difference between an experienced physical therapist and an expert therapist with a similar number of years of experience can surely be found in the professional development path taken by each practitioner. Our experts, goal oriented and hungry for knowledge, all pursued advanced training to enhance their knowledge and skills as therapists in their specialty areas. They sought to learn from many sources: continuing education, colleagues within and external to the profession, mentors, formal education programs, residencies, participation in professional organizations, and self-structured learning activities. Practitioners can model these behaviors with a similar array of learning opportunities in almost any setting. Perhaps the most valuable learning resource is right under their noses every day: patients. To consider required work (i.e., treating patients)

15

the most valuable learning asset requires an intentional change of perspective for some therapists. Some may simply need a little push that reminds them that they can do a better job with their patients and encourages them to investigate how that might happen. Collaborative case conferences with practitioners of varied years of experience, all critiquing the same case, can work well to explicate the varied approaches to patients. The profession needs more dialogue that elucidates the preferred practice for similar groups of patients.

For some, biographies are fascinating. These short professional biographies whet our appetite for more information on expert therapists in specialties not covered by this study, international practitioners in physical therapy, promising novice practitioners, and promising students. Each of our careers holds wisdom from which we could all benefit, had we the mechanism to collect it. We each have patients to thank for gracing us with this wisdom, and we vow to pass it along to our colleagues so that they might be of greater service to their patients. This study of expert practice in physical therapy is intended to pass the wisdom of the experts in our profession on to students and practitioners of all types.

Perhaps the most motivating aspect of the stories of these experts is the continued great joy that they express in their chosen profession. Their passion for knowledge, reflection on clinical decision making, rigor in perfecting practice, and virtues were all rewarded by finding joy in their daily lives. As Margaret Burke-White noted, "Work is something you can count on as a trusting life-long friend who never deserts you" (10). As with all friendships, friendship with the practice of physical therapy develops because of the effort put into it, and it rewards us each day for that effort.

One wonders if, in the next century, physical therapy will continue to attract similarly capable candidates into physical therapy. These experts are 12 individuals who are fully satisfied with their careers as they have defined them. As physical therapy continues to mature, the role of the physical therapist will follow the paths blazed by these expert practitioners. This increasing autonomy should enhance the ability to attract capable new entrants to the profession who will expect a career filled with intellectual challenges, respect of professional peers, and the potential for committed patient advocacy.

REFERENCES

1. Jette DU, Bacon K, Batty C, et al. Evidence-based practice: beliefs, attitudes, knowledge, and behaviors of physical therapists. *Phys Ther.* 2003;83:786–805.
2. Watts NT. Task analysis and division of responsibility in physical therapy. *Phys Ther.* 1971;51:23–35.
3. The Center for Gerontology and Health Care Research, Brown Medical School. *Continuity of care.* Available at http://www.chcr.brown.edu/pcoc/Contin.htm. Accessed February 8, 2006.
4. Sternberg R. Abilities are forms of developing expertise. *Educ Res.* 1998;28(4):11–20.
5. Sahrmann S. Moving precisely? Or taking the path of least resistance? *Phys Ther.* 1998;12:8–18.
6. Purtilo R. Moral courage in time of change: visions for the future. *J Phys Ther Ed.* 2000;14(3):4–6.
7. Purtilo R, Jensen G, Royeen C (eds). *Educating for moral action: a sourcebook for health and rehabilitation needs.* Philadelphia: FA Davis, 2004.
8. Glaser JW. *Three realms of ethics: individual, institutional, societal, theoretical model and case studies.* Lanham, MD: Rowman & Littlefield; 1994.
9. Hack, L. On disparity. in R Purtilo, G Jensen, C Royeen (eds). *Educating for moral action: a sourcebook for health and rehabilitation needs.* Philadelphia: FA Davis 2004.
10. Partnow E (ed). *The quotable woman.* Philadelphia: Running Press; 1991.

Appendix

OBSERVATION OF CLINICAL PRACTICE AND EPISODES OF CARE INTERVIEWS

Data collection is nothing more than asking, watching, and reviewing (1).

The discussion of what data to collect drew heavily on our experience in gathering qualitative data in busy clinic settings. In our previous two studies, our primary data gathering tool was based on the researcher being engaged in nonparticipant observation of the therapist working with a patient (2,3). We received many questions from peers about the potential effect of our presence in the confined clinical spaces in which the therapists were working. For this study, we decided to use a video camera to provide a less obtrusive method of recording therapist–patient interactions.

A second concern from our previous work was how to capture a therapist's thinking and clinical reasoning process in a way that was consistent with the moment-to-moment decision making that occurs in clinical practice. This was achieved by replaying the videotapes for the therapists and asking them to describe what they were thinking during their work with their patients. This process was extremely beneficial: We were amazed to discover how much we had missed and misinterpreted when we had based our data only on nonparticipant observation and a follow-up interview. We were provided with a view of how expert therapists discovered information, hunched, felt, speculated, risked, and challenged their own thinking about patients.

The next question was how many treatment sessions to videotape. Using a video camera for all patient visits would be impossible. Discussions resulted in defining an episode of care that included all the visits received by a patient during a single episode or up to 3 months of care for patients with chronic impairments. A video camera was used to record at least three patient treatment sessions for each of the 12 patients studied: 1) the initial patient examination, 2) at least once during ongoing treatment, and 3) the last visit (discharge). These videotapes were replayed for the therapist and used as the basis for debriefing interviews that focused on knowledge and clinical reasoning processes the therapist used during the treatment sessions. The following questions were used as an interview guide for conducting debriefing interviews with therapists:

1. What were you thinking about as you completed your evaluation of the patient? What is your diagnosis? What evidence did you use? How do you know what information to focus on? Where did you learn that? Where will you go next?

2. Talk about what is going on with this patient. What is your prognosis? How did you reach that conclusion? What evidence did you use? How did you know to use that evidence? Where did you learn that?

3. Talk about your most difficult problem with this patient. How did you identify the problem? What evidence did you use? What was your strategy for solving the problem? How did you learn to do this?

4. Describe how you went about making clinical decisions with this patient. What is your approach? Describe an example as we go through the tape.

5. Is this process of making a decision different for you now compared with when you were a novice clinician? What are the differences?

6. What do you think your best patient care skills are? What knowledge do you draw on as you execute these skills? (Look at video for specific examples.)

7. How do you know you have been effective in your evaluation and treatment of this patient?

8. What would you tell a student about how to go about decision making in this patient care environment? Would what you tell a student differ from what you actually do? How would it be different and why?

Each researcher spent a minimum of half a day observing the daily practice of each therapist in her or his practice environment. These observations provided an initial understanding of various practice settings and allowed us to build a rapport with the therapists.

Professional Development Interview

The professional development interview was used to provide insight into therapists' conceptions of their work—that is, what they value; what they know (aspects of craft knowledge); where, when, and how they acquired their knowledge; how their knowledge and decision-making processes changed (transformed) over time; and what events stimulated changes (4). Before the professional development interview, we obtained a copy of the therapist's professional résumé. Information from résumés was organized into categories (e.g., education, clinical experience, and involvement in professional activities). These categories were placed on note cards, and each therapist was asked to sort the résumé cards into one of three categories to provide a self-assessment of the important events in his or her professional development. This information was used to guide subsequent interviews.

The first category included those events that were considered most important in affecting the therapist's growth into expertise. The second category included those events that were considered somewhat important, and the third category contained those events considered least important in the therapist's growth into expertise. As the therapists sorted the résumé cards, they were asked to talk about how each résumé item affected their thinking about physical therapy and how they practiced, both positively and negatively. During and subsequent to sorting the résumé cards, the following professional development interview questions based on collective résumé items were posed:

1. Talk about experiences that have affected how you think about physical therapy and how you practice.
2. After résumé categories have been sorted, talk about each of the categories you have grouped. Why have you grouped these together? What is meaningful about this course (or person, experience, and so forth)? (This is done for each of the categories [e.g., education, clinical experiences, and mentors].)
3. How has your knowledge of physical therapy changed over time? How has your knowledge of your specialty area changed over time? Describe an example. To what do you attribute these changes?
4. What aspects of your clinical knowledge have changed the most over time? What are the sources for your clinical knowledge?
5. How did you acquire your present decision-making style? How has this style changed over the years? Describe an example. What do you believe accounts for these changes?
6. What do you consider to be the milestones in your learning that have led to your becoming the clinician you are today?
7. What advice would you give new graduates wanting to become experts in your area of practice?

Clinical Exemplars

The third data collection strategy involved creating and discussing one or more clinical exemplars. We adopted a strategy from Benner, who described the use of exemplars in interpretive research with nurses (5,6). The purpose of clinical exemplars was to provide an in-depth example of a critical event in professional development. Exemplars can be situations that stand out as the pinnacle of good physical therapy practice, situations memorable because they taught the therapist something new, or situations in which the therapist clearly made a difference. The expert clinicians were fascinated by the use of clinical exemplars, and many delighted in providing a number of clinical exemplars that demonstrated both the struggles and wonderful moments of discovery associated with growth into expertise. The following text, taken from Benner (6), describes how the clinical exemplars were prepared:

> Have the informant tell her or his story in a narrative first person reporting style. Oral reporting of the exemplar is preferred because the oral tradition is less linear than writing. It is natural during the telling of a story for the person to include actual dialogue along with feelings, musing, concerns, speculation and interpretations.
>
> Tape record the exemplar, transcribe the tape and return it to your informant. The informant will then review the written exemplar, edit it and fill in the missing details. The informant will be thinking about the meaning of the exemplar from the time of the first telling until she or he reviews the transcribed copy. Thus in reviewing the written exemplar, the informant may be able to add more specific or accurate dialogue, a clearer portrayal of specific events as well as related thoughts and feelings. At this time the informant may also be about to give you information that will help you interpret how the exemplar "triangulates" with other aspects of professional growth.

DOCUMENT ANALYSIS

The fourth data collection strategy involved reviewing documents. These documents included any professional writings, patient documentation in medical records, and written communication with insurers or other health professionals.

ENVIRONMENT AND ARTIFACTS

The fifth data collection strategy concentrated on generating thorough descriptions of practice environments, including treatment and teaching equipment, arrangement of treatment and office space, and objects on walls (e.g., pictures, blackboards, bulletin boards). These data were used to help understand the context of the therapist's practice and provide specific data to illustrate and triangulate information the therapist reported about his or her style of practice. For example, the use of modality equipment was observed to be minimal, and using space and furniture to allow a focus on functional activities was evident.

MEMOS

The sixth and final data collection strategy incorporated the use of memos. Memos are a way to "catch the thoughts of the researcher on the fly" (7). These were ongoing memos written by a researcher immediately after observing or interviewing a therapist. These memos allowed us to capture initial thoughts and interpretations and were used to move systematically from empirical data to concepts. While recording our thoughts, other questions also arose about additional data needed to confirm an observation or interpretation. These questions were written out and used in follow-up interviews with the therapists. The memos were shared with other members of the research team to help clarify what we were seeing and interpreting to allow us to think carefully about how personal or professional bias might be interfering with what we were observing and how we were making sense of it. In other words, the memos helped keep us honest and on course.

REFERENCES

1. Wolcott HF. *Transferring qualitative data: description, analysis and interpretation.* Thousand Oaks, CA: Sage, 1994.
2. Jensen GM, Shepard KF, Hack LM. The novice versus the experienced clinician: insights into the work of the physical therapist. *Phys Ther.* 1990;70:314–323.
3. Jensen GM, Shepard KF, Gwyer J, Hack LM. Attribute dimensions that distinguish master and novice physical therapy clinicians in orthopedic settings. *Phys Ther.* 1992;72:711–722.
4. Grossman PL. *The making of a teacher: teacher knowledge and teacher education.* New York: Teachers College Press, 1990.
5. Benner P, Tanner CA, Chesla CA. *Expertise in nursing practice.* New York: Springer, 1996.
6. Benner P, Wrubel J. *The primacy of caring: stress and coping in health and illness.* Menlo Park, CA: Addison-Wesley, 1989.
7. Miles M, Huberman AM. *Qualitative data analysis: a sourcebook of new methods,* ed 2. Thousand Oaks, CA: Sage Publications, 1992.

Index